Physical Rehabilitation
Outcome Measures

A Guide to Enhanced
Clinical Decision Making

Second Edition

Physical Rehabilitation Outcome Measures

A Guide to Enhanced Clinical Decision Making

Second Edition

Elspeth Finch, BScP & OT, MHSc
Associate Professor (Part Time)
School of Rehabilitation Science
McMaster University
Hamilton, Ontario

Dina Brooks, BSc(PT), MSc, PhD
Assistant Professor
Department of Physical Therapy
University of Toronto
Toronto, Ontario

Paul W. Stratford, PT, MSc
Associate Professor
School of Rehabilitation Science
McMaster University
Hamilton, Ontario

Nancy E. Mayo, BSc(PT), MSc, PhD
James McGill Professor
Department of Medicine
School of Physical and Occupational Therapy
McGill University
Division of Clinical Epidemiology
McGill University Health Center
Montreal, Quebec

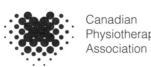

Canadian
Physiotherapy
Association

Association
canadienne de
physiothérapie

BC Decker Inc
P.O. Box 620, LCD 1
Hamilton, Ontario L8N 3K7
Tel: 905-522-7017; 1-800-568-7281
Fax: 905-522-7839; 1-888-311-4987
e-mail: info@bcdecker.com
www.bcdecker.com

ISBN 1–55009–220–0 (BC Decker Inc)
ISBN 0-7817-4241-2 (Lippincott, Williams & Wilkins)
Printed in Canada

Sales and Distribution

Canada
Canadian Physiotherapy Association
2345 Yonge Street, Suite 410
Toronto, Ontario M4P 2E5
Tel: 416-932-1888
Fax: 416-932-9708
e-mail: information@physiotherapy.ca
Website: www.physiotherapy.ca

United States
Lippincott, Williams & Wilkins
351 West Camden Street
Baltimore, MD 21201-2436
227 East Washington Square
Philadelphia, PA 19106
Tel: 1-800-368-3030; 301-714-2324
Fax: 301-824-7390
Website: www.LWW.com

Foreign Rights
John Scott & Company
International Publishers' Agency
P.O. Box 878
Kimberton, PA 19442
Tel: 610-827-1640
Fax: 610-827-1671
e-mail: jsco@voicenet.com

Argentina
CLM (Cuspide Libros Medicos)
Av. Córdoba 2067 – (1120)
Buenos Aires, Argentina
Tel: (5411) 4961-0042/(5411) 4964-0848
Fax: (5411) 4963-7988
e-mail: clm@cuspide.com

Japan
Igaku-Shoin Ltd.
Foreign Publications Department
3-24-17 Hongo
Bunkyo-ku, Tokyo
Japan 113-8719
Tel: 3 3817 5680
Fax: 3 3815 6776
e-mail: fd@igaku-shoin.co.jp

U.K., Europe, Scandinavia, Middle East
Elsevier Science
Customer Service Department
Foots Cray High Street
Sidcup, Kent
DA14 5HP, UK
Tel: 44 (0) 208 308 5760
Fax: 44 (0) 181 308 5702
e-mail: cservice@harcourt.com

Singapore, Malaysia, Thailand, Philippines, Indonesia, Vietnam, Pacific Rim, Korea
Elsevier Science Asia
583 Orchard Road
#09/01, Forum
Singapore 238884
Tel: 65-737-3593
Fax: 65-753-2145

Australia, New Zealand
Elsevier Science Australia
Customer Service Department
STM Division
Locked Bag 16
St. Peters, New South Wales, 2044
Australia
Tel: 61 02 9517-8999
Fax: 61 02 9517-2249
e-mail: stmp@harcourt.com.au
Website: www.harcourt.com.au

Mexico and Central America
ETM SA de CV
Calle de Tula 59
Colonia Condesa
06140 Mexico DF, Mexico
Tel: 52-5-5553-6657
Fax: 52-5-5211-8468
e-mail: editoresdetextosmex@prodigy.net.mx

Brazil
Tecmedd
Av. Maurílio Biagi, 2850
City Ribeirão Preto – SP – CEP: 14021-000
Tel: 0800 992236
Fax: (16) 3993-9000
e-mail: tecmedd@tecmedd.com.br

Encomium

The gestation and birth of this beautiful new book inevitably brings back warm and proud memories of its older and labor-weary sibling that was born in 1994.[1] To that "child," I had a paternal attachment as its editor. Now, my role is to be proud honorary grand-uncle of this fine book and what a fine book it is! Reading it has been a thrill and not work at all, and writing this foreword is truly an honor.

In 1994, our book was desperately needed and it well served many rehabilitation therapy clinicians and researchers and their students. This new book will rapidly set the scene for a dramatic enhancement of problem-based learning by students and evidence-based practice by *all* rehabilitation clinicians and associates. These now include more than physical and occupational therapists. Woe be to rehabilitation physicians and surgeons, nurses, psychologists, speech-language pathologists, exercise physiologists, kinesiologists, social workers, rehabilitation administrators, and litigation lawyers who are not well versed in its messages. Any of the above list of people are at risk if they fail to learn the principles in the following pages. Many of you must learn to *apply the details* as well.

John V. Basmajian, OC, O Ont, MD, FRCPC, FRCP (Glasg., Edin., Austral.)
Professor Emeritus
School of Rehabilitation Science
McMaster University
Hamilton, Ontario

---

[1] Cole B, Finch E, Gowland C, Mayo N. In: Basmajian J, editor. Physical rehabilitation outcome measures. Toronto (ON): Health and Welfare Canada and Canadian Physiotherapy Association; 1994.

Foreword

Somewhere near the close of the twentieth century rehabilitation professions became acutely aware that we were providing services to our patients based primarily on tradition and anecdote, which when challenged both internally and externally, we could not justify by sound theory rooted in scientific evidence. We are not alone in this predicament. Along with many other health professions, the physical rehabilitation field is responding to the dilemma of inadequate evidence. This guide is an important part of that response.

The second edition of *Physical Rehabilitation Outcome Measures: A Guide to Enhanced Clinical Decision Making* arrives as the landscape in physical rehabilitation has changed radically. Calls for "evidence-based practice" in the health professions are heard all around us. Clinicians are under increasing pressure to base their practice more firmly on "evidence," and the rehabilitation professions are increasingly being called upon to differentiate the impact of services they provide from the natural course of recovery following the onset of disease or injury. In the face of mounting pressures to demonstrate that what they do "works," researchers and clinicians within the rehabilitation professions are aggressively pursuing clinical outcomes research. Outcomes management has been described by its proponents as the technology of patient experience designed to assist making more rational medical care-related choices based on better insight into the effect of these choices on the patient's life. The goal of outcome research is to provide scientific evidence to guide the choice of effective health care decisions made by all who participate in health care—patients, providers, policy makers, and third party payers. Today, outcomes research findings are being used in medicine, and increasingly in physical rehabilitation, to form evidence-based decisions regarding clinical practice.

This guide provides the clinician, student, faculty member, and researcher with a valuable and easily accessible source of critical information on outcomes tools and instruments. Rehabilitation researchers can use it as a helpful summary of information about the latest measurement instruments to conduct high-quality, clinically relevant outcomes research. It will assist academic faculties that are being asked to train a future generation of rehabilitation professionals who have the skills to be critical consumers of the growing body of scientific literature to manage their patients. Clinicians will find it a convenient source of information to help them stay current with the ever-changing methods being used in rehabilitation outcomes research.

Although there is a growing awareness of the range of outcome measures available today and a growing sophistication that methodologic criteria contemporary measures should meet, descriptions of measurement instruments and methods are widely scattered in the medical, social science, and methodologic journals. Few articles compare instruments and methods to help the reader do a comparative evaluation for a particular target population or application. Although some excellent book length sources on medical outcome instruments exist, none is written specifically for a physical rehabilitation audience. The second edition of this book goes a long way toward filling this gap.

Chapters 1 to 6 provide the reader with an excellent summary of the major analytic issues that a rehabilitation professional must address in selecting among available outcome instruments: differentiating among outcome concepts relevant to rehabilitation; choosing a measure; evaluating measurement properties; and distinguishing between application of outcome measures in individual clients and rehabilitation programs. This first section of the book provides the student or novice outcomes researcher with an excellent introduction to these critical issues, and the more experienced rehabilitation professional with a concise review of the basic principles of outcome assessment.

The heart of the book contains a careful and comprehensive compendium of a wide range of outcome measures used in physical rehabilitation. Outcome concepts covered include body functions, activity restrictions, and participation limitations with a preference for those that are true outcome measures with an ability to measure change over time in an individual or group of clients. Important information is provided to the potential user on the conceptual basis of each instrument, psychometric properties, interpretability, and administrative characteristics.

Readers of *Physical Rehabilitation Outcome Measures* will come away impressed by the progress made over the past 20 years in developing and evaluating outcome instruments that are relevant for the critical evaluation physical rehabilitation. The careful reader will also come away with a deeper understanding of the shortcomings of current outcome methodology and the remaining challenges that the field of physical rehabilitation must address if we are to successfully solve the dilemma of inadequate evidence and create a solid foundation on which to build evidence-based practice in physical rehabilitation.

Alan M. Jette, PT, PhD
Professor and Dean
Sargent College of Health and
    Rehabilitation Sciences
Boston University
Boston, Massachusetts

Preface

The first edition of *Physical Rehabilitation Outcome Measures* provided a user-friendly manual to promote and facilitate the efficient use of measures by rehabilitation clinicians to enhance decision making. At the time it met a need for those who wanted to get started using outcome measures to enhance client care. A recent survey found that in 1998, 90% of respondents were familiar with the first edition of this book and 46% had used it in the previous 6 months.[1] The second edition includes substantial additional text in response to the changes that have occurred during the last 8 years in the familiarity with the use of outcome measures among rehabilitation professionals. As for the first edition, the target readers of the second edition are rehabilitation clinicians and students in rehabilitation programs. In addition, it will be of interest to rehabilitation researchers who are choosing outcome measures for clinical studies. As students were avid buyers and users of the first edition along with their graduate colleagues, we considered their needs as well as those of the clinician when planning the measures to review and the description of the process of outcome evaluation. Thus, readers should be selective about the sections most useful to them considering background knowledge and the stage they are at in addressing outcome evaluation of clients.

In Chapter 2, we have outlined how to develop an outcome measurement plan. Suggestions are provided on how to determine the most relevant attributes or constructs to measure when considering outcomes affected by rehabilitation. Many rehabilitation professionals are confident in their ability to measure what is relevant to their clients.[1] This chapter provides a framework for those clinicians to consider the constructs they measure at present and may provide some additional suggestions for others they may not have considered. It may also provide a method of thinking through the alternatives for those who are less confident in knowing what to measure, particularly if there are insufficient resources to monitor all aspects of change in individual clients or in client groups. A well-devised outcome measurement plan will increase the likelihood that outcome data will assist in making decisions about individual clients, groups of clients, and rehabilitation programs.

Chapter 3 reviews the steps of how to choose the outcome measure that best fits the client population, the purpose of the outcome evaluation, and the intended use of the outcome data. It suggests how to identify a range of potential measures and then narrow that list based on the measurement properties important for an outcome measure and the clinical feasibility of using the measure in the proposed clinical setting. Steps are outlined about how to test the measure(s), incorporate them into an outcome measurement plan, and evaluate the process of collecting and using outcome data.

Chapter 4 is a reference on measurement properties and the terms used in the reviews of measures found later in the text. It describes reliability and validity and explains the terms used for the subcategories of these terms. At present, the terminology used in describing sensitivity to change is in transition and therefore the terms—construct validity, sensitivity to change, and responsiveness—have somewhat different meanings depending on the author and the text. This chapter attempts to sort out these differing concepts. In this edition, we have chosen to use the more recent

---

[1] Kay TM, Myers AM, Huijbregts MPJ. How far have we come since 1992? A comparative survey of physiotherapists' use of outcome measures. Physiother Can 2001;53:268–75, 281

terminology, which may not be familiar to some readers, in the belief that this will be the terminology of choice within the next few years. This chapter also addresses the concept of clinically important change and how it differs for an individual and a group.

Chapter 5 addresses the application of outcome measures to individual clients and may well be the most useful chapter in the book for clinicians. It poses questions asked when assessing an individual client's outcome and demonstrates how outcome data can assist in answering these questions. The most appropriate reassessment interval is considered and the link is made between assessing outcomes, establishing goals, and documenting findings on the individual client. Ways to use outcome data to enhance the care of clients are presented.

Chapter 6 demonstrates how outcome data can be used in client program planning and evaluation. The choice of measures considered suitable for program evaluation is outlined and how the outcome data can be interpreted and used in decision making related to the program is demonstrated using a clinical example.

The template for reviewing a measure that can be used by readers is on page 64. Although it is similar to the one used in the first edition, the terminology has been revised in keeping with the terms we have used in this edition. Next, reviews of over 70 measures are provided. In response to reader feedback from the first edition, on the accompanying CD-ROM we have included as many of these measures as we could obtain permission to copy, as well as a list of important references for each. We have also included contact information, current at the time of publication, for obtaining more information on each measure. The measures are sequenced by name alphabetically. In addition, on pages 66–69, we have provided a list of the measures by client population and by construct measured to enable readers to find a measure (a) if the name of the measure is known, (b) if the name is unknown but the client population is the focus of the search, or (c) if the construct to be measured is the primary interest.

The Appendix includes an information extraction form and critical appraisal form for measurement studies.

ACKNOWLEDGMENTS

Many readers have asked for an updated version of the original "red book," and to them we are grateful for the push to take on this challenge. The Canadian Physiotherapy Association (CPA), under the leadership of Dianne Parker-Taillon, former Director, Education Practice & Research, and Margaret Parent, Director, Communications, has taken an active part in putting together the plan and the finances to produce, publish, and market the new edition.

The authors' group—Elspeth Finch, MHSc, McMaster University; Dina Brooks, PhD, University of Toronto; Paul Stratford, MSc, McMaster University; and Nancy Mayo, PhD, McGill University—took on the responsibility for the text and overseeing the process of the choice and review of measures. Although we had assistance from the many people mentioned here, the final decisions about content were ours. Throughout many teleconferences and meetings, the aspects of the first edition that needed change were identified and the level of complexity for the new edition was decided. Each author brought a perspective and ideas that contributed to the new edition in a way that we hope will result in as much success as the first edition enjoyed. The thought and work that the authors put into this project on top of their usual commitments are a tribute to their dedication to rehabilitation and to the advancement of patient care.

The adjustments to the template were drafted and the proposed measures to be reviewed were discussed with our advisory group listed on page xi.

They have provided advice to the authors on the choice of measures, reviews of measures, statistical terminology, and various other topics as the need arose throughout the project. Their assistance has been invaluable, and we thank them for their willingness to share their expertise.

Katrina Schmitz of KSR Consulting acted as project manager, under contract with the CPA, and has been invaluable to the authors in keeping us organized, arranging meetings and teleconferences, reminding us of deadlines, maintaining contacts, and obtaining information from advisors, reviewers, developers, and publishers. Her contribution to the success of the project has been immense. The CPA also contracted BC Decker Inc of Hamilton, Ontario, to publish the book and market it outside Canada. They have helped to produce a book that builds on the original edition but provides the reader with current information in a format that is comprehensive and accessible. In particular, we wish to thank Brian Decker, Charmaine Sherlock, Associate Medical Editor, and Paula Presutti, Production Manager of BC Decker Inc, who have worked with the authors to guide us through the many decisions needed to produce a book that meets the readers' needs.

We are most grateful to John Basmajian, MD, McMaster University, for writing the encomium, and to Alan Jette, PhD, Sargent College of Health and Rehabilitation Sciences, Boston University, USA, for writing the foreword to this edition. Dr. Basmajian, who edited the first edition of the book, has been a valued advisor and supporter from the beginning, and we are delighted to have his contribution to the second edition. Dr. Jette's work on outcome measurement is held in high esteem internationally, and we are most appreciative of his willingness to contribute the foreword to this edition.

Many people have participated in reviewing the measures. For this edition, we invited those familiar with the measures—the developers themselves, users, or graduate students working with advisors—to be reviewers. In this way, we have attempted to obtain the most current, accurate information about the measures we have chosen to include. We are deeply indebted to those listed on page xi, who worked diligently to provide comprehensive and accurate information within the length and time limits needed to meet publication requirements and to the CPA for providing them with an honorarium as a token of our appreciation.

Elspeth Finch
June 2002

Advisors

Jill Binkley; PT, MClSc; Appalachian Physical Therapy; Dahlonega, GA

Catherine Dean; PT, PhD; The University of Sydney; NSW, Australia

Gordon Guyatt; MD; McMaster University; Hamilton, ON

Mary Law; OT, PhD; McMaster University; Hamilton, ON

Daniel Riddle; PT, PhD; Virginia Commonwealth University; Richmond, VA

Christina H. Stenström; PT, PhD; Karolinska Institutet; Huddinge, Sweden

Sharon Wood-Dauphinee; PT, PhD; McGill University; Montreal, QC, Canada

Reviewers

Sara Ahmed; PT, MSc (PhD candidate); McGill University; Montreal, QC, Canada

Dorcas Beaton; OT, PhD; Institute for Work and Health; Toronto, ON, Canada

Katherine Berg; PT, PhD; McGill University; Montreal, QC, Canada

Jill Binkley; PT, MClSc; Appalachian Physical Therapy; Dahlonega, GA, USA

Catharine Bradley; BScPT; The Hospital for Sick Children; Toronto, ON, Canada

Dina Brooks; PT, PhD; University of Toronto; Toronto, ON, Canada

Suzann K Campbell; PT, PhD, University of Illinois at Chicago; Chicago, IL, USA

Geneviève Côté-Leblanc; OTR (MSc candidate); McGill University; Montreal, QC, Canada

Elsie Culham; PT, PhD, Queen's University; Kingston, ON, Canada

Johanna Darrah; PT, PhD; University of Alberta; Edmonton, AB, Canada

Johanne Desrosiers; OT, PhD; Université de Sherbrooke; Sherbrooke, QC, Canada

Kari Elliott; MSc (PT); Home Care; Edmonton, AB, Canada

Laura-Beth Falter; PT, MSc (Rehab); University of Toronto; Toronto, ON, Canada

Lois Finch; PT, MSc (PhD candidate); McGill University; Montreal, QC, Canada

Carolyn (Kelley) Gowland; PT, MHSc; McMaster University; Hamilton, ON, Canada

Johanne Higgins; OT, MSc; Royal Victoria Hospital; Montreal, QC, Canada

Maria Huijbregts; PT, MHSc; Baycrest Centre for Geriatric Care; Toronto, ON, Canada

Gayatri Kembhavi; MSc (PT); University of Alberta; Edmonton, AB, Canada

Deborah Kennedy; BSc (PT) (MSc candidate); Orthopaedic & Arthritic Institute of Sunnybrook and Women's College Health Sciences Centre; Toronto, ON, Canada

Jacek A. Kopec; MD, PhD; University of British Columbia; Vancouver, BC, Canada

Mylène Kosseim; OT, MBA (PhD candidate); McGill University; Montreal, QC, Canada

Sydney Lineker; PT, MSc; The Arthritis Society; Toronto, ON, Canada

Sunita Mathur; PT, MSc; University of British Columbia, Vancouver, BC, Canada

Nancy Mayo; PT, PhD; McGill University; Montreal, QC, Canada

Brenda McGibbon Lammi; BHSc (OT) (MSc candidate); McMaster University; Hamilton, ON, Canada

M. Ellen Newbold; PT, MSc; St. Michael's Hospital; Toronto, ON, Canada

Ulrika Öberg; PT, PhD; Eksjö-Nässjö Hospital; Eksjö, Sweden

Tom Overend; PT, PhD; University of Western Ontario; London, ON, Canada

Sonia Pagura; PT, MSc; Orthopaedic & Arthritic Institute of Sunnybrook and Women's College Health Sciences Centre; Toronto, ON, Canada

James Pencharz; BSc (Kin); University of Toronto; Toronto, ON, Canada

Lise Poissant; OT, PhD; McGill University; Montreal, QC, Canada

Darlene Reid; PT, PhD; University of British Columbia; Vancouver, BC, Canada

Lori Roxborough; PT/OT, MSc; Children's and Women's Health Centre of British Columbia; Vancouver, BC, Canada

Dianne Russell; BSc (Kin), MSc; McMaster University; Hamilton, ON, Canada

Nancy Salbach; PT, MSc (PhD candidate); McGill University; Montreal, QC, Canada

Holger Schünemann; MD, PhD; University at Buffalo; Buffalo, NY, USA

Alexander B. Scott; BSc (PT) (MSc candidate); University of British Columbia; Vancouver, BC, Canada

Louise Seaby; PT, MSc; Ottawa, ON, Canada

Sherra Solway; PT, MSc; Institute for Work & Health; Toronto, ON, Canada

Greg Spadoni; BHSc (PT), (MSc candidate); McMaster University; Hamilton, ON, Canada

Christina H. Stenström; PT, PhD; Karolinska Institutet; Huddinge, Sweden

Paul Stratford; PT, MSc; McMaster University; Hamilton, ON, Canada

Jessie VanSwearingen; PhD, PT; University of Pittsburgh; Pittsburgh, PA, USA

Adriana Venturini; PT, MSc; Montreal Neurological Hospital; Montreal, QC, Canada

Jean Wessel; PT, PhD; McMaster University; Hamilton, ON, Canada

Kelly Westlake; PT, MSc (PhD candidate); Queen's University; Kingston, ON, Canada

Carole White; RN, MSc (PhD candidate); McGill University; Montreal, QC, Canada

Sharon Wood-Dauphinee; PT, PhD; McGill University; Montreal, QC, Canada

Virginia Wright; PT, MSc (PhD candidate); Bloorview MacMillan Children's Centre; Toronto, ON, Canada

Nancy Young; PT, PhD; The Hospital for Sick Children; Toronto, ON, Canada

Contents

PART I

Principles in Outcome Measurement

CHAPTER 1

Outcome Measurement in Rehabilitation

The first edition of *Physical Rehabilitation Outcome Measures*, published in 1994, responded to a need among rehabilitation professionals for a text to help them grapple with the concept of outcome measures and how to start using them in clinical practice. In the early 1990s, the emphasis in health care was on quality management, and the process of providing care had undergone considerable attention. Outcome measurement was in its infancy. As a result, much of the first edition stated and argued the case for the need for outcome measurement and strived to change attitudes toward what was then a new challenge.

A survey of Canadian physiotherapists and physiotherapy directors, done in 1992, informed the authors of the first edition about the state of outcome measurement at that time.[1] It explored what respondents understood about standardized measures, what measures they were using, what barriers they perceived to outcome measurement, and what assistance they felt they needed to move ahead. At that time, there was a limited use of outcome measures, and the major barriers to their use were a lack of knowledge of available instruments and their properties and the time needed to implement outcome measures.

In 1998, Kay and colleagues conducted a comparable survey of staff therapists and professional practice leaders in five university-affiliated Toronto hospitals.[2] The samples were somewhat different in the two surveys; in 1992, 20% of respondents used at least one published outcome measure and identified it, whereas, in 1998, 97% of the sample used at least one of a provided list of 22 outcome measures. Although there appears to be at least increased familiarity with outcome measures over the 6 intervening years, Kay et al[2] concluded that it is unclear from the two surveys to what extent the use of outcome measures in clinical practice has increased. It is clear that even in 1998, a number of respondents do not use them systematically and efficiently as part of a total outcome evaluation plan to enhance clinical decision making. Major barriers reported by respondents were similar in both surveys and included lack of time and lack of knowledge about measures.

In the 1998 survey[2] and a follow-up focus group study,[3] respondents' confidence in various aspects of the choice and use of outcome measures was explored. Respondents were relatively confident with what to measure and how to administer, score, and track progress with measures; they were less confident in how to choose the best measure and how to use the information provided by the measures.[2,3]

The first edition of this book and educational workshops on outcome measurement given during the 1990s focused on the need for and benefit to using outcome measures, the desired measurement properties of an outcome measure, and how to choose and administer a measure. Most physiotherapists now accept the need for outcome measurement and are comfortable administering measures and using them to track an individual client's progress. However, they now need more clinically useful information about competing measures, more practical ways to use outcome data in decision making about their individual clients and in planning and evaluating patient programs, and better understanding of how to implement a systematic plan for outcome evaluation.[2,3] This confirms our decision in this edition to concentrate more on elaborating the process of finding and evaluating outcome measures appropriate for a specific need and providing examples of how outcome data can be used to make decisions that enhance the care of individual clients and client programs.

Although rehabilitation may target impairments, activity limitations, or restrictions in participation as well as environmental factors, the outcome of these interventions is usually best seen by the client in terms of his/her ability to perform an activity or participate with his/her family or community in some desired role. Impairment outcome data do not correlate highly with activity (disability) and participation (handicap) outcome data. For this reason, outcome measures that determine the level of the client's ability to be active and participate in life as he/she wishes are usually more useful to the client and the health care practitioner in determining if the intervention has been effective. We have based our construct terminology on the recent *International Classification of Functioning, Disability and Health* (ICF) proposed by the World Health Organization.[4] Definitions of frequently used terms can be found in the glossary on page 270. Further information can be found at *http://www.who.int/icf*.

We have included a wider range of measures than the first edition and have concentrated on measures in the activity and participation categories of the ICF framework, although we have also included some impairment, quality of life, and patient satisfaction measures that have particular relevance to clients. We have also tried to include measures that are suitable for a wider range of client populations than was attempted in the first edition. The choice of the measures to include was a difficult one; inevitably, we had to leave out some to keep the book at a manageable length. To clarify what is understood by a standardized published outcome measure, we set an arbitrary requirement that each measure reviewed should have at least two related published articles in peer-reviewed journals so that there would be a reasonable level of information available about the measurement proper-

ties and method of administration and scoring. Modified versions of measures are included only if they have been shown to be superior to the original versions, although, in some cases, these versions are mentioned in the reviews so that readers can seek further information about them if they wish to do so.

We have predominantly included measures that are true outcome measures, that is, they have measurement properties that enhance their ability to measure change over time in an individual or group.[5] These are also called evaluative measures, the purpose of which is primarily to evaluate the effect of an intervention. They are designed to maximize the measurement properties important for this purpose: test–retest reliability, longitudinal construct validity, and responsiveness. The few exceptions to this emphasis have been reviewed either because they are frequently used in clinical practice as outcome measures or are measures that may be suitable for that purpose in particular client populations once their ability to measure change has been formally examined.

Measures may also be designed for other purposes such as discriminating among clients on a particular construct or predicting an outcome in the future based on the results of measuring a construct at an earlier point in time. The measurement properties for these will emphasize somewhat different strengths to suit their purposes. For example, a discriminative measure should emphasize good cross-sectional validity, whereas a predictive measure should have good predictive criterion validity.[5] As a result, a measure that is developed for one of these purposes may not have the psychometric properties suitable for the purpose of evaluating outcome.

Another important and complex issue we considered in this new edition was language and cultural adaptation of outcome measures. In the reviews of each measure, we have indicated the languages in which the measure is available and if the measure has been validated in the language. This information has been difficult to obtain for some measures so may not be comprehensive. It will provide those readers interested in obtaining a measure in a language other than English with an indication of whether it is available but should not imply that a standardized procedure for validation has been followed.

Culture, language, and geography should all be considered when using a measure in a setting different from the one in which it is developed.[6] When measures are used cross-culturally, there is a standardized procedure by which they must be translated and validated.[6] First, a person familiar with both languages and the construct being measured translates the measure into the target language. Then another translator not involved in the initial step translates the measure from the target to the original language to ensure that the true meaning of the items has been retained. A multidisciplinary committee should then consider modifications to ensure equivalence of the original and new versions. The measure in the target language must next be validated to test its psychometric properties by pretesting and adapting the weighting of scores where necessary.[6,7] When proposing to use a measure in a different language from the one in which it was developed, a description of the process by which it was translated, culturally adapted, and validated should be sought in the literature. This will allow the potential user to judge to what extent the ideal procedure has been followed and therefore the degree of confidence with which the measure can be used in the new setting.[6] It should also provide the user with guidance about whether comparison of scores from the two versions is possible.[6]

As with any publication, the level of complexity the authors choose to use is a difficult decision based on the needs of the target audience. We have made a conscious decision to substantially increase the level of complexity of this edition compared with the first one, based on the increased knowledge of our readers, both clinicians and students, over the past 8 years. For some, this may present a challenge. Whatever the level of comfort with employing a systematic evaluation plan, we ask readers to use the parts of the text that facilitate the search for and selection of outcome measures and their interpretation to enhance clinical decision making. Whatever ideas or methods are gained by using this text, we hope that they will stimulate and further your use of outcome measures in enhancing patient care.

REFERENCES

1. Cole B, Finch E, Gowland C, Mayo N. In: Basmajian J, editor. Physical rehabilitation outcome measures. Toronto (ON): Health and Welfare Canada and Canadian Physiotherapy Association; 1994.
2. Kay TM, Myers AM, Huijbregts MPJ. How far have we come since 1992? A comparative survey of physiotherapists' use of outcome measures. Physiother Can 2001;53:268–75, 281.
3. Huijbregts MPJ, Myers AM, Kay TM, Gavin TS. Systematic outcome measurement in clinical practice: challenges experienced by physiotherapists. Physiother Can 2002;54:25–31.
4. ICF International Classification of Functioning, Disability and Health [online]. 2001 [cited 2002 Feb 4]. Available from: http://www.who.int/icf. Geneva: World Health Organization.
5. Kirshner B, Guyatt G. A methodological framework for assessing health indices. J Chron Dis 1985;38:27–36.
6. Guillemin F. Cross-cultural adaptation and validation of health status measures. Scand J Rheumatol 1995; 24:61–3.
7. Streiner DL, Norman GR. Health measurement scales: a practical guide to their development and use. Oxford (UK): Oxford University Press; 1989. p. 17–8.

CHAPTER 2

How to Choose Outcomes Relevant to the Client and the Rehabilitation Program

Although the majority of rehabilitation professionals have now been exposed to the need to use objective, reliable, and valid measures to evaluate the clients they treat and the programs they offer, there is often confusion as to what outcomes should be measured. The wider availability of good measurement tools has added to the confusion because the outcomes chosen for measurement are often driven by the measures that are at hand. The purpose of this chapter is to outline how to devise a measurement plan for the evaluation of outcomes relevant for clinical practice, research, and program evaluation. This chapter deals with what should be measured before proceeding with how.

LEARNING OUTCOMES AND OBJECTIVES

At the completion of this chapter, the reader will be able to:

1. Name the principal outcomes that are relevant in rehabilitation;
2. Identify the components of rehabilitation care that need to be evaluated;
3. Identify those outcomes that are impacted on by the therapeutic strategy, intervention, or program offered; and
4. List outcomes that would be the most likely to be impacted by treatment and the least likely to be affected by extraneous variables.

MEASUREMENT PARADIGMS THAT WILL HELP IN CHOOSING THE RELEVANT OUTCOMES TO MEASURE

A large number of outcomes are relevant to the evaluation of physical rehabilitation. Some of these outcomes relate to the immediate consequences of the client's condition and the immediate impact of therapy; other outcomes relate to consequences that are more remote in time. For example, a person who is experiencing joint pain may not be able to walk more than a short distance, and, in the long term, this will interfere with his/her participation in usual activities and quality of life. In other words, the consequences of even a relatively circumscribed condition can be far reaching. A therapist treating this client would therefore be interested in measuring the effect of his/her treatment on many of these consequences—pain, range of motion, strength, mobility, walking endurance, speed of movement, ability to play sports, and quality of life, to name a few. As it is clearly not feasible to measure all of these outcomes, how should the choice be made of which outcomes to measure? Once the outcome is chosen, the next step would be to choose a measure of the outcome. Guidelines for taking this next step are outlined in Chapter 3.

There are several measurement paradigms that are helpful in organizing outcomes with respect to the various health effects experienced by clients and the short-, medium-, and long-term effects of therapy. Three that are most relevant to the evaluation of physical rehabilitation are (1) the World Health Organization's (WHO) International Classification of the Consequences of Disease, Impairment, Disability and Handicap (ICIDH),[1] newly termed International Classification of Functioning, Disability and Health (ICF)*[2]; (2) health-related quality of life (HRQL); and (3) cost.

For the past few years, the WHO has been revising the ICIDH, and the three original dimensions, impairment, disability, and handicap, have been reclassified into two domains: (1) body structure and function and (2) activity and participation. Two umbrella terms, *functioning* and *disability,* are used to refer to performance or capacity in these domains. Functioning refers to all body functions, activities, and participation; any alteration in functioning in terms of performance or capacity—impairments, activity limitations, and participation restrictions—is termed *disability.* (For more information, see <http://www.who.int/icf/>).

Body structures and functions are closely related. Consider these examples: the eye is a structure, and seeing is the function associated with it; a joint is a structure, and mobility is its function. Poor vision and limitation of joint mobility would, therefore, be impairments. The brain is a very complex structure and has many functions. Common impairments associated with neurologic dysfunction include altered motor control, sensation, memory, and cognition.

An activity is defined as the performance of a task or action. Although it is impossible to list all activities, one may easily imagine a variety of activities that would be impacted on by an impairment in body structure or function, for example, activities of daily living, walking, writing, doing household tasks, driving a car, and doing personal activities such as painting or playing a musical instrument. Activity limitation would be manifested by a change in the performance and capacity of that activity for that person. Someone who has no capacity to play the piano would not be considered to have an activity limitation. Consider the situation of a person who plays the piano as a leisure activity and who has a hand injury. He/she may still be able to play the piano, but the quality of the performance is altered; in this situation, he/she would be considered to have an activity limitation. If that person was, instead, a professional piano player, the activity limitation would also lead to a participation restriction. Because the capacity or performance is altered, the person is considered to have a disability.

The third dimension established by the ICF refers to the *participation* of an individual and his/her involvement in life situations. When an individual faces problems from physical, social, or attitudinal sources, he/she is said to experience restricted participation. Both the activity and participation dimensions are affected by contextual factors that include both environmental and personal factors. Participation also refers to involvement, that is, being engaged in meaningful, fulfilling, and satisfying activities that are socially or culturally expected of a person. Examples would include family, social, and work-related roles. Table 2–1 gives examples of specific constructs that would fit under the broad rubrics of impairment, activity, and participation.

A second paradigm is quality of life or, in the context of the health field, HRQL recently defined as "the value assigned to duration of life as modified by impairments, functional status, perceptions and opportunities influenced by disease, injury, treatment and policy."[3] The construct of HRQL is broad and encompasses domains related to physical, mental (emotional and cognitive), social, and role functioning, as

---

*This classification, revised from the original ICIDH, was initially referred to as ICIDH-2. In May 2001, the World Health Assembly adopted ICF as its acronym.

TABLE 2–1 Constructs Describing Impairment, Activity, and Participation at the Physical Level Using ICF Terminology

Impairment	Activity	Participation
Pain	Changing body position	Relationships
Altered Mobility of joint	Carrying, moving, handling objects	Community life
Altered Muscle power	Walking and moving	Recreation and leisure
Altered Muscle tone	Self-care	Education
Altered Gait pattern	Household tasks	Work
Altered Respiration functions (lung volume, etc.)	Interpersonal interactions	Economic
Altered Vestibular function	Conversation	Assisting others

ICF = International Classification of Functioning, Disability and Health.

well as an individual's perception of health and well-being.[4] Within the construct of HRQL, it is common to distinguish between *generic*† and *disease-specific* HRQL. Generic HRQL is the term used to incorporate those aspects of HRQL that are relevant to all health states, including ostensibly healthy individuals. A particular feature of generic HRQL is that it is also relevant to the general population, and measures of this construct are often included in national population health surveys. Disease-specific HRQL refers to those aspects of HRQL that reflect the impact of a specific illness or injury.

A construct related to HRQL is the concept of utility, defined as the value, between 0 and 1, representing the strength of preference an individual has for a given multidimensional health state. The closer the value is to 1, the more the health state is seen as being the best possible one.[5] When linked to life expectancy, utility values lead to quality-adjusted life-years.[6] A key feature of utility is that it summarizes information about many health domains by one number, hence the term multidimensional. In this way, gains (or losses) in one domain can be offset by losses (or gains) in another domain. For example, following a total hip replacement, an individual may have gained through pain reduction but may have lost strength. Nevertheless, there is a positive net gain in health status because absence of pain is of more "utility" than having strength. The utility values for a given health state come from surveying the general population and not usually people with the condition. The respondent from the general population is asked to imagine he/she is in this health state and indicate on a scale from 0 to 1 where this health state lies. With these values, it is possible to evaluate the various changes in health state in relation to the resources required to produce that improvement in health state.

This leads to the third measurement paradigm, cost—a construct that is becoming increasingly important in the context of the rehabilitation community. Two types of costs are relevant: direct costs to the health care system for resources consumed as part of the treatment or program and indirect costs to the client and family as a result of participating in the treatment or program. Whereas few practicing rehabilitation professionals will use cost as a primary outcome, managers will use cost as an outcome and potentially relate costs to the more familiar client-based outcomes. Thus, it is crucial that the most relevant outcomes are selected as these will be the out-

---

†The term "generic" does not apply only to the measurement of HRQL. Measures of constructs other than HRQL can be generic or disease specific, but when applied to these measures, the term generic usually means that the measure was not developed to assess a particular condition but would be used across conditions (eg, a "generic" functional status measure). For further discussion about generic vs specific measures, see Chap. 3.

comes that are evaluated against cost in a cost-effectiveness analysis.[7]

The relationships between these three paradigms are depicted in Figure 2–1. This diagram shows that the constructs of body structure and function, activity, and participation have overlapping elements. Health-related quality of life is a more encompassing paradigm that includes components of the ICF model but is much broader and underlies the other constructs. Utility is a part of HRQL, but it also has its own distinct component, that of preference for a particular health state. Cost is omnipresent and can both influence and be influenced by the other paradigms. There are important costs associated with impairments in body structure and function, activity limitation, participation restriction, low HRQL, and health states that have a low preference rating. On the other hand, the cost of care or services may be a barrier to achieving good outcomes in the other paradigms.

WHAT COMPONENTS OF REHABILITATION ARE BEING EVALUATED?

The choice of outcome also depends on what aspect of rehabilitation care is being evaluated. Health professionals in the rehabilitation field offer a variety of clinical modalities or therapeutic approaches to their clients; therefore, structuring a measurement plan could be quite complex.

Instead of thinking about a measurement plan, modality by modality, it is useful to think about what consequence of the disease or injury is being targeted by the modality or therapeutic approach and measure the outcome for each consequence. The ICF has moved away from a *consequence of disease* classification to a *components of health* classification. Some aspects of rehabilitation care are intended to impact at a cellular, organ, or tissue level or, using the ICF terminology, body structure and function. For example, cooling targets the tissue level. Other aspects of care target an individual's ability to carry out certain activities. Gait training would target walking ability. Taken globally, rehabilitation targets an individual's capacity to participate in community, family, and societal roles. Clearly, each one of these different aspects of rehabilitation care would need to be evaluated using a different set of outcomes.

A new way of thinking about what we do in therapy and how our actions interact with outcomes requires some more focused terminology. Rehabilitation modalities, approaches,

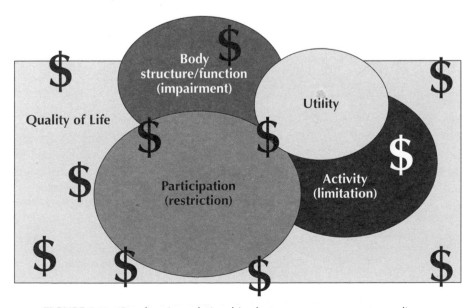

FIGURE 2–1 Overlapping relationships between measurement paradigms.

or techniques that seek to normalize body structure or function will be termed *strategies*. If the desire on the part of the therapist is to evaluate the impact of a strategy, then outcomes that relate to the target tissue, organ, or system would be the most relevant to choose—impairments. Examples of strategies include biofeedback, body-weight support, constraint-induced forced use, the application of an orthosis, and physical modalities such as ice, heat, cold laser, ultrasound, and electrical stimulation.

It is rare that rehabilitation would comprise a single strategy to target one aspect of body structure and function. Often multiple approaches or techniques (strategies) are combined into a rehabilitation *intervention* with the aim of normalizing an individual's performance or capacity for activity. Therefore, interventions comprise a number of strategies and would be evaluated on outcomes related to activity. Gait training, for example, could comprise strategies such as body-weight support, an orthosis, biofeedback, repetition, practice, and balance training. The sum impact of these strategies is to normalize walking. The outcome of walking can be evaluated using different measures, each one focusing on a different aspect of walking (eg, speed, distance, safety).

In some cases, there is limitation in one activity only; in this case, the rehabilitation intervention targets that activity. A knee injury could conceivably interfere mainly with the activity of walking. But such an injury may also affect sitting endurance, transfers from sitting to standing, and stair climbing and result in deconditioning and mental anguish. When the particular illness or injury impacts widely, resulting in limitations in several activities, and produces subsequent restriction in role participation—consider that the client with a knee injury is a football player—the client would need to be offered interventions that target each of the areas in which limitation and restriction are seen.

Rehabilitation *programs* encompass many interventions in order to impact globally on an individual's capacity to perform usual activities and participate fully. For example, a rehabilitation program for traumatic brain injury will comprise interventions designed to improve walking, self-care, memory, writing, reading, speaking, self-esteem, etc. An outcome that encompasses the impact of all of these components would be ideal for the evaluation of a program. Such outcomes could be drawn from the measurement paradigms of participation, HRQL, or utility. Figure 2–2 illustrates these components and the relevant outcomes.

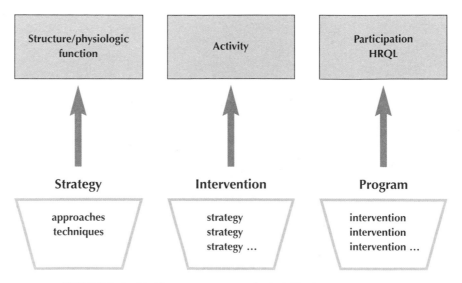

FIGURE 2–2 Linking components of rehabilitation to ourcomes.

MATCHING OUTCOMES TO REHABILITATION TARGETS

An outcome is a characteristic or construct that is expected to change owing to the strategy, intervention, or program. The ideal outcome would be the construct that is most impacted on by the strategy, intervention, or program that is being offered and least affected by outside influences. However, the outcome must also be relevant for the target—organ, individual, or group—and able to be summarized for the purposes of generalizing the results to the appropriate level—individual, group, or population. This is quite important considering that the information on your client may be used to ascertain whether the rehabilitation program is meeting expectations for the group of clients that is being served. If the outcomes are difficult to summarize for a group of individuals, then this may not be the best choice of outcome.

Table 2–2 summarizes the targets of rehabilitation and indicates those constructs that are the most relevant for each of the targets.

When rehabilitation clients are being offered specific strategies designed to impact on the target organ, tissue, or system, constructs at the level of impairment are most common. Activity could be assessed, particularly if movement of the body as a whole is the target or to relate the change at the impairment level to a change in activity.

When clients are being offered rehabilitation interventions (a group of strategies), it is usually most relevant to measure activity, although including measures of impairment would help to isolate what contributed to the change in activity. Interventions target the whole person; thus, it is plausible that there would be an observable effect on the extent to which a person takes up roles that are usual for him/her and thereby reintegrates into normal family and community living. Disease-specific HRQL is a relevant outcome when the intervention contains a sufficient number of efficacious strategies that could impact on perceptions of well-being.

When the aim is to evaluate the impact of a program, impairment outcomes are no longer relevant because it is difficult to summarize impairment-level variables for groups of individuals; for example, how is muscle strength or range of motion aggregated for a

TABLE 2–2 Matching Rehabilitation Targets to Constructs

	Target	Construct	Summary Level
Strategy	*Cell, tissue, organ, system*	**Primary:** *impairment* **Secondary:** *activity*	*Individual*
Example: muscle strengthening	Muscle	**Primary:** strength of quadriceps **Secondary:** number of step-ups in a minute	Strength of the lower extremity of an individual
Intervention	*Individual*	**Primary:** *activity* **Secondary:** *participation, specific HRQL*	*Group*
Example: gait training	Person with a stroke	**Primary:** walking quality, speed, and endurance **Secondary:** IADL, community activity; stroke-specific HRQL	Group of persons admitted for inpatient stroke rehabilitation
Program	*Groups*	**Primary:** *participation, disease-specific HRQL* **Secondary:** *activity, generic HRQL, utility, health service use, cost*	*Population*
Example: home-based stroke rehabilitation program	Group of persons with stroke in your hospital	**Primary:** community activity, family roles, stroke-specific HRQL **Secondary:** ADL, walking, IADL, generic HRQL, health status, resource use, cost	Population of persons hospitalized with stroke

HRQL = health-related quality of life; IADL = instrumental activities of daily living such as taking own medications, using the telephone, meal preparation, shopping, housework, etc.; ADL = activities of daily living.

group of persons or a population? There are also challenges for summarizing these constructs at an individual level, considering that the strength may be measured for many muscles and range of motion for many joints.

As programs are usually designed to normalize an individual's participation in usual roles and relationships, measures of participation would need to be included. However, it is only when the impact of programs is being evaluated that the constructs of generic HRQL, utility, and cost are relevant. This is because programs ideally target all of the resulting health states and are offered widely, with few restrictions as to who can be treated. Measures that reflect society's values for outcome and cost are relevant to evaluate as sometimes it is necessary to make a decision as to which programs will continue to be supported and which will not. Measures that cross disease boundaries are essential. For example, if your hospital has received extra funding to develop a rehabilitation program in the area of pediatrics, it may be difficult to choose between a program for cerebral palsy, rheumatoid arthritis, or autism. It is only by evaluating outcomes that cross these condition-specific boundaries that it would be possible to judge which program produces the most benefit at the least cost. By relating values on generic measures of HRQL, utility, and participation to program costs, it is now possible to make an informed decision as to which area would provide the greatest impact at the least cost. As society bears the cost of these programs, the outcomes need to be relevant to its citizens. Generic measures, developed for use in ostensibly healthy persons, are the relevant measures.

In thinking about matching outcomes to rehabilitation targets, it is as important to think about what not to include as it is to think about what should be included. For example, would it be relevant to evaluate the impact of a strategy beyond the tissue level and include a measure, for example, of HRQL? After all, one might say that, by reducing pain, it is very likely that the client will walk better, be able to return to sports and recreational activities, and, consequently, have better HRQL. Including additional measures may not be advantageous in this situation because the pain reduction may not have had a dramatic impact on walking if the disuse had produced serious weakness. The inability to walk may also have resulted in deconditioning, preventing the return to athletics. The disappointment experienced by the client when, magically, he/she could not do the desired activities may be reflected in paradoxically poorer HRQL. It would not be the fairest evaluation of the impact of the chosen strategy to provide data on outcomes that are quite distant from the targeted consequence. An even worse scenario might be imagined if the client, immediately after feeling pain relief, rushed off to the squash court to participate in a vigorous game of squash, only to damage another part of the body because he/she had become seriously deconditioned for this sport because of the pain. How would you interpret the outcomes—pain relief was successful—client on crutches. Of course, in an ideal world, this client would not have been offered only a pain relief strategy. A competent therapist would have evaluated other aspects of this client's condition and treated them all, including the deconditioning. Then, of course, several strategies are being combined, and together, as an intervention, these may have enough potency to impact on the construct of HRQL (condition specific). In the real world, however, once the pain has been relieved, this client may not be back for further therapy. Evaluate close to what you treat as the primary outcome. Include a more distant outcome to help with summarizing the impact to groups of persons, but if you evaluate too far from your primary impact level, you may have paradoxical responses: all of the people with good outcomes may no longer be attending therapy and are unavailable for further evaluation, and all of those still in pain continue to attend and are available for further outcome measurement.

The moral of the story is to measure where the impact of your strategy, intervention, or program is the strongest. Here is where research may be helpful; use results from research studies to show that improvement in one health component has future benefit for other components. You do not necessarily have to measure this outcome; having evidence supporting its relationship to your outcome is sufficient. The concept of "evidence based" extends beyond "practice"; here, it is important to have formulated an "evidence-based" outcome measurement plan.

CHOOSING AMONG COMPETING CONSTRUCTS

Within these broad domains of impairment, activity, and participation, there are a range of related constructs. Some examples are given in Table 2–1.

Clearly, it is not feasible to measure all of these constructs or outcomes in one individual. For example, consider a rehabilitation program for occupationally induced back pain. By definition, the program is multifaceted, providing specific exercises targeting muscle strength, endurance, and flexibility; strategies to reduce pain and improve conditioning; and education on how to prevent further back strain. Other members of the team may provide psychological counseling and pharmacologic agents. What would be the most appropriate outcome or outcomes to measure? Each of the different components of the program could be evaluated independently. For example, the exercise component could be evaluated by improvements in pain, muscle strength and endurance, and flexibility. The conditioning component could be evaluated by aerobic capacity. The combined effect of these strategies could also be evaluated through the measurement of various activities such as walking, carrying, climbing, and manipulating objects.

However, the outcome that is the most desirable and toward which all members of the team are striving would probably be return to work. The disadvantage with return to work as an outcome is that there may be many reasons outside the control of the rehabilitation program that may prevent an individual from returning to work. The work environment may have changed or the job may no longer exist for economic reasons. Therefore, in this example, an activity measure for low back pain that has been shown to predict an eventual return to work would be a good outcome measure to choose. The fact that back-related disability has been shown to predict an eventual return to work explains why it was a good outcome to choose to evaluate a low back pain management program even though the all-encompassing outcome of this program is return to work. Chapter 3 deals with how to choose from among many measures the one best suited to your clientele, setting, etc.

Although it is most desirable to choose an outcome that is the most affected by the strategy, intervention, or program to which the client is exposed, it is wisest to choose an outcome that is least affected by variables outside the control of the service providers and yet still under the direct influence of therapy that is being offered.

In selecting an outcome to measure, clinicians must also consider the time frame for the measurement strategy. Although the ultimate end point of rehabilitation services is reintegration and optimal HRQL, these outcomes may not be realized until long after the index event or therapy and therefore may not be relevant in the immediate post-acute time period. Consider an individual recovering from stroke. During the early rehabilitation phase, the person may still be hospitalized; thus, asking about household management, community travel, roles, and HRQL would not be appropriate as the individual would not yet have had the opportunity to participate in these types of roles. However, there are other outcomes that are relevant to the specific time frame when therapy is being offered that are associated with future community reintegration and HRQL. These intermediate outcomes would be ideal to measure early on in the therapeutic encounter. An outcome that predicts other important outcomes in the future, such as HRQL, return to work, hospitalization, institutionalization, or death, would be useful to measure when rehabilitation is being offered early on in the course of recovery. Measuring these later outcomes may also be quite costly as an organized follow-up would have to be in place.

This chapter has outlined the critical thinking that needs to take place in making the first step toward formulating an outcome measurement plan—choosing the relevant and appropriate outcomes. The following points were presented in this chapter:

- An outcome is a characteristic or construct that is expected to change owing to the provision of a strategy, intervention, or program.
- The outcomes that are relevant in rehabilitation are numerous and relate to body structure and function, activity, participation, HRQL, utility, and cost.
- The measurement plan will depend on the targets of the rehabilitation components: body structure or function, activity, and participation.
- The measurement plan will depend on whether a rehabilitation strategy, intervention, or program is being evaluated.
- Outcomes related to body structure and function can be summarized for an individual but not for a group.
- Outcomes of activity and participation relate to the individual but can also be interpreted for a group.
- Choose an outcome most affected by the therapeutic strategy, intervention, or program offered.
- Choose an outcome least affected by variables outside your control.
- Choose outcomes that are known to be associated with future beneficial end points.

REFERENCES

1. World Health Organization. International Classification of Impairments, Disabilities, and Handicaps: a manual of classification relating to the consequences of disease. Geneva: World Health Organization; 1980.
2. ICIDH-2 International Classification of Functioning, Disability and Health. Prefinal draft. Geneva: World Health Organization; 2001.
3. Patrick DL, Erickson P. Health status and health policy. New York: Oxford University Press; 1993.
4. Fitzpatrick R, Fletcher A, Gore S, Jones D, Spiegelhalter D, Cox D. Quality of life measures in health care. I: Applications and issues in assessment. BMJ 1992; 305:1074–7.
5. Torrance GW. Utility approach to measuring health-related quality of life. J Chron Dis 1987;40:593–600.
6. Kaplan RM. Assessment for estimating quality-adjusted life-years. In: Sloan F, editor. Valuing health care. New York: Cambridge University Press; 1995.
7. Drummond MF, O'Brien BJ, Stoddart GF, Torrance GW. Methods for the economic evaluation of health care programs. New York: Oxford University Press; 1997.

CHAPTER 3

How to Choose a Measure for the Relevant Outcome(s)

LEARNING OUTCOMES AND OBJECTIVES

At the completion of this chapter, the reader will be able to

1. Specifically describe the construct to be measured;
2. Identify the measurement purpose;
3. Define the client population;
4. Identify a range of potential measures and select the best ones based on measurement properties, feasibility, and use in similar populations;
5. Identify when a combination of measures may be required;
6. Plan and conduct a pilot test of the best measure(s);
7. Incorporate the selected measure(s) in an outcome measurement plan; and
8. Evaluate the collection and use of outcome data.

Now we come to the heart of the matter: choosing one or more outcome measures to meet your needs and administering the measure within a complete outcome measurement plan. Chapter 2 outlined how to go about identifying the relevant constructs to track the client's progress toward reducing the consequences of his/her condition. This chapter describes considerations in choosing appropriate outcome measures related to that construct and in administering the measures to obtain accurate, complete data for decision making. To read more about applying this process to individual clients, see Chapter 5; to read more about this process used for groups in program evaluation, see Chapter 6.

SPECIFICALLY DESCRIBING THE OUTCOME YOU ARE MEASURING

The outcome(s) or construct(s) identified as the target of your rehabilitation strategy, intervention, or program will need to be refined to consider what exact aspects of the outcome are important to this particular client within his/her environment and to identify an indicator of the outcome. For example, if your rehabilitation care is targeting reducing impairments of the lower extremity and increasing use of the lower extremity in daily activities, you have probably identified ambulation as an important indicator of outcome. You next need to consider whether speed, distance walked, use of aids, level of assistance, and/or safety are the aspects of walking you expect to change with your strategy or intervention. Another consideration is the environment in which you expect your client's ambulation to change and where he/she will usually be ambulating (eg, inside the home, outside on city streets, or outside in a rural community). You will then want to consider the environment in which you will achieve the most accurate and meaningful measurement of your client's ability.[1] For example, do you need to measure the outcome in the client's natural environment, or can it be done in a structured setting such as the outpatient department or the area surrounding the treatment facility?

IDENTIFYING YOUR MEASUREMENT PURPOSE

In most cases, you will be measuring the effect of the care you are providing in similar clients. However, the measures taken may have to serve several purposes simultaneously. You may need to make decisions about whether an individual client is progressing satisfactorily or consider a change in the therapeutic approach. You will need to communicate progress to the clients in a way that is meaningful and motivational to them (see Chapter 5 for further discussion). Health professionals also need to communicate progress to other members of the health care team; therefore, the measurement must have meaning in this wider context. Additionally, the measurements of outcome may be used to make decisions about the effectiveness of a comprehensive rehabilitation program offered to a group of clients (see Chapter 6 for further discussion).

As there are multiple purposes for which a measurement plan may be used, it is worth thinking about why you want to measure an outcome and what you want to do with the information you gain, even if, on the surface, it seems self-evident. It may help you make a decision to use an outcome measure that truly meets your needs rather than one that is most readily available or popular among health care providers at the moment. For example, if most of your clients are part of a multidisciplinary program, you may choose to include a measure that is easily interpretable by other health professionals.

As was outlined in Chapter 1, it is important to keep in mind that you must still focus on measurement tools that were primarily developed for evaluative purposes, that is, to track change over time. Some measures that are commonly used clinically because of their simplicity and interpretability across many disciplines may, in fact, be discriminative measures that are used to distinguish those individuals who have different levels of that construct (eg, Rankin Index, Mini-Mental State Examination) or predictive measures that are used to classify people according to a criterion that may exist now or in the future.

For example, the Mini-Mental State Examination is designed as a screening test for cognitive loss and might be used to identify potential participants for a rehabilitation program designed for clients with little or no cognitive loss. It would not be used to evaluate the effectiveness of the program. Another example is the use of percussion to identify an area of lung consolidation; it would not be used as an evaluative measure to assess a client's progress.

DEFINING THE CLIENT POPULATION

The client population you are targeting for your strategy, intervention, or program will affect the measure you choose. So the next task is to define your clients as clearly as you can. How old are they? Are they men only or women only? Have they some chronic limitation of activity or restriction in participation that is unlikely to change? The specific characteristics of your clients will have an impact on the measures that will be suitable for your purpose and on the normative or customary values you can use to interpret your data.

CHOOSING POTENTIAL MEASURES SUITED TO YOUR PURPOSE

Now you are ready to consider the types of measures that may be most appropriate for the construct you are measuring, why you want to measure it, and your client population. At this point, it helps to consider which health domains are important for the construct you are measuring. The International Classification of Functioning, Disability and Health (ICF) classifies body functions and structures along body systems.[2] At the activity and participation levels, health domains such as mobility, self-care, communication, learning and applying knowledge, domestic life, interpersonal interactions and relationships, and community, social, and civic life are identified.[2] You may want to consider an outcome measure that addresses one or several of these systems and domains.

Outcome measures can be classified by focus (generic or specific as to condition, region, or patient) and by mode of administration: performance (viewed performance) or self-report (self-completed, interviewer completed, or surrogate completed).[3,4] See Table 3–1 for some examples of these classifications. Although it may be clear that one type of measure suits your purpose best, there may be an advantage in combining the use of two types of measures to reflect the broader aspect of a construct in which you are interested.

CLASSIFICATION BY FOCUS: GENERIC VERSUS SPECIFIC MEASURES

Generic measures were originally developed as comprehensive measures for use in a general, ostensibly healthy, population. They can also be used to assess and compare client populations with different levels of disablement.[3,4] They may be unidimensional, primarily addressing physical function (eg, Barthel Index, gait speed), or multidimensional, addressing social and community life in conjunction with physical function (eg, 36-Item Short-Form Health Survey [SF-36], Sickness Impact Profile). For some authors, their key characteristic is their use in ostensibly healthy populations; for others, interested in comparing groups with different conditions, their comprehensiveness may be the most important attribute.[3–5]

This ability of a generic measure to allow comparisons to be made between people with different conditions or different consequences of the disease or injury is an important asset.[3,5] An additional advantage is that they are likely to have normative data associated with them, as well as values for typical groups of persons with various diseases, health states, or other characteristics, such as age, sex, and race.[6] Generic measures often have been developed and demonstrated to have good measurement properties, a necessary feature of all health measures (these properties are outlined in Chapter 4).

A potential disadvantage of generic measures is that they may be less sensitive to change than specific measures. When only a few items of the generic measure can potentially change, progress in these key items will be masked by the lack of change in those items not affected by the intervention.[3,4] They may also have ceiling and floor effects, limiting their ability to reflect change at either the high or low end of the construct they are measuring.[4] For example, the SF-36 includes several items reflecting relatively high physical function (walking a mile). An item such as this is unlikely to change in clients with chronic conditions such as chronic obstructive pulmonary disease (COPD) who, after an intervention, may have progressed only as far as to be able to dress and use the bathroom independently.[7] In addition, they also tend to have less face validity (makes sense to the person taking or administering the test) in that the client or health professional may think they are too general to accurately reflect the effect of the intervention.

TABLE 3–1   Examples of Different Types of Measures

Mode of Administration	Type of Measure	
	Generic	Specific
Self-report	SF-36	RMQ
Performance	FIM	DASH

SF-36 = 36-Item Short-Form Health Survey; RMQ = Roland-Morris Questionnaire; FIM = Functional Independence Measure; DASH = Disabilities of the Arm, Shoulder and Hand.

Specific measures may be specific to a disease, condition, region, or client. They are designed for a specific client population having the condition or those having a disability in one part of the body; therefore, comparisons are limited to other clients within the same population. The items or tasks are specific to the problems of that client population; therefore, the measures tend to have greater face validity than generic measures.[8] They also may be more responsive in that client group; most of the item scores are likely to change if the problem(s) is alleviated by a strategy, intervention, or program, which then translates to a greater change in summary scores.[3] Because of their narrower focus, they may, however, miss measuring an unanticipated effect of a treatment (eg, change in overall mental well-being or self-esteem).[8]

Measures that are specific to the client, such as the Canadian Occupational Performance Measure and the Patient-Specific Functional Scale, are examples of a method of tailoring the measure to the domains and constructs important to an individual client. In these measures, the respondent is asked to identify key indicators (eg, activities) that are important to him/her within a domain (eg, domestic life). These activities then become the items on which the respondent is measured within that domain. The items will be somewhat different from one respondent to another but relevant to the individual client. These measures are based on the belief that equivalent questions within a domain that are pertinent to the individual will result in as good or better standardization of information than the exact same wording used for everyone, which is open to different relevance and interpretation from one individual to another.[9] Although the concept of an individualized measure is appealing, clients often need assistance in providing meaningful responses; the influence of the persons assisting becomes a potential source of bias. In addition, if the areas of concern change over time, it is difficult to summarize improvement.

CLASSIFICATION BY MODE OF ADMINISTRATION: PERFORMANCE VERSUS SELF-REPORT MEASURES

Performance measures could also be called viewed performance because someone else, usually a health professional, is viewing the performance of the test and measuring it in some way. In rehabilitation, physical performance measures are frequently used. These measures test the client's actual performance of an activity in a given environment at a given point in time, whether it is walking 30 meters on an indoor uncarpeted surface or a more complex task of standing up, walking 3 meters, turning around, returning to the chair, turning, and sitting down. The tasks can be measured by timing the task, measuring the distance over which the task can be performed in a given time, observing the performance and judging on a predefined scale the amount of assistance needed or the safety with which the task is performed, or other ways of measuring the person's ability to perform the activity. Because performance measures may involve the use of equipment to measure the level of performance, they have traditionally been considered as providing more accurate data than self-report measures.[9,10]

Viewed performance measures, like other types of measures, have sources of inaccuracy. Different viewers may apply the equipment differently (eg, a stopwatch) or rate the client's performance somewhat differently. Another factor to consider is that the test situation may not reflect conditions in which the client must perform on a day-to-day basis.[11] The results on a performance measure are also influenced by practice, fatigue, and effort. Many of these tests will involve several trials, and only one of these trials (usually the last) is used, or a summary of the several trials is calculated. If the effort put into the test changes over time, the performance on the measure may also change, making it necessary to assess the effort of the client—a difficult challenge. This is why many of these tests have detailed instructions to optimize performance, and these must be followed to produce meaningful information. These factors together influence the amount of time it takes to collect accurate data on performance and thus will impact on the cost of using the measure.

Of course, some constructs, such as pain or health-related quality of life (HRQL), cannot be rated using viewed performance, in which case, a self-report measure is appropriate. Clients may complete self-report measures themselves in a health care facility under supervision or by using a mailed version at home (self-completed), or the measures may be administered by an interviewer, either in person or by telephone, who completes the questionnaire based on the client's responses (interviewer completed).[3] Sometimes a surrogate respondent (eg, a family member) completes these measures on behalf of the client if he/she is unable to do so.[3] A self-report measure is particularly useful to measure constructs that cannot be observed with performance (eg, pain, energy level). They can also be used in conjunction with performance measures to explore the relationship between the client's perception of his/her performance in a customary setting from his/her capacity in an ideal environment.[9,11]

There are advantages and disadvantages to the various ways in which these measures can be administered that impact on cost and complete collection of data. The self-completed measure requires few resources, but there is a greater likelihood of a low response rate and missed items.[3] If the measure is self-completed in a health care facility under supervision rather than at home, this may offset some of the difficulties. The interviewer-administered measure results in a high response rate with few missing items, but it costs more to administer, and respondents may not be willing to report problems.[3]

SEARCHING FOR A RANGE OF POTENTIAL MEASURES

One of the purposes of this book is to optimize your search for potential outcome measures to meet your needs. Although this book has focused on including those measures most widely used and evaluated for physical rehabilitation clients, there are many other outcome measures that could not be included in this text. You may also need to widen your search to meet the needs of other types of clients. In addition, as time goes on, new measures will emerge, and you will need a way of identifying and evaluating them.

Probably the most often used sources of information on measures are colleagues or experts in your area of practice. However, the published literature will be the most consistent and comprehensive source to identify measures that are being developed in a rigorous and scientific manner.

Searching the published literature can be a daunting task. You will need a way to connect to the electronic sources of information. Your medical library is your best bet because it will subscribe to many useful electronic collections of literature and have computers that can access these collections. In addition, librarians will be helpful in guiding you in the search, and even an experienced navigator will benefit from their knowledge. If you cannot easily get to a medical library and are connected to the Internet at home or in the office, you can get to one electronic source of literature, MED-LINE, using PubMed, which is a search engine. But let us start with the assumption that you have access to all of the electronic sources through your library.

There are several ways in which you can approach searching, depending on what information you already have. Here are some scenarios:

1. *You want to measure a particular construct, and you need to know what mea-*

sures are available. There is a very good database providing information on instruments called Health and Psychosocial Instruments. By typing in the construct you want to measure, you will be given a description of the tests that measure this construct and the relevant references.

2. *You have the name of the measure you are interested in.* You can search other sources using the name of the instrument in the search strategy. A good place to start for literature related to rehabilitation is an electronic database called CINAHL (Citation Index of Allied Health Literature). The major advantage of this database is that the indexing system includes not only the title and abstract but also all of the measurement instruments listed in an article. So if you are looking for references on the Functional Independence Measure (FIM), you will be given all references that had this term (key word) that not only referred to the FIM in the title or abstract but also those articles that used it as a measure in the study but may not have mentioned this in the abstract. No other database has this feature. You can use this same search strategy to search the well-known database called MEDLINE, but the name of the measure must have been in the title or the abstract for it to identify the article.

3. *You know the name of the author of the primary article on the measure you want to investigate.* The best electronic information source about authors is the Web of Science database. To search, you enter the author's name (no spaces, hyphens, or apostrophes) and the year of the publication. You will be given a listing of all of the articles that cited, in the reference list, the article that refers to the measure of interest. Science Citation Index will do the same job, allowing you to look for citations of the author in which you are interested, but you cannot go any further. Web of Science, like its name, can take you to other articles listed in the reference lists

and then to other reference lists and so on. Be careful not to get lost.

4. *You have a list of articles that mentioned the instrument you want to investigate.* How do you identify those articles that described the instrument and its psychometric properties? CINAHL and MEDLINE (but not the Web of Science) will let you search jointly using other key words to narrow down the list. Words like "psychometric properties" are helpful, as well as "reliability," "validity," or "responsiveness," as these are the terms commonly used in studies of the instrument itself. Use all of these terms to make sure you identify all articles on the measurement properties. You can also ask if these measurement terms are the "primary" or "secondary" focus of the article. This is helpful for instruments that have a large number of references like the FIM or the SF-36.

These are four suggestions about how to start a literature search, but, of course, each one has many more features that cannot be described here. The best way is to try this out yourself with the help of your librarian if you are a novice searcher. The Physiotherapy Evidence Database (PEDro) is another database that you may find useful. McKibbon[12] has written a helpful text that includes a compact disc and provides good information on potential search strategies as well as some examples and key words that you could use in your own searches. At this point, you are trying to find as many potential measures as possible before you start the process of narrowing down your choice.

REDUCING YOUR LIST OF POTENTIAL MEASURES

Consider Measurement Properties

The original article describing the early development of the measure will state the purpose of the measure. You are particularly interested in those designed as evaluative or outcome measures and less interested if they were designed as discriminative or predictive measures. Some measures designed primarily as discriminative or predictive measures have also been used as evaluative measures, but the measurement properties that are needed for evaluation may not be well developed in measures that have not been designed as outcome measures.

Next, examine the measurement properties (ie, reliability and validity) of your list of potential measures. This is important to consider before you look at feasibility so that you exclude, at an early stage, measures that do not have strong measurement properties. No matter how quick and cheap tests are to administer, without good measurement properties they will not be a strong basis of information for decision making. The critical properties are test–retest reliability, longitudinal validity/sensitivity to change, and interpretability. It may help to turn to Chapter 4 to read more about these properties so that you can better evaluate the information you find in the articles. You can also look at the reviews of any of your chosen measures that are included in this text or use the template on page 64 to conduct your own review if the measure you are interested in is not found here. The Appendix and related material on the CD-ROM will be of assistance in extracting information from and critically appraising a measurement study.

Now you can start ranking your list of potential measures. You want a measure that has high test–retest reliability. Experts vary in what they consider an adequate level of reliability.[9,13–15] Without relatively high reliability, you will not be able to have confidence that an observed change in values is a true change and not measurement error. Similarly, it is important that a measure has a high level of sensitivity to change or longitudinal construct validity. At this point, start to put your potential measures in order based on whether their measurement properties are good or poor or there is no information available about some of the important properties. Chapter 4 provides background on different ways in which reliability, sensitivity to

change, or longitudinal validity of a measure can be expressed. The Appendix and related material on the CD-ROM will be of assistance in extracting information from and critically appraising a measurement study. This will help you interpret the information you find in the articles on the measure as well as interpret the data from the evaluations of your own clients.

A set of values using the same measure on healthy individuals or on individuals with the same disability as your client population and identified as low, middle, or high functioning is very useful. The availability of these normative or comparative values will help you interpret the evaluations you make on your clients.

Another useful feature to look for in an instrument is the minimum number of points (or measurement units) that needs to change before an individual can detect this change or that has some clinical meaning; this is called the minimal clinically important difference (MCID). You will find more information on this concept in Chapter 4. Unfortunately, comparison values and MCID values will not always be available. Those measures for which they are available should be moved higher on your list of potential measures. You may wish to rank your list of measures according to their measurement properties by putting them in categories of good and moderate measurement properties. Those with poor measurement properties should probably be discarded at this point.

Consider Feasibility

Next look at your list of potential measures for feasibility of administration. Consider the cost of the measures including any training necessary for administering and scoring the measure, cost of equipment and supplies, mailing or interviewer costs, and any other direct or indirect costs of obtaining the measure. Next consider the time it would take to administer and score the test and how often the test needs to be administered to fulfill your purpose, tracking the progress of your client over time. If the test is administered weekly over an average treatment time of 6 weeks, the cost and time will obviously be greater than if the test is administered at admission and discharge only. Time is considered one of the major barriers to the use of outcome measures; therefore, strategies to decrease the time it takes to administer the measures are important.

Respondent burden, the time and difficulty the measure imposes on the client, is another consideration in choosing a feasible outcome measure.[11] Face validity and interpretability also influence how health professionals will administer and use the data gained in clinical decision making. Those administering the measures must value and use the information they gain; otherwise, they will not feel it is worthwhile taking time away from client treatment to administer the measures.

These considerations may allow you to reorder your list of potential measures, retaining those measures with good measurement properties and feasibility of administration at the top of your list. Be careful to reorder according to feasibility within the categories of good and moderate measurement properties. Feasibility difficulties may sometimes be overcome by creative administrative strategies, but a measure with poor measurement properties needs to be redesigned or modified and then retested—a very lengthy process—before it can be used with confidence.

Consider Use in Similar Populations

Identify those measures at the top of your list that have been used with populations similar to the group with which you are intending to use it. If the measure has not been used with a population similar to yours, consider its use in the population closest to yours in terms of age, gender, disability, etc. Are the populations close enough to gain something from the experience of these authors? Examine carefully the reports of these studies to see if you can learn the strengths and weaknesses of the measure so that you can maximize the strengths and minimize the weaknesses where possible.

When reading the study report, you should pay attention to the amount of missing data as a source of potential bias. Sometimes you have to be very observant to notice that data are missing by looking carefully at the tables and at the footnotes that often follow tables. The research report should indicate how many subjects contributed the data at each evaluation, and if this number fluctuates from one evaluation to another, data are missing. Some measures also have more missing data in some populations than in others. The Timed Up and Go (TUG) test will have missing data for persons who are unable to walk. If this is a considerable part of your population, you may wish to rethink using such a measure. Because it is a timed test, when someone cannot do the activity, the time is infinite. Other measures of the same or similar constructs that have a natural "0" value when someone cannot complete the test (eg, gait speed) may be more appropriate. Therefore, the scaling of the measure is another important consideration when choosing the best measure for you and your clients.

It is also possible to contact the authors/ developers to discuss their views on the measure and its use in your population. If the author is someone you do not know, you could ask your librarian for assistance in obtaining the current contact information of the person. This step may also allow you to decide between two measures with similar measurement properties and feasibility.

IDENTIFY WHEN A COMBINATION OF MEASURES MAY BE REQUIRED

It is sometimes useful to combine the use of generic and specific measures,[5,8] depending on how you plan to use the data. For example, in clients with COPD, the use of the SF-36, a generic self-completed measure, together with the Chronic Respiratory Disease Questionnaire (CRQ), a disease-specific interviewer-completed questionnaire, will allow you to evaluate HRQL as well as dyspnea, fatigue, emotional function, and coping following treatment. Thus, you could compare HRQL in clients with COPD with individuals who have other diseases, as well as comparing changes found in dyspnea, fatigue, emotional function, and coping in your clients with other individuals with COPD.

On the other hand, if it is unlikely that you will use the information from the generic HRQL measure in any current decision-making process, then do not collect it just because the measure is available. There may be hidden dangers to having too much data. For example, if the program is very unlikely to impact on generic HRQL (or another particular outcome), and you have meticulously collected these data, the information may be used in a way that is disadvantageous to you—showing that your program did not improve this outcome when perhaps another program did. Make sure that your strategy, intervention, or program is seen in the best light as reflected through the measurement plan that is ideally tailored to your treatment and your clients' outcomes.

Consider whether your picture of the construct of interest in your clients will be enhanced by the use of both performance and self-report measures. If so, is it feasible for you to use several measures given the cost and time it takes to administer and score the measure and the respondent burden involved? This decision depends on your measurement purpose and resources and is a balance between what is ideal and what is possible. Only you can make this decision and live with the results.

PILOT TEST YOUR POTENTIAL OUTCOME MEASURE(S)

Pilot testing the outcome measures you are considering using is well worth the time and effort. It allows you to consider all aspects of administering and scoring the test and using the data as you intend. Choose a small number of clients in your population to use in the pilot test and obtain any equipment or supplies needed. Train several health care practitioners in the use of the test, frequency of administra-

tion, and scoring and interpretation, providing them with any comparative data you can find from healthy populations or clients with disabilities similar to your own. Gather data and score a small number of clients, keeping close track of the time taken for each step. The group of health professionals administering, scoring, and using the data for decision making can work together to streamline the process and explore various uses for the data in clinical decision making for individuals and groups. Read Chapters 5 and 6 on individual and group clinical decision making to explore the possibilities of using the data from the measures you have chosen. Set a date to finalize your decision about the outcome measures you will use.

CONFIRM THE OUTCOME MEASURES MOST SUITABLE FOR YOUR PURPOSE AND YOUR POPULATION

Reconsider all aspects of the process you have used in narrowing down your choice of outcome measures. Have you searched all sources to identify potential outcome measures? Are the measurement properties of your chosen measures good? Is it feasible to use the measure(s), and do you have the resources to do so? Do the measures suit your population? Are the data you plan to gather useful in individual and group decision making? Will use of the measures enhance your ability to provide high-quality care to your clients in a cost-efficient way? If you can answer yes to these questions, you are ready to implement these measures.

IMPLEMENT A COMPLETE OUTCOME MEASUREMENT PLAN

Your attention now needs to shift to strategies to facilitate the accurate and complete collection of the data on all clients who fit the requirements for use of the measures. This includes with whom the measures should be used, how frequently they should be used, instructions for administering the test(s), guidelines for scoring the measure and how to handle missing data, how to provide feedback to the client, and how to interpret the data for decision making. Methods for compiling scores of groups of clients and providing feedback to the users and other interested parties should be addressed at an early stage. Often simple graphs of scores with attached explanations of interpretability are helpful to those who need a quick assessment of how these clients are doing. You may want to provide more detailed information to those who can use the details in their decision making. Attention at this stage to providing feedback to those who are interested and can use the information increases the likelihood that people will be supportive of the efforts to implement a change in practice.

Set specific times to evaluate the process of measuring outcomes and using the data. Ensure that the data are being used in a way that enhances patient care and look for strategies to improve efficiency while maintaining or improving quality.

This process of choosing suitable outcome measures to provide information on the desired effect of your interventions involves time and effort. The result in terms of data useful for decision making is worth the process. Starting to use an outcome measure you have heard about without considering what it will do for you and how to maximize its usefulness and minimize the time it takes may result in health care providers resenting the time involved and unconsciously subverting the process. This ends in frustration for everyone. There is great potential return for using appropriate outcome measures for clients, health care providers, health care administrators, and funders. It is worth doing well.

SUMMARY

The following are steps to consider when choosing a measure:

- Describe the outcome of interest as specifically as possible and identify an indicator

of this outcome suitable in your client population.

- Clarify your intended purpose. Measures designed for evaluative purposes are likely to have characteristics necessary for good outcome measures.
- Clearly define the client population in which you are interested.
- Identify what combination of performance, self-report, generic, and specific measures would best suit your purpose.
- Search for as many potential measures you can find that meet your criteria, find reviews of them in this text, or complete one yourself based on the review template; do a literature search for articles about the measure.
- Group your measures in categories of those with good measurement properties and those with moderate measurement properties. Eliminate those with poor measurement properties unless you have no alternatives.
- Consider the feasibility of the measures with good measurement properties.
- Determine which measures at the top of your list have been used in populations similar to yours; examine the strengths and weaknesses of the measure in the reported studies.
- Consider the advantages and burden of using a combination of measures and decide which best suits your purpose and resources.
- Pilot test potential measures with a group of clinician colleagues and explore uses for the data.
- Review the reasons for your choice of measures and confirm that you have made the best choice for your purpose and resources.
- Make and implement a complete outcome measurement plan so that it can be used for individual client decision making, summarizing data for group decision making, and providing relevant feedback.
- Evaluate the process at set time frames to detect and solve problems.
- It is worthwhile to collect and use outcome data well.

REFERENCES

1. Kane RL. Looking for physical therapy outcomes. Phys Ther 1994;74:425–9.

2. ICF International Classification of Functioning, Disability and Health [online]. 2001 [cited 2002 Feb 4]. Available from: http://www.who.int/icf. Geneva: World Health Organization.

3. Guyatt GH, Feeny DH, Patrick DL. Measuring health-related quality of life. Ann Intern Med 1993;118:622–9.

4. Maciejewski M. Generic measures. In: Kane RL, editor. Understanding health care outcomes research. Gaithersburg (MD): Aspen; 1997. p. 19–52.

5. Kantz ME, Harris WJ, Levitshy K, Ware JE Jr, Davies AR. Methods for assessing condition-specific and generic functional status outcomes after total knee replacement. Med Care 1992; 30 Suppl 5:MS240–52.

6. Patrick DL, Deyo RA. Generic and disease-specific measures in assessing health status and quality of life. Med Care 1989;27 Suppl 3:S217–32.

7. Mawson S. What is the SF-36 and can it measure the outcome of physiotherapy? Physiotherapy 1995;81:208–12.

8. Atherly A. Condition-specific measures. In: Kane RL, editor. Understanding health care outcomes research. Gaithersburg (MD): Aspen; 1997. p. 53–66.

9. McDowell I, Newell C. Measuring health: a guide to rating scales and questionnaires. 2nd ed. New York: Oxford University Press; 1996. p. 12–27, 41–42.

10. Deyo RA, Carter WB. Strategies for improving and expanding the application of health status measures in clinical settings. Med Care 1992;30 Suppl 5:MS176–86.

11. Studenski S, Duncan PW. Measuring rehabilitation outcomes. Geriatr Rehabil 1993;9:823–30.

12. McKibbon A. PDQ evidence-based principles and practice. Hamilton (ON): BC Decker; 1999.

13. Law M. Measurement in occupational therapy: scientific criteria for evaluation. Can J Occup Ther 1987;54:133–8.

14. Rondinelli RD, Katz RT. Impairment rating and disability evaluation. Philadelphia: WB Saunders; 2000 p. 40–1.

15. Domholdt E. Physical therapy research: principles and applications. 2nd ed. Philadelphia: WB Saunders; 2000. p. 234.

CHAPTER 4

Why Measurement Properties Are Important

LEARNING OUTCOMES AND OBJECTIVES

At the completion of this chapter, the reader will be able to

1. Explain the concepts of reliability and validity;
2. Identify two essential components of a reliable measure;
3. Distinguish between cross-sectional and longitudinal validity;
4. Explain the following types of validity: face, content, criterion, and construct;
5. Explain the essential features associated with the following forms of construct validity: convergent, known group, and discriminant;
6. Compare single- and multigroup longitudinal validity coefficients;
7. Compare three methods for estimating true and clinically important change; and
8. Explain why an estimate of clinically important change for an individual is likely to differ from an estimate of clinically important change for a group.

SCALING ISSUES

Levels of Measurement

It is generally agreed that there are four levels of measurement: nominal, ordinal, interval, and ratio. Nominal scales are represented by categories, with no hierarchy among response options (eg, gender, geographic region, and race). Ordinal scales demonstrate an obvious order or hierarchy among response options; however, the spacing among the responses is not viewed as being equal. Level of education

expressed in the following format, high school, junior college, undergraduate university degree, and graduate degree, is an example of an ordinal scale. The response options for interval scales are equally spaced; however, the scale does not have a meaningful zero value. The classic example of an interval scale is that of temperature measured in degrees Celsius. Although the difference in temperature between 10 and 20 degrees Celsius is the same as the difference in temperature between 35 and 45 degrees Celsius, a temperature of zero Celsius does not signify no temperature; this is reserved for zero degrees Kelvin. Moreover, a temperature of 40 degrees Celsius is not twice that of 20 degrees Celsius. By analogy, it is unlikely that a score of zero on a particular health-related quality of life measure indicates no quality of life. For this reason, most self-report measures are at best considered to represent interval scales. Ratio scales have equal spacing between response options and possess a meaningful zero. In our previous example, temperature measured in degrees Kelvin represents a ratio scale.

Being able to distinguish among the different levels of measurement is important for two reasons. First, the level of measurement of a scale dictates the mathematical operations that can be performed. For example, to add response options across items, the scale must be interval or ratio; to multiply, divide, or create percentages, the scale must be ratio. Often scales that by a strict definition would be considered ordinal are treated as being interval. Many psychometricians accept this practice if the following conditions are met.[1] First, the scale developers should provide evidence that steps were taken to ensure that the spacing between the adjectives associated with the scale points is approximately equal. Second, the scale should have a minimum of seven response options. When the measure is made up of multiple items, fewer response options per item are acceptable. Finally, the distribution of responses provided by those to whom the measure is applied should be consistent with a normal distribution. Most of the measures presented in this text fulfill the requirements of an interval scale. For this reason, we consider reliability and validity indexes that are applicable to interval and ratio scales.

Floor and Ceiling Effects

A useful measure must provide room on the scale for clients to demonstrate improvement and deterioration. Suppose that when a measure is administered, clients' responses cluster at the more negative health state end of the scale. In this situation, the measure cannot detect deterioration in these individuals. This is referred to as a floor effect. Conversely, if clients' responses cluster near the more positive health state end of the scale, there is no room to detect improvement. This is referred to as a ceiling effect. Thus, a clinically useful measure must not demonstrate ceiling or floor effects.

For a measure to be useful, it must provide accurate and meaningful results to clinicians and researchers. Accuracy is determined by a measure's measurement properties. These properties include reliability, validity, and the ability of a measure to detect change. To be meaningful, a measure's score or change score must provide a clinician or researcher with a vivid representation of a client's or group's current health state and, when applicable, whether a client or group has changed since the previous assessment. In this chapter, we review the terminology used to describe a measure's measurement properties and provide illustrations of methods commonly used to give meaning to a measure's change score.

RELIABILITY

Reliability Defined

A reliable measure must fulfill two requirements. First, a reliable measure must provide consistent values with small errors of measurement.[1] Consider the example in which two force measuring devices, such as two handheld dynamometers, are being compared. It would seem reasonable that the device yielding the smallest difference between replicate measurements on a client who truly has not changed would be the preferred measure. However, consider the situation in which one device is broken and always reads the same value. Clearly, this device would yield the smallest difference between replicate measurements—the difference is zero—however, this device would not be clinically useful in distinguishing clients with normal grip strength from clients with compromised grip strength. For this reason, a reliable measure must demonstrate more than consistency. The second requirement is that a reliable measure is capable of differentiating among the clients on whom the measurements are being applied.[1] Thus, for a measure to be declared reliable, it must demonstrate both consistency and the ability to differentiate among the objects of measurement. In the clinical setting, the objects of measurement are usually clients, and throughout this chapter we will apply the term clients to represent the objects of measurement.

Two Expressions of Reliability

Relative Reliability

Given that there are two components of reliability—the ability to differentiate among clients and consistency—it makes sense that a measure's reliability is often summarized in two ways. The term relative reliability is used to describe a measure's ability to distinguish among clients. This coefficient is typically based on Classical Test Theory's interpretation of reliability[2,3]:

Relative reliability coefficient =

$$\frac{\text{true variance}}{\text{observed (total) variance}} =$$

$$\frac{\text{true variance}}{\text{true variance} + \text{error variance}}$$

or in the clinical setting

Relative reliability coefficient =

$$\frac{\text{between-client variance}}{\text{between-client variance} + \text{within-client variance}}$$

In brief, Classical Test Theory defines reliability as the ratio of true variance to observed or total variance. Variance is the statistical term that is used to describe the variability in the data. The true variance represents the extent to which clients' average scores differ. This is also referred to as between-client variance. The error variance represents the extent to which replicate measures within a client differ. For obvious reasons, this is also termed within-client variance. There are no units associated with the relative reliability coefficient. Moreover, when expressed in this format, the relative reliability coefficient is an intraclass correlation coefficient. Typically, intraclass correlation coefficients vary from 0 to 1, with higher values representing higher reliability.

Some investigators—usually in the more distant past—have used Pearson's correlation coefficient as a reliability index. This coefficient does not represent the true variance divided by the observed variance; rather, it describes the association between duplicate measures. The use of Pearson's correlation coefficient as a measure of reliability is limited in two ways. First, it is not sensitive to systematic differences between measures. For example, if the second measure performed on clients as part of a reliability study differed in the same way for each client (eg, exactly half of the first measure), Pearson's coefficient would be 1; however, the intraclass correlation coefficient would be less than 1. A second shortcoming is that Pearson's correlation coef-

ficient is suitable when there are only two replicate measures: the analysis used to calculate the intraclass correlation coefficient can handle two or more replicate measures. As a final note, the value of Pearson's correlation coefficient will approximate the value of the intraclass correlation coefficient when there is no systematic difference between the duplicate measures (ie, the mean scores for the first and second measures are the same).

Absolute Reliability

The second method of representing the reliability of a measure is to express the measurement error in the same units as the original measurement. For this reason, the term absolute reliability is applied and the standard error of measurement (SEM)—not to be confused with the standard error of the mean—is used to quantify the absolute reliability of a measure in the same units as the original measurement.[3] Typically, investigators have reported a single SEM for a measure. However, some investigators have acknowledged that the amount of error varies depending on where the client's score is on the scale and have reported conditional standard errors of measurement (CSEM).[4] Typically, the CSEM is greatest at the mid region of the scale and gets progressively smaller toward the extremes of the scale range.

Although there are several algebraically equivalent methods for calculating the SEM, perhaps the most conceptually appealing description is that of the square root of the error or within-client variance:

$$\text{SEM} = \sqrt{\text{within-client variance}}$$

Sample calculations for the intraclass correlation coefficient and SEM are provided in the Appendix of this chapter.

Types of Reliability

This section examines three types of reliability that impact most frequently on clinical practice and clinical research. Emphasis is placed on the interpretation of clients' scores.

Internal Consistency

Internal consistency studies are based on parallel assessments of clients at an instant in time.[3] This form of reliability is applicable when multi-item measures are summarized into a single score. Estimates of internal consistency are most often associated with questionnaires; however, they also apply to multi-item performance tests. The internal consistency of a test is important for three reasons. First, it assesses the homogeneity of items. Second, it provides an index of a test's ability to differentiate among clients at an instant in time. Third, the internal consistency coefficient is used to calculate the SEM that is associated with a measure's score at an instant in time. Frequently reported internal consistency coefficients include the following: the split-half coefficient, item-item total correlation, Kuder-Richardson 20 and 21 coefficients, and coefficent alpha (α).[1] Of these, coefficient α is reported most frequently, and it is for this reason that we will elaborate on this coefficient. Internal consistency coefficients can take on values from 0 to 1. Higher values represent higher levels of internal consistency.

Conceptually, coefficient α can be thought of as the average correlation, corrected for test length, of all possible split-half correlation coefficients.[1] A split-half correlation coefficient is obtained by dividing the test items into two halves and calculating the correlation between the halves. Although providing specific details is beyond the scope of this book, coefficient α is a Shrout and Fleiss Type 3,k intraclass correlation coefficient, where k is equal to the number of test items.[5]

Test–Retest Reliability

Test–retest reliability studies are based on parallel assessments of clients on different occasions.[3] These studies provide information about the stability of clients' responses over time. The typical study design involves two or more assessments over an interval when clients are believed to be stable with respect to the attribute of interest. Once again, the intraclass correlation coefficient serves as the index of relative reliability and the SEM provides a representation of absolute reliability. Whereas the interpretation of error estimates based on coefficient α are specific to an instant in time, error estimates derived from test–retest reliability studies can be generalized over a time interval equal to that applied in the test–retest reliability study. Later in this section, we will see that the results from test–retest reliability studies can also be used to assist in determining whether a client has changed over time.

Interrater Reliability

Interrater reliability studies are based on parallel assessments by different raters.[3] These studies are of interest when raters are part of the measurement process. For example, interrater reliability would be of interest when assessing attributes that require hands-on assessments or observational skills to arrive at clients' scores. Depending on how the study is constructed, sources of error may be specific to the raters or may include error attributed to clients and raters. For example, consider the case in which all raters observe the same client performance. Here the raters are the only source of error. However, if each rater observed a different performance on the same client, both the raters and the clients would contribute to the error. One design is not to be preferred over the other; rather, it is the goal of the study and the research question of interest that dictate the more appropriate design.

In summary, it is important to appreciate that although reliability is a determinant of validity, reliability alone is insufficient to ensure the validity of a measure.

VALIDITY

A measure is valid to the extent that it assesses what it is intended to measure.[6] Accordingly, validity is not an all or none property but rather a matter of degree.[6] Consistent with this concept is the notion that knowledge of a measure's validity is constantly evolving as new information becomes available. Traditionally, validity has been divided into the following topics: face validity, content validity, construct validity, and criterion validity. More recently, additional terms have been applied to distinguish among different approaches for assessing the construct validity of a measure.

Face Validity

Quite simply, face validity considers whether a measure appears to be measuring what it is intended to measure.[7] For example, if the goal of a measure is to assess lower extremity functional status, one would expect to see items concerning walking, standing, running, and negotiating stairs. However, if a measure designed to assess lower extremity functional status focused primarily on upper extremity tasks or inquired about emotional well-being, one would question its face validity.

Content Validity

Content validity exists to the extent that a measure is composed of a comprehensive sample of items that completely assess the domain of interest.[1,6] Once again, if the goal is to measure lower extremity functional status, one would expect a set of activities that cover all aspects of lower extremity function. Simply measuring a client's walking distance in two minutes or asking clients about their ability to climb a flight of stairs is not a comprehensive set of lower extremity items: they sample only a select aspect of the spectrum of activities associated with lower extremity function.

Criterion Validity

Criterion validity examines the extent to which a measure provides results that are consistent with a gold standard.[1,6] For example, if one is interested in determining the validity of manual muscle testing, the results from a manual muscle test could be compared with results from an assessment using a dynamometer that does not involve the assessor to physically interact with the client. In this example, the dynamometer's results represent the gold standard. Typically, criterion validity is divided into concurrent validity and predictive validity.[6] As the name suggests, concurrent validity compares the measure's result to the gold standard's result that is obtained at approximately the same point in time. The manual muscle testing and dynamometer illustration is an example of concurrent criterion validity. Predictive validity examines a measure's ability to predict some subsequent criterion event. One example would be the use of the Berg Balance Test to predict falls over the following 6 weeks. In this example, the criterion standard would be whether the patient fell over the next 6 weeks.

Construct Validity

For some attributes such as pain and health-related quality of life, no criterion standard exists. It is usually insufficient to depend on face and content validity alone. In the absence of a gold standard, a construct validation process is applied. Construct validation involves forming theories about the attribute of interest and then assessing the extent to which the measure under investigation provides results that are consistent with the theories.[1] For example, several theories applied to the construct validation of functional status measures in clients with low back pain include[8]:

1. Clients who are off work because of their low back pain are more disabled than clients who are able to work with low back pain.
2. Clients who have low back pain and pain radiating into the lower extremity are more disabled than clients who present with back pain only.
3. Clients presenting with acute low back pain are more disabled than clients with longer-standing episodes of back pain.

A more recent interpretation of construct validation is that it is not restricted to testing theories; rather, it includes all aspects of validity (ie, face, content, and criterion).[6]

Cross-sectional and Longitudinal Validity

Some authors point out that if a measure is intended to assess an attribute at a single point in time and to detect change over time, in both instances, the issue is one of validity.[9] Here the validation of a measure at a single point in time would apply a concurrent assessment with a comparison standard. However, we have seen previously that the term concurrent validity has been traditionally used to represent an aspect of criterion validity.[1,6] This poses a problem because criterion or gold standards do not exist for attributes such as health-related quality of life, pain, and functional status. To avoid confusion with the term concurrent validity as it applies to criterion validity, the terms cross sectional validity and longitudinal validity have been applied within the realm of construct validation to distinguish between measures taken at a single point in time (cross-sectional) and measures that relate to change scores (longitudinal).[10–13] Moreover, the terms convergent validity, known group validity, and discriminant validity have been applied to help distinguish among the various strategies for assessing construct validation. These strategies apply equally well to cross-sectional and longitudinal validation designs.

Convergent Validity

This form of validity examines the extent to which a measure's result agrees with the result of another measure that is believed to be assessing the same attribute.[1,6] If the comparison measure is the gold standard, this would represent criterion validity; however, if the comparison standard is not the gold standard, this would represent construct validity.

Cross-sectional example. The results from the measure of interest obtained at a single point in time should demonstrate a moderately high correlation with the results from a second measure that has been validated previously for the same purpose.

Longitudinal example. The assessment of change by the measure of interest should demonstrate a moderately high correlation with the results of change from a second measure that has been validated previously for the same purpose.

Correlation coefficients are often used to quantify the convergent validity of a measure.

Known Group Validity

Known group validity refers to a validation process that examines two or more distinct groups.[10,14] The groups are conceived during the design of a study to represent different levels of the attribute of interest.

Cross-sectional example. Clients with acute low back pain will have lower functional status levels than clients with subacute low back pain.

Longitudinal example. The functional status of clients with acute low back pain will change more over a 1-week interval than will the functional status of clients with subacute low back pain.

T-tests for independent sample means, analysis of variance (ANOVA), and analysis of covariance (ANCOVA) are often used to provide a statistical test of known group validity.

Discriminant Validity

Usually, measures are designed to assess a specific attribute (eg, pain, balance, upper extremity functional status). Accordingly, one would expect a measure designed for a specific purpose to perform better when assessing the attribute of interest than it would if used to assess other attributes. If a measure correlated highly with a spectrum of attributes, a possible interpretation is that the measure is assessing a general concept (eg, overall well-being) rather than the specific attribute of interest. Discriminant validity examines the extent to which a measure correlates with measures of attributes that are different from the attribute the measure is intended to assess.[1,6]

Cross-sectional example. Clients' scores on a lower extremity functional status measure will correlate more highly with the physical functional subscale scores from a generic health status measure than with the emotional subscale scores from the generic measure.

Longitudinal example. Clients' change scores on a lower extremity functional status measure will correlate more highly with the physical functional subscale change scores from a generic measure than with the emotional subscale change scores from the generic measure.

Once again, correlation coefficients are frequently used to indicate the discriminant validity of a measure.

Sensitivity to Change and Responsiveness: A Brief Historical Perspective

Over the past two decades, authors have applied the terms sensitivity to change and responsiveness inconsistently. Kirshner and Guyatt were the first to define responsiveness as "the power of the test to detect a clinically important difference."[12] Within Kirshner and Guyatt's framework, responsiveness is one of three properties associated with an evaluative measure. The other two properties are reliability and longitudinal construct validity. Hays and Hadorn suggested that if the goal of a measure is to detect clinically important change, then the issue is one of validity, and it is unnatural to suggest that a measure can be responsive but not valid.[9] Other authors have noted that the terms sensitivity to change and responsiveness are often used interchangeably.[1] Recently, in an attempt to add clarity to this jargon issue, Liang suggested the following definitions for the terms sensitivity to change and responsiveness.[13] Liang defined sensitivity to change as "the ability of an instrument to measure change in the state regardless of whether it is relevant or meaningful to the decision maker. Sensitivity to change is a necessary but insufficient condition for responsiveness."[13] Responsiveness is defined as

> the ability of an instrument to measure a meaningful or clinically important change in a clinical state . . . It implies a change

that is noticeably, appreciably different that is of value to the patient (or physician). The change may allow the individual to perform some essential task or to perform tasks more efficiently or with less pain or difficulty. These changes also should exceed variation that can be attributed to chance.[13]

We find Liang's definitions attractive for two reasons. First, they offer a distinct meaning to each term. Second, although Liang's definition of responsiveness is consistent with the spirit of Kirshner and Guyatt's definition, it does not make what some would consider an inappropriate distinction between important change and validity. However, at the time this book was written, scholars continued to debate jargon and methods for classifying change.

Of the many methods proposed, the most comprehensive is that provided by Beaton and colleagues.[15] Their classification system considers three domains. The first is whether the unit of interest is an individual client or a group. The second domain addresses the mechanism for estimating change. Three options are provided: between individual or group, within individual or group, and both between and within. The third domain has five options and reflects the type of change or difference: minimum potential change, minimum detectable change, observed change in a population, observed change in those estimated to have changed, and observed change in those estimated to have changed an important amount.

Longitudinal Validity

We use the term longitudinal validity in reference to a measure's ability to detect change without considering whether the change is important. Applied in this manner, our use of the term longitudinal validity is consistent with Liang's definition for sensitivity to change. Throughout this text, a measure's longitudinal validity will be summarized as a coefficient, series of coefficients, or a formal statistical test. Examples of frequently applied longitudinal validity coefficients include the standardized response mean, the effect size, Norman's intraclass correlation coefficients, Pearson's and Spearman's correlation coefficients, and area under receiver operating characteristic (ROC) curves.

Longitudinal Validity Coefficients (Sensitivity to Change Coefficients)

Longitudinal validity coefficients are unitless indexes representing a measure's ability to detect change. Although their values, other than zero, have little meaning when expressed in isolation, they are useful for making relative comparisons between measures. We will divide these coefficients into single-group and multi-group indexes.[16]

Single-group indexes. As the name suggests, single-group indexes are obtained from a study design that examines one group that is presumed to have changed over the course of the study. An illustration of a single group design is shown in Figure 4–1.

Effect size. The effect size (ES) is calculated by dividing the mean change by the standard deviation of the baseline scores.[17] There is no upper limit associated with this coefficient:

$$ES = \frac{mean\ change}{standard\ deviation\ of\ baseline\ scores}$$

$$ES = \frac{(mean\ follow\text{-}up\ score) - (mean\ baseline\ score)}{standard\ deviation\ of\ baseline\ scores}$$

Standardized response mean. The standardized response mean (SRM) is calculated by dividing the mean change by the standard deviation of the change scores.[18] There is no upper limit associated with this coefficient:

$$SRM = \frac{mean\ change}{standard\ deviation\ of\ change\ scores}$$

$$SRM = \frac{(mean\ follow\text{-}up\ score) - (mean\ baseline\ score)}{standard\ deviation\ of\ change\ scores}$$

Multigroup indexes. Because multigroup indexes are based not only on a measure's ability to detect change but also on its ability to identify different levels of change, multigroup indexes are often viewed as being more rigorous than single-group indexes.[16] Multigroup indexes are derived from studies in which two or more groups that are expected to change by different amounts are examined. An example of a two-group study is shown in Figure 4–2.

A number of multigroup change indexes or coefficients exist. We will begin by describing methods suitable for two groups and then consider methods appropriate for more than two groups.

Diagnosing change and the area under a receiver operating characteristic curve as a longitudinal validity coefficient. This analysis is appropriate when two groups of clients are being investigated. Often the two groups represent clients who have and have not changed an important amount; however, the groups could represent stable clients and clients who truly change. Because gold standards do not exist for either important change or true change, a construct rather than a criterion validation standard is applied.

The intent of the ROC curve analysis is to evaluate a measure's ability to differentiate clients in the two groups. For the purpose of this section, we will assume that the goal is to differentiate between clients who have improved an important amount and clients

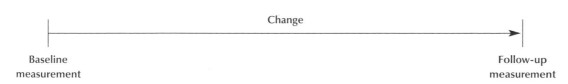

Change

Baseline measurement

Follow-up measurement

FIGURE 4–1 Illustration of a single-group design.

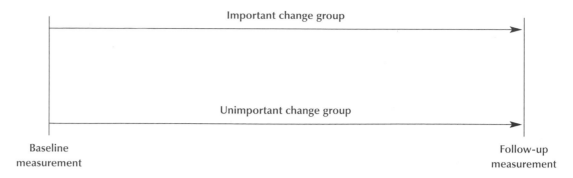

FIGURE 4–2 Illustration of a two-group design.

who have not improved an important amount. From a clinical perspective, this challenge can be viewed as diagnosing important improvement.[19,20] The goals are to identify a measure's ability to detect important improvement and to determine the change score that best differentiates clients who have and have not improved an important amount. The latter issue is one of responsiveness, and it will be addressed in the subsequent section on interpretability.

A ROC curve is constructed by plotting sensitivity against one minus specificity.[19,20] Within the context of our example of change, sensitivity represents the number of clients the measure correctly identifies as having improved an important amount divided by all clients who truly improved an important amount. Specificity is defined as those clients whom the measure correctly identifies as not having improved an important amount divided by all clients who truly did not improve an important amount. A sample 2 × 2 table is shown in Table 4–1. In this example, the sensitivity and specificity values are 0.81 and 0.80, respectively.

In Table 4–1, we have used 3.5 as the cutoff value. To generate a ROC curve, a number of 2 × 2 tables are generated using different

cutoff values for each table, and sensitivity and specificity values are calculated for each table. Table 4–2 presents sensitivity and one minus specificity values calculated for the Back Ouch Scale (BOS) score using a number of cutoff values. The BOS is a hypothetical measure created for this example.

The sensitivity and specificity values shown in Table 4–2 were plotted to produce the ROC curve illustrated in Figure 4–3. The sensitivity to change coefficient is the area under the curve (AUC) and represents the area beneath the solid curved line in Figure 4–3. The area under a ROC curve can vary from 0 to 1 (1 being the total area available). In this example, the AUC is 0.83. To assist in the interpretation of this value, an AUC of 0.50 indicates that the measure does no better than chance in correctly identifying clients as having changed or not. This is indicated by the diagonal line in Figure 4–3.

Guyatt's Change Index. This index also uses information from two groups of clients. One group is composed of clients who have changed an important amount, and the second group consists of unchanged or stable clients. Guyatt's Change Index (GCI) is defined as the minimal clinically important difference (MCID),

TABLE 4–1 Example of a 2 × 2 Table for the Back Ouch Scale (BOS)

BOS Change Score	Important Improvement		Total
	Yes	No	
≥ 3.5	81	20	101
< 3.5	19	80	99
Total	100	100	200

TABLE 4–2   Change Score, Sensitivity, and 1 – Specificity for Back Ouch Scale

Change Score	Sensitivity	1 – Specificity
–3.0	1.00	1.00
–2.0	1.00	0.94
–1.0	0.99	0.86
0.0	0.97	0.60
1.5	0.92	0.49
2.5	0.90	0.43
3.5	0.81	0.20
4.5	0.60	0.08
5.5	0.42	0.02
6.5	0.32	0.00
7.5	0.22	0.00
8.5	0.19	0.00
9.5	0.00	0.00

often represented as the mean change in the important change group, divided by the standard deviation of the change scores in the stable client group.[21] There is no upper limit associated with this coefficient:

$$GCI = \frac{\text{minimal clinically important difference}}{\text{standard deviation of change in stable clients}}$$

Norman's S coefficients. Norman has proposed two longitudinal validity coefficients. One coefficient is based on a repeated measures ANOVA; the other is calculated from the results of ANCOVA.[1,22] Both are intraclass correlation coefficients and can take on values from 0 to 1. An S statistic of 0 indicates that a measure cannot discriminate among groups that have truly changed by different amounts, whereas an S value of 1 reflects a measure that discriminates perfectly among groups that changed by different amounts.

Norman's repeated measures S coefficient. As the name suggests, this coefficient is calculated from the results of a repeated measures ANOVA. Norman's S_{repeat} is defined as the variance owing to the group × time interaction term divided by the sum of the group × time interaction and the error variances.[22] The

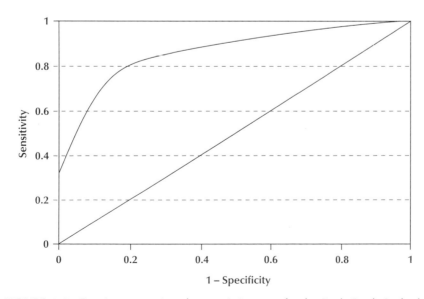

FIGURE 4–3   Receiver operating characteristic curve for the Back Ouch Scale data.

group × time interaction assesses the extent to which the groups change by different amounts.

Norman's ANCOVA S coefficient. This coefficient is based on the results from an ANCOVA that examines the between-group difference in follow-up scores having adjusted for baseline scores. Norman S_{ANCOVA} is defined as the group variance in follow-up scores, having adjusted for baseline differences, divided by the sum of the group variance in follow-up scores, having adjusted for baseline differences, plus the error variance.[22]

Correlation coefficient. Some studies do not attempt to identify distinct subgroups but rather acknowledge that it is possible for clients to display many levels of change. When this condition exists, a multilevel comparison standard quantified on an ordinal or interval scale is applied. The longitudinal validity index is defined by the correlation between the comparison standard's rating of change and the measure's change score (ie, the difference between baseline and follow-up scores).[8,11,16]

Interpretability

For a measure to be clinically useful, its scores must have meaning to clinicians. This includes the interpretation of a score value at a single point in time and change scores assessed over time. We use the word interpretability to cover both of these concepts. Where possible, we will attempt to report four values that relate to the interpretability of a measure: the first and second make reference to a client's score at a single point in time; the third and fourth reflect change. The first value will be the typical, customary, or normal value for the population of interest. Although some measures, such as the SF-36, have population values, many measures do not. The second value, as a confidence interval for a client's score, provides insight into the error associated with a client's score at a point in time. The third value, minimal detectable change, expresses the error associated with a change score (eg, previous assessment's value – current assess-ment's value) and provides an insight into whether a client has truly changed. The fourth and final value reflects the magnitude of the MCID. A change in a client that meets or exceeds the MCID is strong evidence that a client has changed an important amount.

Responsiveness as It Applies to the Interpretability of Change Scores

Applying Liang's terminology, responsiveness addresses clinically important change.[13] However, before considering responsiveness, it is important to recall that Liang cautions, "Sensitivity to change is a necessary but insufficient condition for responsiveness."[13] Given that one accepts that a measure must be sensitive to change before it can be responsive, the next question is, "What constitutes clinical importance?" To some, important change is any change greater than measurement error; to others, it represents a change that has value to the client. Yet others add further complexity to the issue by forcing us to consider the risk and consequences of adverse effects as we attempt to define the magnitude of a clinically important change. Finally, several investigators have suggested that the size of an important change is related to a client's current functional status level. For example, to achieve a clinically important improvement, clients who have a lower functional status level may need to undergo a greater change than clients with a higher functional status level. Because there is no singularly agreed on definition or method for estimating clinically important change, we will consider two types of change from two perspectives. The two types of change are true change—this represents the lower limit of detectable change—and clinically important change by whatever definition those reporting the results apply. Goldsmith and colleagues have shown that the magnitude of clinically important change for an individual is substantially greater than the size of a clinically important between-group difference.[23] Accordingly, when considering the interpretability of a measure's change score, we will distinguish between methods used to estimate responsiveness indexes for individual client and group estimates. We will consider the individual client perspective first.

Individual client perspective. Typically, investigators have applied one of three methods for estimating change scores. Each approach can be used to estimate either true change or important change; however, the sample composition will differ depending on the attribute of interest. Table 4–3 summarizes the group composition for these methods.

For example, if one applies Method 1 and the goal is to estimate true change, only stable clients are investigated. On the other hand, if the goal is to estimate important improvement, only clients not achieving an important improvement are studied. Note that the latter sample will include both stable clients and clients who have changed but not by an important amount. For the purpose of illustration, we provide examples of the three methods as they pertain to the estimation of important change. Once again, we will consider the hypothetical BOS mentioned previously.

Method 1. This approach is similar to a test–retest reliability study; however, the sample composition consists of clients who have not achieved an important improvement. Change scores are obtained, and a multiple of the standard deviation of the change score is used as the estimate of important improvement. Typically, one chooses a probability level associated with a client having a low probability of being from the distribution of clients who have not improved an important amount. For example, some investigators have used the 95% confidence interval; however, the choice is purely arbitrary. To illustrate this method, let us assume that the standard deviation of the change scores for the BOS when applied to clients with low back pain who have not improved an important amount is 2.7 BOS points. When the data are consistent with a normal distribution, the one-sided 95% confidence interval is obtained by multiplying this value by the corresponding z value (z = 1.65). Assuming that the average improvement in clients who have not improved an important amount is 1 BOS point, the upper one-sided 5% confidence estimate is 1 + 4.5 BOS points. The value 4.5 is the product of the standard deviation of the change scores, 2.7 BOS points, and the z value (1.65). Accordingly, an improvement of 5.5 or more BOS points would be considered an important improvement. The interpretation is that there is less than a 5% chance that a client displaying an improvement of 5.5 or more BOS points is from a group of clients who have not improved an important amount. It is important to stress that the interpretation is not that the client has a 95% chance of having improved an important amount. This method is illustrated in Figure 4–4.

Method 2. This approach is similar to Method 1; however, in this case, only clients who have improved an important amount are included. For the purpose of illustration, we will assume that the distribution of change scores for this group is consistent with a normal distribution. Because this group of clients has improved an important amount, we are interested in identifying a change score that has a relatively high probability of being associated with this group of clients. In this example, we will choose the lower one-sided 80% confidence level (the z value is −0.84). If the mean change for this group was 8.0 BOS points and the standard deviation of the change scores was

TABLE 4–3 Group Composition for Three Classification Methods Used to Quantify True Change and Important Change

Method	Estimating True Change	Estimating Important Change
1	Stable clients	Clients not achieving an important change
2	Changed clients	Clients achieving an important change
3	Stable and changed clients	Clients achieving and not achieving an important change

5.0 BOS points, the lower one-sided 80% confidence value is 3.8 (ie, 8.0 – 4.2). Thus, clients who display improvement scores greater than 3.8 BOS points will be labeled as having improved an important amount. This method is illustrated in Figure 4–5.

Method 3. This method includes clients who have and have not improved an important amount. An estimate of important improvement is obtained by applying the diagnostic approach that was described previously in the Sensitivity to Change section. However, rather than stopping once the sensitivity to change coefficient (AUC) has been calculated, one applies the data used to generate the ROC curve to identify the improvement score on the measure of interest that best classifies clients as having or not having improved an important amount. This value is referred to as the cutoff score. Typically, there are three ways to select a cutoff score: rule in an important improvement, rule out an important improvement, and maximize the correct classification of clients. In this example, we will apply the last approach. Specifically, this choice simultaneously maximizes sensitivity and specificity. The cutoff score is identified as the improvement score that was used to identify the data point on the ROC curve closest to the top left corner of the curve. Applying this approach, clients with BOS improvement scores greater than 3.5 are deemed to have improved an important amount. This method is illustrated in Figure 4–6.

Minimal clinically important difference: between-group perspective. Methods 1 to 3 are used to estimate an important improvement when an individual client is the unit of interest. As such, their results are of interest to clinicians. Clinical researchers are also interested in knowing the magnitude of a clinically important difference; however, rather than being interested in an important within-client difference, researchers are interested in knowing the magnitude of an important between-group difference. Researchers apply this knowledge to estimate sample size for clinical trials and to

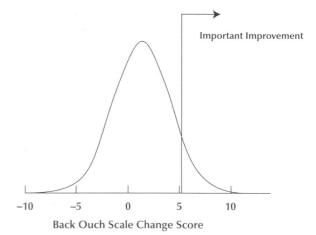

FIGURE 4–4 Estimate of important improvement using Method 1.

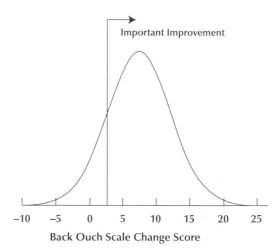

FIGURE 4–5 Estimate of important improvement using Method 2.

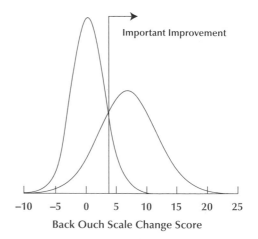

FIGURE 4–6 Estimate of important improvement using Method 3.

judge whether statistically significant findings are clinically important. The work of Goldsmith and colleagues suggests that the magnitude of an important between-group difference is approximately 40% of that of an important within-client change.[23] Although work exploring within-client and between-group differences is in its infancy, a possible explanation for this finding is related to differences in the group composition of clients used to estimate important within-client and between-group differences. In Methods 1 and 2, the groups were homogeneous: they were composed of clients who improved an important amount or clients who did not. However, when considering an important between-group difference for clinical trial applications, the groups are typically composed of clients receiving different interventions. Rather than assuming that all clients in one group will respond the same way (eg, those receiving the placebo will not improve an important amount) and that all those in the second group will respond in another way (eg, improve an important amount), it is reasonable to believe that some clients in the control group will improve an important amount and that some clients in the experimental group will not

improve an important amount. The consequence of this heterogeneity is that there will be much more overlapping of the distributions used to estimate a between-group difference compared with the overlapping of the distributions used to estimate an important within-client improvement (Method 3). For this reason, the mean difference between groups—this is the usual method of quantifying a between-group difference—will be smaller than the difference between the groups used to estimate a within-client improvement. Figure 4–7 illustrates the mean between-group difference.

SUMMARY

- A reliable measure must demonstrate the ability to differentiate among clients and provide consistent values on repeated assessments.
- The intraclass correlation coefficient is often used to quantify relative reliability.
- The SEM or a multiple of it is frequently used to express the absolute reliability of a measure in scale points.
- Several types of reliability exist, including internal consistency, test–retest reliability, and interrater reliability.

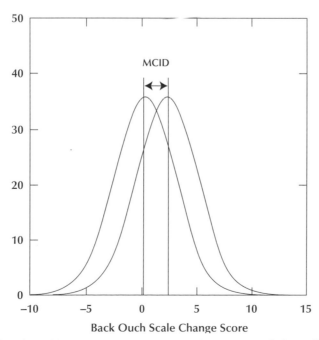

FIGURE 4–7 Group estimation of important improvement. MCID = minimal clinically important difference.

- Reliability is a prerequisite of validity, but reliability does not ensure validity.
- Validity addresses the extent to which a measure assesses what it is intended to measure.
- Traditionally, validity has been subdivided into the following terms: face, content, construct, and criterion validity.
- The terms convergent, known group, and discriminant validity are being used more frequently to add further descriptive clarity to construct validity.
- The terms cross-sectional and longitudinal validity have been applied more recently to describe the validity of a measure at a single point in time and the ability of a measure to detect change over time.
- Different authors have applied the terms sensitivity to change and responsiveness differently.
- Longitudinal validity (sensitivity to change) examines the ability of a measure to detect change without making reference to whether the change is clinically important.
- Responsiveness focuses on clinically important change and contributes to the interpretability of a measure.
- The MCID for a group of clients is substantially less than for an individual client.
- The MCID may vary depending on a client's level of disability or the risk of an adverse effect associated with the proposed intervention.

APPENDIX

Reliability Coefficient Calculations

Relative and absolute reliability coefficients can be calculated from information provided in an ANOVA table. The following vignette is used to illustrate the calculations.

Suppose that an investigator was interested in assessing the test–retest reliability of the Three-Step Performance Measure (a hypothetical measure). The unit of measurement for this test is distance in meters. Ten patients recovering from ankle sprains were tested on two occasions separated by 48 hours. The data are shown in Table 4–4 and the results from the analysis of variance are reported in Table 4–5.

Relative Reliability Calculation

$$R = \frac{\text{between-client variance}}{\text{between-client variance} + \text{within-client variance}} = \frac{\sigma_B^2}{\sigma_B^2 + \sigma_W^2}$$

$$R = \frac{23.05}{23.05 + 1.76}$$

$$R = 0.93$$

TABLE 4–4   Three-Step Patient Data Recorded in Meters

Patient	Time 1	Time 2	Difference
1	16.20	17.90	−1.70
2	5.90	4.40	1.50
3	10.80	8.70	2.10
4	17.20	17.60	−0.40
5	8.00	6.30	1.70
6	12.70	12.80	−0.10
7	4.50	7.20	−2.70
8	19.60	16.60	3.00
9	10.30	12.70	−2.40
10	14.70	15.40	−0.70
Mean	11.99	11.96	0.03
SD	4.99	4.99	1.98

TABLE 4–5 Analysis of Variance Table and Variance Component Calculations

Source	DF	SS	MS	Variance Components
Between clients	9	430.62	47.85	$\sigma_B^2 = \dfrac{MSB - MSW}{k} = \dfrac{47.85 - 1.76}{2} = 23.05$
Within clients	10	17.57	1.76	$\sigma_W^2 = MSW = 1.76$
Total	19			$\sigma_B^2 + \sigma_W^2 = 24.81$

k is equal to the number of measurements on a patient.

Absolute Reliability Calculation

$$SEM = \sqrt{\text{within-client variance}} = \sqrt{MSW}$$

$$SEM = \sqrt{1.76}$$

$$SEM = 1.33 \text{ meters}$$

The interpretation of 1 SEM is that there is a 68% chance that a client's true score will be within 1.33 meters of the measured value.

REFERENCES

1. Streiner DL, Norman GR. Health measurement scales: a practical guide to their development and use. Oxford: Oxford University Press; 1995.

2. Nunnally JC. Psychometric theory. Toronto: McGraw-Hill, 1978.

3. Feldt LS, Brennan RL. Reliability. In: Linn RL, editor. Educational measurement. Phoenix: Oryx Press; 1993. p. 105–46.

4. Lord FM. Standard errors of measurement at different score levels. J Educ Measurement 1984;21:239–43.

5. Shrout PE, Fleiss JL. Intraclass correlations: uses in assessing rater reliability. Psychol Bull 1979;86:420–8.

6. Messick S. Validity. In: Linn RL, editor. Educational measurement. Phoenix: Oryx Press; 1993. p. 13–103.

7. McDowell I, Newell C. Measuring health: a guide to rating scales and questionnaires. 2nd ed. New York: Oxford University Press; 1996.

8. Kopec JA, Esdaile JM, Abrahamowicz M, Abenhaim L, Wood-Dauphinee S, Lamping DL, et al. The Quebec Back Pain Disability Scale: measurement properties. Spine 1995;20:341–52.

9. Hays RD, Hadorn D. Responsiveness to change: an aspect of validity, not a separate dimension. Qual Life Res 1992;1:73–5.

10. Ware JE, Kosinski M, Keller SD. A 12-item short-form health survey. Med Care 1998;34:220–33.

11. Deyo RA, Diehr P, Patrick DL. Reproducibility and responsiveness of health status measure. Statistics and strategies for evaluation. Controlled Clin Trials 1991;12 Suppl 4:142S–58S.

12. Kirshner B, Guyatt G. A methodological framework for assessing health indices. J Chron Dis 1985;38:27–36.

13. Liang MH. Longitudinal construct validity: establishment of clinical meaning in patient evaluative instruments. Med Care 2000;38 Suppl II:II-84–90.

14. Kerlinger FN. Foundations of behavioral research. New York: Holt, Rinehart and Winston; 1964.

15. Beaton DE, Bombardier C, Katz JN, Wright JG, Wells G, Boers M, et al. Looking for important change/differences in studies of responsiveness. J Rheumatol 2001;28:400–5.

16. Stratford PW, Binkley JM, Riddle DL. Health status measures: strategies and analytic methods for assessing change scores. Phys Ther 1996;76:1109–23.

17. Kazis LE, Anderson JJ, Meenan RF. Effect sizes for interpreting changes in health status. Med Care 1989;27 Suppl 3:S178–89.

18. Liang MH, Larson MG, Cullen KE, Schwartz JA. Comparative measurement efficiency and sensitivity of five health status instruments for arthritis research. Arthritis Rheum 1985;28:542–7.

19. Deyo RA, Centor RM. Assessing the responsiveness of functional scales to clinical change: an analogy to diagnostic test performance. J Chron Dis 1986;39:897–906.

20. Stratford PW. Diagnosing patient change: impact of reassessment interval. Physiother Can 2000;52:225–8.

21. Guyatt G, Walter S, Norman G. Measuring change over time: assessing the usefulness of evaluative instruments. J Chron Dis 1987;40:171–8.

22. Norman GR. Issues in the use of change scores in randomized trials. J Clin Epidemiol 1989;42:1097–105.

23. Goldsmith CH, Boers M, Bombardier C, Tugwell P. Criteria for clinically important changes in outcomes: development, scoring and evaluation of rheumatoid arthritis patient and trial profiles. J Rheumatol 1993; 20:561–5.

CHAPTER 5

How Outcome Measures Can Be Used to Enhance Clinical Decision Making about Individual Clients

LEARNING OUTCOMES AND OBJECTIVES

At the completion of this chapter, the reader will be able to

1. Compare the benefits and barriers associated with activity and participation measures;
2. Pose three questions that require answers when assessing a client's outcome;
3. Describe the importance of selecting the most appropriate reassessment interval; and
4. Structure an efficient approach for establishing goals, assessing client outcomes, and documenting the findings in the medical record.

ACTIVITY AND PARTICIPATION MEASURES

For decades, clinicians have measured impairments (eg, strength and range of motion) and planned interventions based on the findings of these measures. More recently, there has been a growing interest in complementing impairment measures with health-related quality of life and activity and participation measures. This trend was first seen in the clinical neuroscience arena and has spread to many other subspecialties.

Although some clinicians have embraced the application of activity and participation measures, other clinicians have questioned the necessity of administering additional measures. The essence of the latter clinicians' concerns is summarized nicely in the following quotation from one of our colleagues: "In order for me to perform additional measures on my patients,

the measures must be efficient to administer and provide more meaningful information than is available from the tests I currently use." This statement demands that proponents of activity and participation measures examine the barriers and benefits associated with the implementation of these measures in busy clinical practice settings. This chapter addresses this issue and demonstrates how the complementary use of activity and participation measures can enhance clinical decision making.

Barriers to the Use of Measures

Barriers to the successful implementation of activity and performance measures fall into two categories: real and perceived. Table 5–1 provides a summary of common myths concerning activity and performance measures.

In addition to these perceived barriers, there are also real barriers that, unless addressed, may impede the use of activity and performance measures. These barriers include the following:

1. *Scores from activity and participation measures often do not have meaning to clinicians.* Clinicians have applied impairment measures for many decades, and the values for these measures have meaning to them. A new measure's value does not have intuitive meaning to a clinician, nor can she/he draw on the experience of more senior colleagues. Accordingly, if researchers do not provide an interpretation of the meaning associated with measured values, there is little incentive for clinicians to take the extra effort to apply these measures. For some measures, investigators have taken

this extra step; however, for many measures, this step has yet to be taken.

2. *Dearth of mentors.* Traditionally, the use of written self-report measures was not taught in clinical programs. Accordingly, some clinical practice opinion leaders are not versed in the use of written self-report measures and have not integrated these measures into clinical practice.

Benefits of Using Participation and Activity Measures

This section offers five benefits associated with providing a comprehensive assessment that includes activity and participation measures:

1. *The only way to gain substantial information about activity and participation is to measure activity and participation.* Because impairment does not tell us very much about activity and participation, the direct application of activity and participation measures represents the most valid method of assessing these domains.

2. *Assessing activity and participation is meaningful to clients and therefore leads to better communication with clients about their change with treatment.* Most clients phrase their reasons for seeking care in terms of activity and role limitations rather than in terms of impairment restrictions. For example, when was the last time a client complained of 108 degrees of knee flexion or an 18-kgf grip strength? Clearly, it is more common for clients to describe their reasons for seeking care in terms of activity and participation limitations (eg, difficulty climbing stairs or the ability to work or participate in recreational events). Thus, by overtly assessing what is important to clients, a better rapport is developed between clinicians and clients.

3. *Assessing activity and participation or client-reported pain represents the only game in town.* For some conditions—plantar fasciitis is one example—observable physical impairments are rare or do not exist. Accordingly, assessing a client's activity and participation levels or reported pain provides the only method for objectifying the presenting complaint and assessing change over time.

4. *Assessing activity and participation is consistent with the directives of numerous professional bodies.* Many professional bodies require clinicians to perform com-

TABLE 5–1 Perceived Barriers: Myth and Reality

Myth	Reality
There is a high correlation between impairment and activity and participation.	Repeatedly, studies have shown that the correlation between physical impairments and activity and participation measures typically varies between 0.2 and 0.5.[1,2] The meaning of a correlation of 0.5 is that knowing about one measure provides 25% of the information about the other measure.
Altering impairment correlates highly with altering activity and participation.	Once again, the correlation between change in impairment and change in activity and participation is also in the order of 0.2 to 0.5.
Activity and participation measures are time consuming to administer.	Although this may be true for some measures, many activity and participation measures can be self-administered in less than 5 minutes.
Activity and participation measures are time consuming for the clinician to score.	This is also true for some measures; however, many newer activity and participation measures can be scored in less than 30 seconds without the use of computational aids.
The measurement properties of impairment measures are superior to the measurement properties of activity and participation measures.	Many studies have shown that the measurement properties of a well-designed activity and participation measure are equal to or better than the measurement properties of impairment measures. Moreover, information concerning a measure's ability to detect change is available for many activity and participation measures but exists for few impairment measures.

prehensive assessments of clients using validated outcome measures. Once again, because of the modest correlation between impairment and activity and participation, a comprehensive assessment in most instances requires the inclusion of impairment, activity, and participation measures. Moreover, in many instances, more is known about the measurement properties of activity and participation measures compared with impairment measures. This is particularly true with respect to longitudinal validity and interpretability, which are critical for measuring outcome.

5. *Providing an assessment of activity and participation is consistent with the mandate of many third-party payers.* More and more, those paying for health care are demanding a meaningful "bang for their buck." Recognizing the modest correlation between impairment and activity and participation, many payers are requiring the use of client-oriented outcome measures that focus on activity and participation.

Clearly, for a measure to be accepted in clinical practice, it must be efficient and provide more information and with greater confidence than is available from current practice.

The following scenario will assist in better understanding the benefits associated with activity and participation measures. Readers are encouraged to take a moment and jot down their responses to the questions. Following an introduction of several important points, we will return to this problem and illustrate how these concepts can be applied to Mr. Smith and our clients in general.

SCENARIO 1: Mr. Smith

Findings from the client's initial assessment. Mr. Smith is a 40-year-old man with low back pain. The discomfort came on 3 weeks ago while he was laying patio stones. The discomfort is located to the right of the midline and extends approximately 10 cm proximal from the iliac crest. Over the first week following the injury, there was a slight reduction in the discomfort; however, there has been little change over the past 2 weeks. Mr. Smith has not experienced low back pain previously. He works in an office, and other than experiencing mild discomfort during the day, his work is unaffected by his back problem. Mr. Smith states that he has cut down on his household and recreational activities.

Take a moment and jot down your responses to the following questions:

What is this client's status today?

How confident are you in your assessment?

When will you reassess this client?

What factors influenced your choice of reassessment interval?

Now consider the following information that was obtained at Mr. Smith's follow-up assessment.

Reassessment. You ask Mr. Smith whether the treatment has been helpful and obtain the following response: "I think so . . . you know my back was quite sore last evening and rather stiff . . . although it felt pretty good this morning when I went for a long walk."

Interpret this dialogue and jot down what you would write in the medical record. Your assessment should include whether Mr. Smith has changed and, if he has, whether the change is important.

How confident are you in your interpretation?

What additional questions would you like to ask this client?

Although we acknowledge that this brief scenario does not contain the amount of information that is available in an actual clinical interaction, it does serve to remind readers of the difficulties encountered when interpreting some clients' responses.

When our colleagues were challenged with this scenario, many stated that when faced with an ambiguous response such as Mr. Smith's, they would ask whether the client had noticed a change since the previous assessment. Although questions that inquire about change are applied frequently in clinical practice, the responses to these questions are suspect for several reasons. First, in many instances, clients have difficulty accurately recalling their previous health status.[3,4] According to Ross's implicit theory of change, clients start with their current state and then work backward and report change in the direction in which they believe it should have occurred.[3] For example, Linton and Melin found that clients with chronic pain recalled their previous pain levels to be worse than they had actually reported at the previous point in time.[5] A second shortcoming is that questions that inquire about change do not provide an absolute representation of a client's state. Accordingly, the answers to these questions do not help clinicians determine whether a client's treatment goals have been met. Finally, questions that ask about change provide a format for clients to provide answers they think their clinicians want to hear. For example, when asked whether they have noticed an improvement, many clients will answer yes. However, this positive response is often followed by a list of activities that the client continues to find difficult or is unable to perform. In summary, the biggest problem associated with questions that ask about change is that because they do not offer an absolute representation of a client's state, it is possible for a client to report continuous improvement without ever reaching the target health state.

INTERPRETING OUTCOME MEASURE RESULTS

Clinical Questions Asked When Assessing a Client's Outcome

Clinicians use measures to assist in planning treatment and to measure the effect of that treatment. Because only a modest correlation exists between impairment and activity and participation measures, a comprehensive assessment demands that all relevant outcomes are assessed and that one measure is not a useful surrogate measure for another. Our main focus in this book is to suggest ways of using outcome measures to assess the attribute of interest at a specific point in time and to evaluate change in clients over time. For example, at a client's initial assessment, a clinician could use a measure such as the Lower Extremity Functional Scale to assess the activity and participation of a client with an ankle sprain. Should the client's activity and/or participation be limited, the clinician is likely to implement an intervention aimed at improving the client in the areas of limitation. Following a course of treatment, the clinician will reassess the client's activity and participation to determine whether a change has occurred and whether the client has reached the goal value in the targeted areas. Three questions clinicians pose and answer daily include the following:

1. What is the client's level of activity and participation today?
2. Have the client's activity and participation truly changed?
3. Have the client's activity and participation changed an important amount?

At the initial assessment, the answer to the first question provides information concerning whether a functional deficiency exists. If the answer is yes, at subsequent assessments, the answer to the first question yields information concerning whether the treatment goals have been met. The answers to the second and third questions are of interest on reassessment. The second question considers whether true change has occurred, and the third question asks whether the change is clinically important. To answer these questions with confidence, clinicians must apply measures that are reliable, valid, and able to detect change. However, in addition to being assured that the coefficients for these measurement properties are sufficiently high to support a measure's use, more information is required for a measure to be a useful clinical decision-making aid. The primary requirement is that a clinician must be able to interpret the meaning of a measure's value.

Conditions That Provide Meaning to Outcome Data

Three conditions must be met for a measured value to be useful to a clinician. First, one must be able to internalize the meaning of the measured value. To illustrate this point, suppose you are told that a client has 116 degrees of knee flexion. Without thinking, most clinicians will instantly picture this joint angle; they know what it is.

Second, a clinician must be able to interpret the measured value's meaning for a specific client. For example, consider the meaning and potential actions you would take for two clients who present with 116 degrees of knee flexion. The first client is a 62 year old who received a total knee joint replacement 6 weeks previously. The second client is an 18-year-old high school student who received an anterior cruciate ligament reconstruction 6 weeks previously. Although, in both instances, the knee joint angle is 116 degrees, the interpretation of this value is different for these clients. For the arthroplasty client, it is likely that 116 degrees of knee flexion would be considered an acceptable amount of knee flexion, and increasing the range of motion would not be a treatment goal. However, for the client with the anterior cruciate ligament reconstruction, 116 degrees of knee flexion would be considered a significant limitation, and an intervention would be implemented to increase this client's range of motion.

The third condition is that, to make meaningful decisions, a clinician must have a sense of the error associated with a measurement. For example, is the true knee flexion range of motion for the first client in our example 116 degrees or is it 116 degrees, plus or minus

so many degrees? Clearly, most readers will choose the latter option. Moreover, when presented with this scenario, many of our colleagues suggested that they believed the error associated with measuring knee flexion is approximately plus or minus 5 degrees. Accordingly, their interpretation of this client's true knee flexion value is between 111 and 121 degrees.

In addition to defining the degree of certainty in a measured value at a single point in time, knowledge of the magnitude of error helps a clinician to interpret whether a client has truly changed since the previous assessment. Consider the client who received the anterior cruciate ligament reconstruction in the previous example. Suppose a mobilization strategy was implemented and the client's knee flexion on reassessment was 121 degrees. Is this apparent improvement of 5 degrees likely to represent a true change in this client, or is it merely a result of inherent variation? One way to answer this question is to consider the error associated with the measures (previous measure and the current measure). Accordingly, one has to factor in the error associated with both measures when judging whether a change has occurred.

The final clinical question forces us to consider whether the amount of change seen in a client is clinically important. However, like beauty, what constitutes a clinically important change may well be in the eye of the beholder. In the Measurement Properties chapter, we learned that the term *responsiveness* is applied frequently to denote clinically important change. We were also introduced to the concept that a client's level of disability and the risk of an adverse effect associated with treatment influence the magnitude of a clinically important difference. Accordingly, it is unlikely that a single value can represent the magnitude of a clinically important change that is applicable to all clients and all clinical situations.[6] Finally, a provision that Liang places on responsiveness is that the value for the minimal clinically important difference must exceed that of measurement error.[7] If this requirement is applied to our client with an anterior cruciate ligament reconstruction, the apparent improvement of 5 degrees does not provide strong evidence that a clinically important change has occurred.

REASSESSMENT INTERVAL

Selecting the Reassessment Interval

Although assessing change may seem like a simple task, it is made difficult in many instances for two reasons. First, none of the tests applied in the clinical setting are 100% accurate. The second reason is a consequence of the first point. Because tests are not 100% accurate, for a clinician to be confident that a true change has occurred, larger changes are required for less accurate tests. However, clients often undergo small changes that are important, and it is for this reason that clinicians must focus on optimizing the accuracy of the clinical decision-making process. The choice of reassessment interval is a crucial part of this process.

Determining the optimal reassessment interval is a topic that has received little attention.[8] The primary goal of the reassessment is to determine whether change has occurred since the previous assessment. For some clients, the anticipated change will be positive, and for other clients, the expected change will be negative. Regardless of whether the predicted change is positive or negative, the same considerations guide the choice of reassessment interval.

Theoretical Considerations When Considering the Reassessment Interval

The framework for establishing the optimal reassessment interval applies diagnostic test methodology; however, rather than diagnosing a disease or functional limitation, the challenge is to identify or distinguish clients who have changed from clients who have not changed.[8] The primary consideration influenc-

ing the optimal reassessment interval is the accuracy of a clinician's impression of when 50% of clients who are similar to the specific client of interest will change. Applying the follow-up assessment at this point will minimize the risk of incorrectly concluding that the client has or has not changed based on the outcome measure's result. When the chance of a client changing within a specified time frame is lower than 50%, one is more likely to incorrectly declare a client as having changed based on the outcome measure's change score. Conversely, when the chance of a client changing within a specified period is higher than 50%, there is a greater risk of incorrectly declaring the client as not having changed.

Practical Considerations When Considering the Reassessment Interval

Having identified the ideal reassessment interval, the next step is to consider the practical issues that will influence the choice of reassessment interval. First, we need to acknowledge that the results from the best prognosis studies and the impressions of the most seasoned clinician of when 50% of clients will change are approximations at best. The crucial issue is that the reassessment interval is not too short or too long as to dramatically increase the chance of incorrectly labeling a client as having changed or not.

The second consideration acknowledges that, in most instances, a client's outcome assessment will include multiple outcome measures (eg, range of motion, strength, pain, activity and participation). Clearly, we do not expect these measures to change at the same rate.[9] For this reason, the specified reassessment interval is likely to vary depending on the outcome measure of interest.

We will now return to Mr. Smith and apply the concepts described in this chapter.

This time we provide Roland-Morris Questionnaire (RMQ) scores and our responses to the questions posed previously.

SCENARIO 1: Mr. Smith—A Reprise

Findings from the client's initial assessment. Mr. Smith is a 40-year-old man with low back pain. The discomfort came on 3 weeks ago while he was laying patio stones. The discomfort is located to the right of the midline and extends approximately 10 cm proximal from the iliac crest. Over the first week following the injury, there was a mild reduction in the discomfort; however, there has been little change over the past 2 weeks. Mr. Smith has not experienced low back pain previously. He works in an office, and other than experiencing mild discomfort during the day, his work is unaffected by his back problem. Mr. Smith states that he has cut down somewhat on his household and recreational activities. You administer several tests and measures and the relevant findings are as follows: activity and participation (RMQ score), 10 of 24; pain (0 to 10 numeric pain rating scale), 4 of 10.

What is this client's status today?

First, we consider the error associated with Mr. Smith's reported RMQ score of 10 of 24. Applying a standard error of measurement of 1.8 RMQ points,[10] the 90% confidence interval for Mr. Smith's score is $10 \pm (1.8 \times 1.65)$ or 10 ± 3. An RMQ score in this range would be expected for a client presenting with subacute nonradiating low back pain.[11,12] Moreover, based on the subject characteristics of clients admitted to low back pain intervention trials, a score in this range suggests that treatment is warranted.[11]

Next, we consider Mr. Smith's pain score of 4 of 10. Using a process similar to that described above, the 90% confidence interval for Mr. Smith's pain score is 4 ± 2 pain points.

How confident are you in your assessment?

Ninety percent based on our confidence intervals.

When will you reassess this client?

We will reassess this client's pain at 1 week and his activity and participation at 2 weeks.

What factors influenced your choice of reassessment interval?

Two factors contributed to our choice of this reassessment interval. The first factor is related to the minimal detectable difference and the minimal clinically important difference. Several studies have shown that a change of 3 pain points and 5 RMQ points represents a true change (ie, 90% of stable clients display retest values less than these values).[10,13–16] The second factor draws on clinical experience. Specifically, it requires us to recall other clients who were similar to Mr. Smith and to estimate the interval when 50% of these clients would improve by the specified values. By estimating the interval over which 50% of clients similar to Mr. Smith would change, we minimize the risk of incorrectly labeling the client as either having changed or not having changed.[8]

Reassessment. At 1 week, you ask Mr. Smith whether the treatment has been helpful and obtain the following response: "I think so . . . you know my back was quite sore last evening and rather stiff . . . although my back felt pretty good this morning when I went for a long walk."

Mr. Smith's 1-week follow-up pain score is 3 of 10. You reassess Mr. Smith at 2 weeks and obtain a pain score of 2 of 10 and an RMQ score of 5 of 24.

Interpret this dialogue and jot down what you would write in the medical record. Your assessment should include whether Mr. Smith has changed and, if he has, whether the change is important.

At 1 week, we concluded that Mr. Smith has not undergone a noticeable change in pain. At 2 weeks, we concluded that Mr. Smith has not undergone a noticeable change in pain; however, he has shown an important improvement in activity and participation.

How confident are you in your interpretation?

Based on the reported minimal detectable change values, we are quite confident in our interpretation.

Efficient Charting: Illustration of a Goal and Outcome Flow Sheet Approach

Maintaining and retrieving information in a timely manner about a client's progress is a recurring challenge in clinical practice. One method that many of our colleagues have found useful is the goal and outcome flow sheet shown in the Appendix to this chapter. This sheet is used to specify measurable goals and client progress. Measurable goals include details concerning the expected outcome and the time interval to meet the goal. Both short- and long-term or terminal goals are recorded. For our example, a checkmark is used to indicate that a short-term goal has been achieved. The word "met" is applied to signify that a terminal goal (ie, no further progress within the realms of active treatment is required) has been achieved. Only measures used to track progress—outcome measures—are recorded. Typically, this sheet is fastened to the inside cover of a client's chart. This affords quick access to the information and provides a summary of the client's progress at a glance. To illustrate the application, Mr. Smith's pain and activity and participation scores are presented in the Appendix and are supplemented with client-specific and impairment measures.

SUMMARY

- This chapter identified a number of benefits and barriers to the use of activity and participation measures.
- Three clinical questions that require answers when assessing a client's outcome are: What is the client's level of activity and participation today? Have the client's activity and participation truly changed? Have the client's activity and participation changed an important amount?
- For outcome measure data to have clinical usefulness, the clinician must understand its meaning for a specific client and have a sense of the error associated with the data.

- The optimal reassessment interval is when 50% of clients with characteristics similar to the client of interest undergo a change. A reassessment interval that is too short increases the chance of incorrectly labeling a client as having changed. A reassessment interval that is too long increases the chance of incorrectly labeling a client as not having changed.
- Forms such as the goal and outcome flow-sheet (see Appendix) provide an efficient method for recording and reviewing a client's status.

REFERENCES

1. Hazard RG, Haugh LD, Green PA, Jones PL. Chronic low back pain: the relationship between patient satisfaction and pain, impairment, and disability outcomes. Spine 1994;19:881–7.
2. Sullivan MS, Shoaf LD, Riddle DL. The relationship of lumbar flexion to disability in patients with low back pain. Phys Ther 2000;80:240–50.
3. Ross M. Relation of implicit theories to the construction of personal histories. Psychol Rev 1989;96:341–57.
4. Norman GR, Stratford P, Regehr G. Methodological problems in the retrospective computation of responsiveness to change: the lesson of Cronbach. J Clin Epidemiol 1997;50:869–79.
5. Linton SJ, Melin L. The accuracy of remembering chronic pain. Pain 1982;13:281–5.
6. Stratford PW, Binkley J, Solomon P, Finch E, Gill C, Moreland J. Defining the minimal level of detectable change for the Roland-Morris Questionnaire. Phys Ther 1996;76:359–65.
7. Liang MH. Longitudinal construct validity: establishment of clinical meaning in patient evaluative instruments. Med Care 2000;38 Suppl II:II-84–90.
8. Stratford PW. Diagnosing patient change: impact of reassessment interval. Physiother Can 2000;52:225–8.
9. Stratford PW, Binkley JM, Watson J, Heath-Jones T. Validation of the LEFS on patients with total joint arthroplasty. Physiother Can 2000;52:97–105, 110.
10. Stratford PW, Finch E, Solomon P, Binkley J, Gill C, Moreland J. Using the Roland-Morris Questionnaire to make decisions about individual patients. Physiother Can 1996;48:107–10.
11. Stratford PW, Binkley JM. Applying the results of self-report measures to individual patients: an example using the Roland Morris Questionnaire. J Orthop Sports Phys Ther 1999;29:232–9.
12. Stratford PW, Binkley JM. A comparison study of

the Back Pain Functional Scale and Roland Morris Questionnaire. J Rheumatol 2000;27:1928–36.

13. Stratford PW, Binkley JM, Riddle DL. Sensitivity to change of the Roland-Morris back pain questionnaire: part 1. Phys Ther 1998;78:1186–96.

14. Riddle DL, Stratford PW, Binkley JM. Sensitivity to change of the Roland-Morris back pain questionnaire: Part II. Phys Ther 1998;78:1197–207.

15. Stratford PW, Riddle DL, Binkley JM. Assessing for changes in a patient's status: a review of current methods and a proposal for a new method of estimating true change. Physiother Can 2001;53:197–204.

16. Stratford PW, Riddle DL, Binkley JM, Spadoni G, Westaway MD, Padfield B. Using the Neck Disability Index to make decisions concerning individual patients. Physiother Can 1999;51:107–12, 119.

APPENDIX

Goal and Outcome Flow Sheet

Client: Mr. Smith Age: 40					
Client-Specific Functional Scale	**Initial Visit**	**1 week**	**2 weeks**	**3 weeks**	**4 weeks**
1. Gardening (/10)	4		7		10
2. Golfing (/10)	3			8	10
Pain Measure					
0 to 10 Numeric Pain Scale	4	3	2	1	0
Condition-Specific Measure					
Roland-Morris Questionnaire (RMQ) (/24)	10		5		1
Impairment Measures					
Beattie Extension (cm)	0.9	1.4	1.7		1.6
Modified Schöber Flexion (cm)	3.1	5.2	6.2		6.3
Goals and Time Frame					
Increase extension to 1.6 cm in 1 week			Met		
Increase flexion to 4.5 cm in 1 week		✓			
Decrease pain to 1 in 1 week				Met	
Decrease RMQ score to 5 in 2 weeks			✓		
Increase gardening to 7 in 2 weeks			✓		
Increase golfing to 6 in 3 weeks (putting and short-iron play)				✓	
Updated Goals and Time Frame					
Increase flexion greater than 6.0 cm (expected normal) by week 3			Met		
Decrease RMQ to less than 2 by week 4					Met
Increase gardening to 10 by week 4					Met
Increase golfing to 9 by week 4					Met

CHAPTER 6

How Outcome Measures Can Be Used to Enhance Decision Making about a Program

LEARNING OUTCOMES AND OBJECTIVES

At the completion of this chapter, the reader will be able to

1. Demonstrate knowledge of the essential steps of program evaluation,
2. Discuss where outcomes fit in the steps of program evaluation,
3. Systematically and logically consider the choice of measures for evaluation of a program, and
4. Demonstrate an understanding of how the data are interpreted and used.

The process of choosing outcome measures is described in Chapters 2 and 3 and is applied to program evaluation in this chapter.

SCENARIO

A year ago, the administration at the rehabilitation hospital where you work allocated some funds to run an outpatient pulmonary rehabilitation program. You started a 6-week program, with a 2-hour session once a week. The program to assist individuals with chronic obstructive pulmonary disease (COPD) in managing their condition is delivered by a nurse and you. The program involves six education sessions and covers the following topics: the pathology of COPD, medications, breathing control, physical activity, nutrition, and energy conservation. In addition, at each weekly visit, the participants spend some time performing a supervised individualized exercise program that consists of stretching, interval training, and strengthening exercises. You would like to assess the effectiveness of the program specifically in terms of its effect on health status and on physical activity and conditioning. How do you proceed?

Background and Definitions

Program refers "to a series of activities supported by a group of resources intended to achieve specific outcomes among particular target groups."[1] Program evaluation is the process of systematically gathering, analyzing, and reporting data about a program and using information to guide decision making.[1,2] It involves examining the merits, worth, or significance of a program.[3]

Different types of evaluation exist and are used in the various stages of the program. Needs assessment and feasibility analysis are usually performed in the program planning stages. Outcome evaluation, process evaluation, and cost analysis are performed during and after program implementation but should be planned during program development. Table 6–1 provides some definitions of the different types of evaluations.

A detailed description of the steps involved in the different analyses and evaluation is beyond the scope of this chapter. We refer the reader to detailed information about this in texts, journals, and Websites.[1–10]

SCENARIO. **What type of evaluation do you need to perform for the scenario at the beginning of the chapter?** *The effectiveness of a program is usually assessed using outcome*

TABLE 6–1   Definitions of Different Types of Analyses

Type of Analysis	What Is It?
Needs assessment	Systematic evaluation of the need for a program, the target audience, nature and scope of existing services[1,2]
Feasibility analysis	Next step after needs assessment; examines the feasibility of the idea for the program[1,2]
Process evaluation	Systematic evaluation of how the program is operating; focuses on program delivery and use[1,2]
Outcome evaluation (also known as summative evaluation and impact evaluation)	Systematic evaluation of the impact of the program to determine whether it meets its objectives[1]
Cost analysis or efficiency evaluation	Appraisal of program costs in relation to program results using a systematic approach[2]

evaluation. It has been recommended that a program should be operational for at least 1 year before an outcome evaluation is performed.[2] This time period ensures the stability of the program in terms of staffing and delivery patterns.[2] However, planning for program evaluation should take place during program development. Process evaluation may be ongoing from the start of the program.[11]

How could other types of evaluation be used for the type of program described in the scenario? If you were considering expansion of the program, needs assessment would be indicated. The purpose would be to guide planning and marketing. Process evaluation would involve collecting data on such things as use and drop out rate, staffing, and the characteristics of clients and of those who drop out. Most programs keep track of these factors. However, more detailed information about the individuals who drop out or barriers to participation may require more detailed data collection. It is often possible to collect process evaluation information as part of outcome evaluation.

Essential Steps in Program Evaluation and Where Measures Fit

Porteous et al[1] developed the Program Evaluation Tool Kit, which presents a decision-oriented model of program evaluation. They present a five-step approach to evaluation as shown in Table 6–2.

Step 1: Focus the Evaluation

This first step consists of identifying the goals of the evaluation, recognizing the stakeholders, and developing a program logic model.

Identifying the purpose. Identifying the purpose of the evaluation is the first step in this process. Table 6–3 lists some potential goals of evaluating a program.

SCENARIO. The primary purpose of the evaluation for the scenario presented is to determine whether the program is meeting its objectives, which are to improve the health status of and physical activity and conditioning in individuals with COPD. Thus, the overall goal is to measure and report achievement.

TABLE 6–2   Steps in Program Evaluation

Step No.	Description of Step	Result
1	Focus the evaluation	Evaluation questions
2	Select methods	Methods and logistic plan
3	Choose Measures	Data collection measures
4	Gather and Analyze Data	Data and findings
5	Make Decision	Decisions

Identify strength and weakness
Improve implementation
Secure funding
Measure and report achievement to date
Make decisions regarding the program

However, program evaluation is often linked to continuing to secure funding for the program. It is unlikely that any health care center or hospital will fund a program that cannot be shown to be meeting its objectives.

Recognizing stakeholders. Recognizing stakeholders and engaging them in the process is an important component in program evaluation. Stakeholders are individuals or groups (both internal and external) who have an interest in the evaluation or who may be involved in making decisions about the program.[1–3] These include those involved in the operation of the program (eg, program staff, volunteers, managers, etc.), those served or affected by the program (eg, clients and their families), and primary users of the evaluation (eg, funding officials, decision makers, administrators).[3]

SCENARIO. The following should be involved in the evaluation of the program:

- *program manager*
- *program staff*
- *epidemiologist or researcher with experience in program evaluation*
- *administrator/funding officials*
- *clients*

Developing a program logic model. A logic model is "a diagram illustrating the main components or activities of a program, the objectives and indicators for each activity, and the connections or linkages between them."[2] A flowchart, map, or table is often used to clarify the program strategies and clearly outlines the program direction.[3] A logic model helps in reviewing the underlying assumptions that may be evaluated through program evaluation and will guide in selection of methods and tools.

Porteous and colleagues[1] provided a simple way to remember the components of the logic model (CAT SOLO = Components, Activities, Target groups, Short-term Outcomes or Objectives, Long-term Outcomes or Objectives). Components of the program are the groups of closely related activities. Activities are "the things that the program does to work toward its desired outcomes"; some of these activities would be interventions. Target groups represent the individuals or groups for whom the program is designed. Short-term Objectives (also referred to as outcomes) are the changes that the program hopes to achieve in the short term. Long-term Objectives are the broader changes that the program hopes to achieve in the long term. Short- and long-term objectives may include target values. For example, you may indicate that a certain proportion of the clients will achieve specific goals.

SCENARIO. Table 6–4 provides a logic model for the program.

Step 2: Select Evaluation Methods

As part of this stage, a data collection plan needs to be developed. Some issues to consider here are the availability of data, the type of data collection needed, who can gather these data or provide them if asked, what is the best design, what is an appropriate sample size, and the time frame for data collection.[1]

Data can be collected in many different ways. These include review of charts, activity logs, attendance sheets, or face-to-face interviews, questionnaires (self-report, telephone), observations, or focus groups.[1] The data can be collected retrospectively (from charts) or prospectively. More complex research designs can also be used such as randomized controlled trials or quasi-experimental or case-controlled designs. Each of these approaches

TABLE 6–4   Logic Model for the Program

Main Components	Referral	Assessment	Physical Conditioning	Education
Activities	Work with respirologists and physicians to recruit clients Write articles in local newspaper to encourage self-referral Send letters about the program	Perform full assessments of clients' health status and physical activity at entry and completion of the program	Develop individualized exercise programs Supervise the program once weekly Encourage physical activities on other days through use of diaries and activity logs	Organize education sessions Facilitate discussion and information sharing Provide educational material on strategies for coping and exercise
Targets	Physicians Respirologists Individuals with COPD Families of individuals with COPD	Individuals with COPD	Individuals with COPD	Individuals with COPD Families of individuals with COPD
Short-term objectives or outcomes	Increase awareness and knowledge of the program	Baseline measure Monitor status Recognize indicators of onset of acute exacerbations	Increase exercise capacity/conditioning Increase regular physical activity	Improve health status Evolve their belief in the positive effect of exercise and education
Long-term objectives or outcomes	Increase enrolment of individuals with COPD in the program	Database of activity level and coping ability and potential for change Provide basis for program evaluation	Decrease the number of acute exacerbations Maintain lung function at a stable level Improve health status	Decrease the number of acute exacerbations Maintain lung function at a stable level Improve health status

COPD = chronic obstructive pulmonary disease.

has advantages and disadvantages. Retrospective chart review is the least desirable option as data may not be recorded consistently from chart to chart, and there is potential for missing data. A prospective pre/post design does not allow for a control group. Therefore, other influences may have an effect on the changes observed, thereby limiting the conclusions that you can make about the program. However, a randomized controlled trial may be difficult to conduct and time consuming. If the interventions have been shown to be effective in the literature, a true control group may not be possible for ethical reasons.

The other consideration is your sample. Do you need to collect data on all of your participants? Can you collect it on a sample? Obviously, data collection for the whole sample provides a better evaluation of the overall program. However, it may not be feasible because of cost or other factors and may be a burden on participants. Therefore, a sample may be more appropriate. If you choose this option, it is critical to ensure that the sample is representative of the participants in terms of gender, age, severity of disease, and other factors. The size of the sample is also dependent on the type of evaluation performed. For an outcome evaluation, a sample of at least 30 is recommended.[2,12]

SCENARIO. You consider two possibilities, a retrospective chart review or a prospective pre/post design, as the most feasible given your resources. If the program has a waiting list, a control group may be used to compare with the rehabilitation group. However, the expense and workload on the clients may limit the use of a control group. Alternatively, the findings could be compared with those of a similar group reported in the literature. Note that, for many of the designs, consent may be needed to access the data and use them for research purposes. The Research Ethics Board at your facility will provide you with guidelines on consent.

For this scenario, 25 clients are enrolled in the 6-week program at one time. To get at least 30 clients,[2,12] you may choose to sequentially sample clients for two sessions over a 12-week period.

Step 3: Choose Measures

Clearly, it is unreasonable to develop high-quality measures in a short time frame. Therefore, existing measures or tools should be sought in the evaluation process. As outlined in Chapter 4, the measurement properties of the measure will determine the accuracy of the results obtained. These properties include reliability, validity, and the ability of a measure to detect change. In addition, you need to consider the need for a performance versus a self-report measure and generic versus specific measures (refer to Chapter 3).

In addition to measurement properties, other features of the measures chosen will influence accuracy and usefulness.[2] These include the following:

1. *Feasibility.* It is more feasible to use existing measures than to develop new ones. Other factors to consider are the time needed to administer the measures and the expertise of the data collector. Refer to Chapter 3 for more discussion about feasibility.
2. *Acceptability.* The demands on the individuals asked to participate need to be considered.
3. *Credibility.* The tools that you choose will have to be credible to the stakeholders in this process.

Goal attainment can be combined with program evaluation whereby one or two goals are chosen for all program participants in addition to goals for individual participants, which may be different. Outcomes that reflect the program goals may only be measured at

the start and end of the program and also, if possible, for follow-up purposes. For more information on goal attainment scaling, refer to Palisano and colleagues.[13]

If the primary method for data collection is focus groups or interviews, specific questions need to be developed and tested. Detailed information on this methodology is beyond the scope of this chapter but is available from other sources.[14–16]

SCENARIO. There are numerous published measures from which to choose how best to assess the health status and physical activity or conditioning in participants with COPD in an outpatient pulmonary rehabilitation program.

Potential measures that may be used to assess the effect of the program on physical activity and conditioning are listed in Table 6–5.[17–22] The advantages and disadvantages of these are outlined.

A functional walk test (eg, a 2-, 6-, or 12-Minute Walk) was chosen as the measure of choice for this evaluation. Timed walk tests measure the ability to undertake physically demanding activities of daily living.[23] Walk tests are objective measures of exercise capacity that can be used to monitor the response to treatment.[17]

How do you choose between the 2-, 6-, and 12-Minute Walk Tests? With respect to the measurement properties, most of the literature focuses on the 6- and 12-Minute Walk Tests.[17] Only the 6-Minute Walk Test has data on responsiveness/sensitivity to change. With respect to feasibility, the 6-Minute Walk Test has a number of advantages. It is better tolerated than the 12-Minute Walk Test in individuals with chronic airway obstruction.[24] It is also more reflective of the requirements of activities of daily living than the 2-Minute Walk Test.[17] Clinically, in individuals with COPD who are community dwellers, a 50-meter change on the 6-minute walk test may be important in the functional mobility of the individual.

TABLE 6–5 Examples of Measures That May Be Used, Their Advantages and Disadvantages

Measure	Advantages	Disadvantages
EXERCISE CAPACITY		
Timed walk tests (2-, 6-, or 12-Minute Walk Test)	Easier to administer than the traditional measures of exercise capacity Feasible for the clients Requires little equipment Employs an activity that is familiar to the clients[17,18]	Only measures one domain of physical activity/conditioning (mainly of the lower extremity)
FITNESS ASSESSMENTS		
Maximal oxygen uptake (VO$_2$ maximum)	Considered the gold standard	Requires specific equipment and medical personnel[19]
Submaximal aerobic testing	Correlates with V$_{O2}$ max More feasible for the client than V$_{O2}$ max	Requires equipment and expertise with the protocols
PHYSICAL ACTIVITY QUESTIONNAIRE (refer to Kriska and Caspersen[22] for a detailed review; two examples listed below)		
Bouchard Three-Day Record[21]	Provides information on physical activity throughout the day for 3 days	Large burden on the client as it involves recording activities for each 15 minutes over 24-hour cycle of 3 consecutive days Not validated in COPD
Modified Activity Questionnaire[22]	Provides information on physical activity throughout the day for 3 days	Not validated in COPD Not appropriate for the pre/post design of 6 weeks duration as it involves recording the number of times per month over the past year that they performed physical activities from a predetermined list

COPD = chronic obstructive pulmonary disease.

There are several measures of health status in individuals with COPD. For a detailed review, the reader is referred to Lacasse and colleagues.[25]

The Chronic Respiratory Disease Questionnaire (CRQ) is developed as an evaluative measure and was considered an appropriate measure for this evaluation. It is a disease-specific interviewer-administered instrument that has four domains: dyspnea (five self-generated items), fatigue (four items), emotional function (seven items), and mastery or the extent to which the individual feels he/she can cope with the disease (four items).[26] Each item is rated using a 7-point Likert scale, with 0 representing no symptoms and 7 showing extreme symptoms. The results are standardized by dividing the score within each domain by the number of items, leading to possible scores of 1 to 7 on all domains.[26] The validity, reliability, and ability to detect change of the CRQ and each of the domains have been well established.[25]

The CRQ was chosen as the measure of choice for this evaluation for several reasons:

1. The measurement properties of the CRQ and each of its domains have been well established and reported.
2. The CRQ is commonly used in the field of COPD.
3. The CRQ is feasible to administer. It requires 20 to 30 minutes on the first interview and 10 minutes on subsequent interviews.

4. *The CRQ provides insight into additional constructs or outcomes such as dyspnea and fatigue.*

The minimal clinically important difference (0.5) is similar for all domains.[26]

Step 4: Gather and Analyze Data

The data collected need to provide a well-rounded view of the program and specifically answer the question of interest. In addition to using standardized measures with good measurement properties, methods of data collection, training of the data collectors, coding, and data management need to be considered to optimize the quality of the data.[3]

Who will collect the data? Examples may include a moderator of a focus group, interviewer for a telephone survey, or a health care professional for pre/post assessments. To maximize consistency, a protocol for data collection should be developed.[1] This would include clear instructions and a standard approach to data collection. Training the data collectors and pretesting the tools and the methodology should also take place before starting the actual evaluation.

It is critical to continuously monitor the data gathering process to ensure quality. For example, if a mail survey is used, the number of surveys returned and those outstanding needs to be monitored and repeat contacts of nonrespondents conducted. If a health care professional is making measurements on clients, keeping track of the number of patients and establishing quality checks are critical.

When summarizing the data, traditional measures of central tendency (mean, median, and mode) or spread (standard deviation, range) are not particularly informative. This is because providing one number to represent a series of measurements results in a considerable loss of information. For example, no one person in the program may ever have had the mean value; the median value says that 50% achieved a higher (or lower) value but is not informative as to whether this is a good or a poor outcome. Given that a target value has been set for the objective, it is more informative to summarize the data in terms of the proportion of individuals who met or exceeded the target value.

SCENARIO. Table 6–6 summarizes the characteristics of the sample at baseline. These measures were obtained by the physical therapist at baseline assessment.

Table 6–7 shows the change in the distance and mastery component of the CRQ before and after the program. There was no statistically significant difference in the distance walked before and after the program (p = 0.3). *However there was a statistically significant difference for all of the components of the CRQ* (p < 0.02).

Another possibly better way to interpret program evaluation data is to assess the proportion of individuals who achieved the objectives (see Table 6–8).

TABLE 6–6 General Characteristics of Sample

Variable	Total Sample (*n* = 40)
Sex	21 females; 19 males
Age (yr)	65.0 ± 6.1
Distance on 6-Minute Walk Test (m)	317.0 ± 81.0
CRQ dyspnea	5.2 ± 1.2
CRQ fatigue	3.5 ± 1.0
CRQ emotional function	4.8 ± 1.1
CRQ mastery	5.8 ± 1.1

Data are presented as mean ± standard deviation.

CRQ = Chronic Respiratory Disease Questionnaire.

TABLE 6–7 Change in Distance Walked in 6 Minutes and Components of the CRQ Between the Beginning and End of the Program

	Mean Change
Distance walked (m)	5.4
CRQ dyspnea	3.0
CRQ fatigue	1.8
CRQ emotional function	2.8
CRQ mastery	2.8

CRQ = Chronic Respiratory Disease Questionnaire.

Step 5: Make Decisions

Once data analysis is complete, the final step is to document the findings and develop recommendations. The type of documentation is dependent on the intended users. For example, the format of a report for accreditation purposes is different compared with a report intended for upper-level management to justify a program and argue for increased resources. Use of graphs may increase the readability of the report and assist in highlighting certain findings. For more detailed information on documenting the results of program evaluation, the reader is referred to Morris and colleagues.[27]

Recommendations are actions for consideration resulting from the evaluation and may include continuation, expansion, discontinuation, or redesign of the program. These recommendations are distinct from judgment regarding the effectiveness of a program.[3] A program may be effective, but the cost/benefit ratio may be such that continuing the program is not possible.

SCENARIO. *Redelmeier and colleagues[28] established that a minimal mean change in 6-Minute Walk Test (6MWT) distance of 54 meters represented a clinically significant change in functional status. They used a COPD population with an average 6MWT distance of 371 meters. Using this criterion, the results from the 6MWT are neither statistically nor clinically significant with respect to exercise capacity. Further, an insignificant proportion of the sample met the criteria for this outcome.*

With respect to the CRQ, the minimal clinically important difference is similar for all domains and was approximately 0.5. A change of 1.0 is considered moderate, and a change of 1.5 is considered large.[26] Thus, the program resulted in a clinically important change for all domains of the CRQ. Furthermore, 75% of the sample met the criteria related to this outcome.

Limitations. *There are a number of limitations of the evaluation process, such as the lack of a control group and the potential influence of confounding variables. Nevertheless, the results indicate that the program resulted in improved health-related quality of life and coping with the disease but no effect on exercise capacity. Comparison of the components of the program to the evidence in the literature may provide further insight into the findings. Synthesis of the lit-*

TABLE 6–8 Percentage of Clients Achieving the Two Objectives for the Programs

Goal	Objective and Target Value	% of Clients Meeting Objective
Increase exercise capacity/conditioning	Improve distance walked in 6 min by 50 m	3
Improve health status	Improve the CRQ score by 0.5 point	75

CRQ = Chronic Respiratory Disease Questionnaire.

erature suggests that exercise training should be a mandatory component of a rehabilitation program but indicates that high-intensity programs optimize the physiologic outcomes.[29] A process evaluation may be needed to examine the components of the exercise program and determine any weaknesses in terms of the intensity or frequency of the aerobic training program.

SUMMARY

- Program evaluation is the process of systematically gathering, analyzing, and reporting data about a program and using information to guide decision making.

- There are different types of evaluation that are performed at different stages in the program evaluation cycle such as feasibility analysis, process evaluation, outcome evaluation, and cost analysis.

- There are five essential steps in program evaluation: focusing the evaluation, selecting the methods, choosing the measures, gathering and analyzing the data, and making decisions.

- A program logic model outlines the main components of the program and the short- and long-term objectives.

- As part of program evaluation, a data collection plan may include chart review, interviews, questionnaires, randomized controlled trials, or quasi-experimental designs. The advantages and disadvantages of these methods must be considered.

- When choosing the measures, measurement properties, feasibility, acceptability, and credibility are considered.

- The data collected need to provide a well-rounded view of the program and specifically answer the question of interest. The quality of the data will be influenced by the measurement properties of the outcome measures, the methods of data collection, training of the data collectors, coding, and data management.

- The final step is to document the findings and develop recommendations tailored to the intended users.

REFERENCES

1. Porteous NL, Sheldrick BJ, Stewart PJ. Program evaluation tool kit. A blue print for public health management. Ottawa (ON): Public Health Research, Education and Development Program, Ottawa-Carleton Health Department; 1997.
2. Myers AM. Program evaluation for exercise leaders. Champaign (IL): Human Kinetics; 1999.
3. U.S. Department of Health and Human Services. Framework for program evaluation in public health. MMWR Morb Mortal Wkly Rep 1999.
4. Herman JL, Morns LL, Fitz-Gibbon CT. Evaluator's handbook. Newbury Park (CA): Sage; 1987.
5. Basic guide to program evaluation by McNamara Carter [online] [cited 2001 July]. Available from: http://www.mapnp.org/library/evaluation/fnl_eval.htm.
6. Hudson J, Mayne J, Thomlinson R. Action-oriented evaluation in organizations. Canadian practices. Toronto (ON): Wall and Emerson; 1992.
7. Morris LL, Fitz-Gibbon CT, Lindheim E. How to measure performance and use tests. Newbury Park (CA): Sage; 1987.
8. Ovretveit J. Evaluating health interventions. Philadelphia: Open University Press; 1998.
9. Community Toolbox [online] [cited 2001 July]. Available from: http://ctb.lsi.ukans.edu/.
10. CDC Evaluation Working Group [online] [cited 2001 July]. Available from: http://www.cdc.gov/eval/index.htm.
11. Weis CH. Evaluation. 2nd ed. Upper Saddle River (NJ): Prentice-Hall; 1992.
12. Mertens DE. Research methods in education and psychology: integrating diversity with quantitative and qualitative approaches. Thousand Oaks (CA): Sage; 1998.
13. Palisano RJ, Haley SM, Brown DA. Goal attainment scaling as a measure of change in infants with motor delays. Phys Ther 1992;72:432–7.
14. Creswell JW. Research design: qualitative and quantitative approaches. Thousand Oaks (CA): Sage; 1994.
15. Patton MQ. How to use qualitative methods in evaluation. Newbury Park (CA): Sage; 1987.
16. Stewart DW, Shamdasani PN. Focus groups theory and practice. Applied Society Research Method Series 20. Newbury Park (CA): Sage; 1990.
17. Solway S, Brooks D, Lacasse Y, Thomas S. A qualitative systematic overview of the measurement properties of functional walk tests used in the cardiorespiratory domain. Chest 2001;119:256–70.

18. Singh S. The use of field walking tests for assessment of functional capacity in patients with chronic airways obstruction. Physiotherapy 1992;78:102–4.

19. American College of Sports Medicine (ACSM)'s health/fitness facility standards and guidelines. 2nd ed. Champaign (IL): Human Kinetics; 1997.

20. Kriska AM, Bennett PH. An epidemiological perspective of the relationship between physical activity and NIDDM: from activity assessment to intervention. Diabetes Metab Rev 1992;8:355–72.

21. Bouchard C, Tremblay A, LeBlanc C, Lortie G, Savard R, Theriault G. A method to assess energy expenditure in children and adults. Am J Clin Nutr 1983;37:461–7.

22. Kriska AM, Caspersen CJ. A collection of physical activity questionnaires for health-related research. Med Sci Sports Exerc 1997;24 Suppl:S1–S205.

23. Guyatt GH, Thompson PJ, Berman LB, Sullivan MJ, Townsend M, Jones NL, et al. How should we measure function in patients with chronic heart and lung disease? J Chron Dis 1985;38:517–24.

24. Butland RJ, Pang J, Gross ER, Woodcock AA, Geddes DM. Two-, six, and twelve-minute walking tests in respiratory disease. BMJ 1982;284:1607–8.

25. Lacasse Y, Wong E, Guyatt G, Goldstein RS. Health status measurement instruments in chronic obstructive pulmonary disease. Can Respir J 1997;4:152–64.

26. Lacasse Y, Wong E, Guyatt G. A systematic overview of the measurement properties of the Chronic Respiratory Questionnaire. Can Respir J 1997;4:131–9.

27. Morris LL, Fitz-Gibbon CT, Freman ME. How to communicate evaluation findings. Newbury Park (CA): Sage; 1987.

28. Redelmeier DA, Bayoumi AM, Goldstein RS, Guyatt GH. Interpreting small differences in functional status: the Six Minute Walk test in chronic lung disease patients. Am J Respir Crit Care Med 1997;155:1278–82.

29. Lacasse Y, Guyatt GH, Goldstein RS. The components of a respiratory rehabilitation program. A systematic overview. Chest 1997;111:1077–88.

PART II

Outcome Measure Reviews

Measure Review Template

Name of Measure:

Developers:

Purpose:

Description:

Conceptual/Theoretical Basis of
Construct Being Measured:

Groups Tested with This Measure:

Languages:

Application/Administration:

Typical Reliability Estimates:

    Internal consistency

    Interrater

    Test-Retest

    Other

Typical Validity Estimates:

    Content

    Criterion

        Concurrent

        Predictive

    Construct

        Cross-Sectional

            Convergent

            Known groups

            Discriminant

        Longitudinal/Sensitivity to Change

            Convergent

            Known Groups

            Discriminant

        Other Validity Coefficients

Interpretability:

    General Population Values
    (Customary or Normative Values)

Typical Responsiveness Estimates

    Individual Patient

    Between Group

Comments:

References:

Measures Listed Alphabetically

Measures Listed by Outcome (Construct)

AMBULATION
Gait Speed
Walk Test—2 minute, 6 minute, 12 minute,
    shuttle, self-paced

BALANCE/POSTURAL CONTROL
Activity-specific Balance Confidence Scale
Berg Balance Scale
Functional Reach Test
Timed Up and Go (TUG)

CLIENT-CENTRED CARE
Canadian Occupational Performance Measure
    (COPM)
Patient Specific Functional Scale (PSFS)
Wascana Client-Centered Care Survey

DEVELOPMENT
Activity Scale for Kids
Alberta Infant Motor Scale
Gross Motor Function Measure (GMFM)
Gross Motor Performance Measure (GMPM)
Peabody Developmental Motor Scales
Pediatric Evaluation of Disability Inventory (PEDI)
Test of Infant Motor Performance (TIMP)
(WeeFIM)® Functional Independence Measure
    for Children

DISABILITY/ACTIVITY
Action Research Arm Test
Activity Scale for Kids
Barthel Index
Box and Block Test
Back Pain Functional Scale
Chedoke-McMaster Stroke Assessment
(DASH) Disabilities of the Arm, Shoulder and Hand
Facial Disability Index
Frenchay Arm Test
Fugl-Meyer Assessment of Sensorimotor Recovery
    After Stroke
(SMAF) Functional Autonomy Measurement System
Gait Speed
Gross Motor Function Measure (GMFM)
Gross Motor Performance Measure (GMPM)
Lower Extremity Activity Profile (LEAP)
Motor Assessment Scale (MAS)

Neck Disability Index (NDI)
OARS-IADL
Oswestry Low Back Pain Disability Questionnaire
Patient Specific Functional Scale (PSFS)
Peabody Developmental Motor Scales
Pediatric Evaluation of Disability Inventory (PEDI)
Quebec Back Pain Disability Scale
Reintegration to Normal Living Index (RNL)
Rivermead Motor Assessment (RMA)
Roland-Morris Questionnaire
(TEMPA) Test d'Évaluation des Membres Supérieurs
    des Personnes Agées
Walk Test—2-Minute, 6-Minute, 12-Minute,
    Self-paced, Shuttle
(WOMAC™) Western Ontario McMaster
    Osteoarthritis Index

DYSPNEA
Dyspnea Index—Baseline/Transitional
Chronic Respiratory Disease Questionnaire
Dyspnea Scale—MRC
Oxygen Cost Diagram
St. George's Respiratory Questionnaire
Visual Analogue Scale (VAS)

FUNCTIONAL STATUS
Action Research Arm Test
Back Pain Functional Scale
Barthel Index
Bath Ankylosing Spondylitis Functional Index
(COVS) Physiotherapy Clinical Outcome
    Variables Scale
Continuing Care Activity Measure (CCAM)
(DASH) Disability of the Arm Shoulder and Hand
Fibromyalgia Impact Questionnaire
Frenchay Arm Test
(SMAF) Functional Autonomy Measurement System
(FIM) Functional Independence Measure
Gross Motor Function Measure (GMFM)
Gross Motor Performance Measure (GMPM)
Gait Speed
Health Utilities Index (HUI Mark2/3)
Lower Extremity Activity Profile (LEAP)
Lower Extremity Functional Scale (LEFS)
Nottingham Health Profile
OARS-IADL

Oxygen Cost Diagram
Patient Specific Functional Scale (PSFS)
Quebec Back Pain Disability Scale
Reintegration to Normal Living Index (RNL)
Roland-Morris Questionnaire
(SIP) Sickness Impact Profile
(TEMPA) Test d'Évaluation des Membres Supérieurs
　　des Personnes Agées
Timed-Stands Test
Timed Up and Go (TUG)
Upper Extremity Functional Scale (UEFS)
WeeFIM®
(WOMAC™) Western Ontario McMaster
　　Osteoarthritis Index

IMPAIRMENT
Chedoke-McMaster Stroke Assessment
Fugl-Meyer Assessment of Sensorimotor Recovery
　　after Stroke

MOBILITY
Action Research Arm Test
Box and Block Test
(COVS) Physiotherapy Clinical Outcome
　　Variables Scale
Continuing Care Activity Measure
Frenchay Arm Test
Fugl-Meyer Assessment of Sensorimotor Recovery
　　After Stroke
Gait speed
Gross Motor Function Measure (GMFM)
Gross Motor Performance Measure (GMPM)
OARS-IADL
Rivermead Motor Assessment (RMA)
(STREAM) Stroke Rehabilitation Assessment
　　of Movement

Timed-Stands Test
Timed Up and Go (TUG)
Walk Test—2-minute, 6-minute, 12-minute,
　　Self-paced, Shuttle

OCCUPATIONAL PERFORMANCE
Canadian Occupational Performance Measure
　　(COPM)

PAIN
Numeric Pain Rating Scale (NPRS)
Visual Analogue Scale for Pain and Dyspnea (VAS)

PERCEIVED EXERTION
Borg's Rating Scale of Perceived Exertion
Oxygen Cost Diagram

QUALITY OF LIFE
Arthritis Impact Measurement Scales
Chronic Respiratory Disease Questionnaire
Child Health Questionnaire
Cystic Fibrosis Questionnaire
(EuroQoL-5D) European Quality of Life Scale
Health Utilities Index (HUI Mark2/3)
Nottingham Health Profile
(SA-SIP30) Stroke-Adapted Sickness Impact Profile
SF-12®
SF-36®
St. George's Respiratory Questionnaire

SELF-EFFICACY/COPING
Activity-Specific Balance Confidence Scale
Arthritis Self-Efficacy Scale
COPD Self-Efficacy Scale
St. George's Respiratory Questionnaire

Measures Listed by Client Population (Area of Practice)

GENERAL REHABILITATION
Activity-specific Balance Confidence Scale
Barthel Index
Berg Balance Scale
Borg's Rating Scale of Perceived Exertion (RPE)
Canadian Occupational Performance Measure (COPM)
(COVS) Physiotherapy Clinical Outcome Variables Scale
(EuroQoL-5D) European Quality of Life Scale
(FIM) Functional Independence Measure
Functional Reach Test
Gait Speed
Health Utilities Index (HUI Mark2/3)
Lower Extremity Activity Profile (LEAP)
Lower Extremity Functional Scale (LEFS)
Nottingham Health Profile
Numeric Pain Rating Scale (NPRS)
OARS-IADL
Patient Specific Functional Scale (PSFS)
Reintegration to Normal Living Index (RNL)
SF-12®
SF-36®
(SIP) Sickness Impact Profile
(TEMPA) Test d'Évaluation des Membres Supérieurs des Personnes Agées
Timed-Stands Test
Timed Up and Go (TUG)
Upper Extremity Functional Scale (UEFS)
Visual Analogue Scale for Pain and Dyspnea (VAS)
Walk Test—2-minute, 6-minute, 12-minute, Self-paced, Shuttle
Wascana Client-Centered Care Survey
(WOMAC™) Western Ontario McMaster Osteoarthritis Index

GERIATRIC
Activity-specific Balance Confidence Scale
Barthel Index
(EuroQoL-5D) European Quality of Life Scale
(SMAF) Functional Autonomy Measurement System
(FIM) Functional Independence Measure
Functional Reach Test
Gait Speed
Health Utilities Index (HUI Mark2/3)
Nottingham Health Profile
OARS-IADL
Reintegration to Normal Living Index (RNL)
(TEMPA) Test d'Évaluation des Membres Supérieurs des Personnes Agées
Timed-Stands Test
Timed Up and Go (TUG)
Walk Test—2-Minute, 6-Minute, 12-Minute, Self-paced, Shuttle

PEDIATRIC
Activity Scale for Kids (ASK)
Alberta Infant Motor Scale (AIMS)
Child Health Questionnaire
Functional Reach Test
Gross Motor Function Measure (GMFM)
Gross Motor Performance Measure (GMPM)
Health Utilities Index (HUI Mark1)
Peabody Developmental Motor Scales
Pediatric Evaluation of Disability Inventory (PEDI)
Test of Infant Motor Performance (TIMP)
(WeeFIM®) Functional Independence Measure for Children

CHRONIC RESPIRATORY OR CARDIAC DISEASE
Chronic Respiratory Disease Questionnaire
COPD Self-Efficacy Scale
Cystic Fibrosis Questionnaire
Dyspnea Index—Baseline/Transitional
Dyspnea Scale—MRC
Borg's Rating Scale of Perceived Exertion (RPE)
Oxygen Cost Diagram
Reintegration to Normal Living Index (RNL)
SF-36®
(SIP) Sickness Impact Profile
St. George's Respiratory Questionnaire
Visual Analogue Scale (VAS)

BACK
Back Pain Functional Scale
(EuroQoL-5D) European Quality of Life Scale
Numerical Pain Rating Scale (NPRS)

Nottingham Health Profile
Oswestry Low Back Pain Disability Questionnaire
Patient Specific Functional Scale (PSFS)
Quebec Back Pain Disability Scale
Roland-Morris Questionnaire
Visual Analogue Scale for Pain and Dyspnea (VAS)

HEAD AND NECK
Facial Disability Index
Neck Disability Index (NDI)
Patient Specific Functional Scale (PSFS)

UPPER EXTREMITY
Action Research Arm Test
Box and Block Test
(DASH) Disabilities of the Arm, Shoulder and Hand
Frenchay Arm Test
Patient Specific Functional Scale (PSFS)
(TEMPA) Test d'Évaluation des Membres Supérieurs
    des Personnes Agées
Upper Extremity Functional Scale (UEFS)

LOWER EXTREMITY
Lower Extremity Activity Profile (LEAP)
Lower Extremity Functional Scale (LEFS)
Patient Specific Functional Scale (PSFS)
Timed-Stands Test
Walk Test—2-Minute, 6-Minute, 12-Minute,
    Self-paced, Shuttle
(WOMAC™) Western Ontario McMaster
    Osteoarthritis Index

RHEUMATOLOGY
Arthritis Impact Measurement Scales
Arthritis Self-Efficacy Scale
Bath Ankylosing Spondylitis Functional Index
(EuroQoL-5D) European Quality of Life Scale
Fibromyalgia Impact Questionnaire
(FIM) Functional Independence Measure
Gait speed

Health Utilities Index (HUI Mark2/3)
Nottingham Health Profile
OARS-IADL
Reintegration to Normal Living Index (RNL)
Timed-Stands Test
Timed Up and Go (TUG)

MULTIPLE SCLEROSIS
(FIM) Functional Independence Measure
Functional Reach Test
Gait speed
Health Utilities Index (HUI Mark2/3)

STROKE
Action Research Arm Test
Barthel Index
Chedoke-McMaster Stroke Assessment
(EuroQoL-5D) European Quality of Life Scale
Frenchay Arm Test
Fugl-Meyer Assessment of Sensorimotor Recovery
    After Stroke
(FIM) Functional Independence Measure
Functional Reach Test
Gait Speed
Health Utilities Index (HUI Mark2/3)
Motor Assessment Scale (MAS)
Nottingham Health Profile
OARS-IADL
Reintegration to Normal Living Index (RNL)
Rivermead Motor Assessment (RMA)
(SA-SIP30) Stroke-Adapted Sickness Impact Profile
(STREAM) Stroke Rehabilitation Assessment of
    Movement
Stroke Impact Scale (SIS)
Timed Up and Go (TUG)
Walk Test—6-Minute

CONTINUING CARE
Continuing Care Activity Measure

Information about Measure Reviews

Abbreviations frequently used

α	Cronbach's alpha coefficient
ANOVA	analysis of variance
CI	confidence interval
Correlations:	
	ICC = intraclass correlation
	r = Pearson product-moment correlation
CSEM	conditional standard error of measurement
ES	effect size
MCID	minimal clinically important difference
MDC	minimal detectable change
RI	Responsiveness Index
SD	standard deviation
SEM	standard error of measurement
SRM	standardized response mean

Bolded references

The bolded references following the measure review provide a starting point if you wish to explore more detailed information about the measure.

Access to measures

Access to the measures is provided in a variety of ways. Some measures can be accessed through a Website address provided which will enable you to obtain or order the most recent version of the measure. Others can be obtained through an e-mail address or Fax number provided by the developer(s). Both will also provide administration guidelines essential to the standardized application of the measure. In other cases, we have included the measure on the CD-ROM with permission of the developer. If you plan to use the measure, it is advisable to contact the developer for administration guidelines and revisions not available at the time of publication. Access information can be found following the references in each review.

Assistance in critically appraising measurement studies

The Appendix on pages 273–280 and associated material on the CD-ROM provide assistance in extracting information from, and critically appraising a measurement study. Dr. Sharon Wood-Dauphinee, McGill University, developed this material and has graciously permitted its inclusion in the text.

ACTIVITY-SPECIFIC BALANCE CONFIDENCE (ABC) SCALE

Developers

Anita M. Myers and Lynda E. Powell,[1-3] Department of Health Studies and Gerontology, University of Waterloo, Waterloo, Ontario, amyers@interlog.com

Purpose

An evaluative measure to assess balance confidence in ambulatory, community-dwelling older adults.

Description

The ABC Scale is a 16-item questionnaire that can be self-administered or administered by face-to-face or telephone interview. Each item describes a specific activity that requires some position change or walking in progressively more difficult situations, ranging from mobility inside the home to walking outside to a parked car, across a parking lot, up and down a ramp, in a crowded mall, etc. Subjects are asked to indicate their level of confidence in doing each activity without losing their balance or becoming unsteady by choosing a percentage point on an 11-point scale from 0 to 100%. Zero percent corresponds to "no confidence," and 100% corresponds to "complete confidence." The ABC Scale was designed to complement Tinetti et al's[4] Falls Efficacy Scale (FES) by providing a wider continuum of activity difficulty and detailed descriptors that would be more suitable for higher-functioning older adults.[1]

Conceptual/Theoretical Basis of Construct Being Measured

The developers of the ABC Scale operationalize "fear of falling" as a continuum of self-confidence that is based on Bandura's theory of self-efficacy. Self-efficacy is defined as an individual's perceptions of his/her capabilities (or self-confidence) within a particular domain of activities.[1] According to Bandura, an individual's cognitive appraisals, regardless of the accuracy, will influence the decision to engage in or avoid particular activities.[1] In other words, someone with a high level of self-efficacy in balancing activities may engage in potentially more hazardous activities (such as standing on a chair) than a person with a low level of self-efficacy. Self-efficacy is amenable to change and situation specific.

Groups Tested with This Measure

Elderly persons living in the community,[1,3] home care users,[3] retirement home residents,[3] persons with osteoarthritis undergoing hip and knee replacements,[3] outpatients with vestibular dysfunction.[5] The measure has also been administered to people with hip fracture undergoing intensive rehabilitation[6] and those with peripheral neuropathy.[7]

Languages

Developed in Canadian English. The measure has been culturally adapted, validated, and tested for reliability in older persons living in the United Kingdom.[8] The measure has been translated, but not formally validated, in Canadian French.[9]

Application/Administration

When administering the ABC Scale, if subjects do not currently do the activity in question, they must try to imagine their confidence level if they had to do the activity. If the subjects normally use assistance or a walking aid to do the activity, they are asked to rate their confidence as if they were using these supports. If subjects qualify their response to items 2, 9, 11, 14, or 15 (ie, different ratings for "up" versus "down" or "onto" versus "off"), separate ratings are solicited, and the lowest confidence rating of the two is used (eg, using stairs). The ABC Scale is scored on an 11-point scale, and ratings must consist of whole numbers (0 to 100). A subject's total score out of 100 can be computed using a calculator by summating the ratings (possible range: 0 to 1,600) and dividing by 16 or the total number of items answered. At least 12 of the 16 items must be answered. The questionnaire takes 5 to 10 minutes to administer.[1]

Typical Reliability Estimates

Internal Consistency

Community-Dwelling Elderly
- Cronbach's alpha = 0.96

- A stepwise deletion of each of the 16 items did not alter the internal consistency. The last item, "walking on icy sidewalks," may be omitted for administration in warmer climates.[1,3]

Interrater
Not applicable

Test–Retest
Community-Dwelling Elderly
- Total ABC scores: $r = 0.92$ (2-week interval).
- Individual item scores: test–retest correlations significant except for car transfers ($r = 0.19$) and walking in the home ($r = 0.36$) (2-week interval).[1]

Typical Validity Estimates

Content
Fifteen clinicians and 12 elderly outpatients were asked to identify activities of daily living "essential to independent living that, while requiring some position change or walking, would be safe and non-hazardous to most seniors." Elderly clients were also asked to identify normal daily activities in which they were afraid of falling. A head-to-head comparison between the ABC Scale and the FES demonstrated that although the FES is suitable for assessing balance confidence in more frail, home-bound seniors, ceiling effects occur for higher-functioning, more mobile seniors. The ABC yields a wider range of scores and more discrimination between low- and high-mobility groups.[1]

Criterion
No gold standard exists for the construct being measured.

Construct—Cross-sectional

Convergent. Among Community-Dwelling Elderly
- Falls Efficacy Scale: $r = 0.84$[1]
- Physical Self-Efficacy Scale (PSES): $r = 0.49$[1]
- Physical abilities subscale score of PSES: $r = 0.63$[1]
- Measures of anterior-posterior sway and medial-lateral sway: $r = 0.37$ to 0.61[2]
- Walking speed: $r = 0.56$[2]
- Frequency of sweeping the floor (classified as daily versus a few times a week versus once a week versus less than once a week) correlated to ABC scores on this item: $r = 0.70$[2]
- Shopping frequency (same classification as above) correlated to a composite score of items 3 to 5, 9 to 12, and 15 that related to shopping: $r = 0.54$[2]
- Total ratings of the extent of difficulty: $r = -0.89$, activity avoidance: $r = -0.92$, and discomfort

experienced for each of the 16 ABC Scale activities: $r = -0.52$[2]
- Age: $r = -0.29$,[3] total number of health problems: $r = -0.30$[3]

Among Retirement Home Residents
- Performance Mobility Assessment: $r = 0.78$[3]
- Timed 'Up and Go': $r = -0.59$[3]

Among Individuals with Osteoarthritis
- Gait speed: $r = 0.60$ to 0.65[3]
- Ratings of function: $r = 0.49$[3]
- Self-reported maximum walking distance: $r = 0.44$[3]
- Pain intensity ratings: $r = -0.35$[3]
- Depression scores: $r = -0.33$[3]

Among Outpatients with Vestibular Dysfunction
- Dizziness Handicap Inventory, $r = -0.64$[5]

Women, with and without Balance Impairment
- Maximum step length: $r = 0.75$[10]
- Rapid step test time: $r = -0.54$[10]

Known Groups. Among Community-Dwelling Elderly
- Persons at a high versus a low level of mobility who were recruited from seniors' centers and a walking club versus home care and day-care agencies, respectively (low defined as requiring personal assistance to leave the home), $p < 0.001$.[1,3] Subjects in the high-mobility group expressed significantly more confidence on every item of the ABC Scale except for item 4 (reach at eye level).[1]
- Persons reporting yes or no to having a fear of falling, $p < 0.001$, and to avoiding activity owing to a fear of falling, $p < 0.001$[2]
- Persons reporting excellent versus good versus fair/poor health status, $p < 0.000$

Among Individuals with Osteoarthritis
- Persons reporting restricted versus not restricted activity levels, $p < 0.01$[3]

Discriminant. Among Community-Dwelling Elderly
- Positive and Negative Affectivity Scale: $r = 0.12$[1]
- General self-presentation subscale score of PSES: $r = 0.03$[1]

Construct—Longitudinal/Sensitivity to Change
Performance on the ABC Scale has been shown to change owing to a fall prevention education plus exercise program with retirement home residents, to hip or knee replacement surgery and therapy in persons with osteoarthritis,[3] to an intensive rehabilitation program for persons with hip fracture,[6] and

to a physical therapy exercise program for individuals with a diagnosis of migraine-related vestibulopathy or vestibular dysfunction with a history of migraine headache.[11]

Convergent. Not available

Known Groups. *Among Community-Dwelling Elderly* Distinguished between persons reporting having suffered a "near fall" in the subsequent year compared with those who did not, $p < 0.001$.[3]

Discriminant. Not available

Other Validity Coefficients
Among Community-Dwelling Elderly
The hierarchicality of the ABC scale was examined using Mokken's Stochastic Cumulative Scaling Program among a sample of community-dwelling elderly. The mean ABC score for the sample was 35.4 (SD 9.4) with a normal distribution. The coefficient of scalability H was 0.59, indicating a "strong" cumulative scale. The coefficient of reliability rho was 0.95, indicating very high reliability. ABC item scores are well distributed across the response categories.[1]

Interpretability

General Population Values
(Customary or Normative Values)
Mean normal values, as well as standard deviations and ranges for the ABC Scale, are reported for older adults participating in a variety of community exercise programs and for persons with various health conditions (eg, diabetes, heart trouble, etc), home care users, and retirement home residents.[3] Developers note that individuals who score in the mid-80s or better on the ABC Scale tend to be highly functioning and already physically active; maintenance of functioning will be the primary objective for this group. For those scoring below 80, there is room for improvement on balance confidence, although incremental improvement is likely to be greater for persons scoring below versus above 80 as demonstrated by three studies.[3]

Typical Responsiveness Estimates
Not available

Comments
It is worthwhile administering the ABC to lower-mobility clients to capture balance confidence in more challenging situations that older adults may attempt if functional abilities improve through various rehabilitative therapies.

References
1. Powell LE, Myers AM. The Activities-specific Balance Confidence (ABC) Scale. J Gerontol A Biol Sci Med Sci 1995;50A: M28–34.
2. Myers AM, Powell LE, Maki BE, Holliday PJ, Brawley LR, Sherk W. Psychological indicators of balance confidence: relationship to actual and perceived abilities. J Gerontol A Biol Sci Med Sci 1996;51:M37–43.
3. Myers AM, Fletcher PC, Myers AH, Sherk W. Discriminative and evaluative properties of the Activities-specific Balance Confidence (ABC) Scale. J Gerontol A Biol Sci Med Sci 1998;53A: M287–94.
4. Tinetti ME, Richman D, Powell L. Falls efficacy as a measure of fear of falling. J Gerontol 1990;45:239–43.
5. Whitney SL, Hudak MT, Marchetti GF. The Activities-specific Balance Confidence Scale and the Dizziness Handicap Inventory: a comparison. J Vestib Res 1999;9:253–9.
6. Petrella RJ, Payne M, Myers A, Overend T, Chesworth B. Physical function and fear of falling after hip fracture rehabilitation in the elderly. Am J Phys Med Rehabil 2000;79:154–60.
7. Richardson JK, Sandman D, Vela S. A focused exercise regimen improves clinical measures of balance in patients with peripheral neuropathy. Arch Phys Med Rehabil 2001;82:205–9.
8. Parry SW, Steen N, Galloway SR, Kenny RA, Bond J. Falls and confidence related quality of life outcome measures in an older British cohort. Postgrad Med J 2001;77:103–8.
9. Simard C, Drouin D. The balance confidence ABC scale: a study with specific ages cohorts. In: 12th International Symposium for adapted physical activity; Spain: 1999. p. 145.
10. Medell JL, Alexander NB. A clinical measure of maximal and rapid stepping in older women. J Gerontol A Biol Sci Med Sci 2000;55:M429–33.
11. Whitney SL, Wrisley DM, Brown KE, Furman JM. Physical therapy for migraine-related vestibulopathy and vestibular dysfunction with history of migraine. Laryngoscope 2000;110:1528–34.

To obtain this measure, contact the developers.

ACTION RESEARCH ARM TEST

Developers

Developed by Lyle[1] based on the Upper Extremity Functional Test (UEFT).[2] In an effort to shorten the administration time, Lyle reduced the original 33 items to 19. Item reduction was based on three factors: (1) low intercorrelation with other items, (2) sufficiently high correlation indicating redundancy, and (3) excessive difficulty of the tasks based on observation during use of the UEFT.

Purpose

This is an evaluative tool measuring specific changes in limb function among individuals who sustained cortical damage resulting in hemiplegia.

Description

This viewed performance test contains 19 items grouped into 4 subtests: grasp, grip, pinch, and gross movement. The items in each subtest are arranged in a hierarchical manner, which was determined through a Guttman scale analysis. The quality of the movements for each item is rated using the following rating system: 0 = no movement possible, 1 = movement partially performed, 2 = movement performed but abnormally, 3 = movement performed normally. To allow for easier distinction between score 2 and 3, Wagenaar et al[3] set time limits for each item based on the performance of 20 healthy elderly subjects.

Conceptual/Theoretical Basis of Construct Being Measured

Although the developers did not refer to a specific theoretical basis for the construct, the objective was to develop a measure that would be sensitive to slight changes and could be used to detect and evaluate highly specific effects in clinical trials.

Groups Tested with This Measure

Individuals who have sustained cortical damage secondary to stroke, traffic or industrial accidents or assaults that resulted in hemiplegia[1]; chronic stroke clients[4]; and acute stroke clients.[5,6]

Language

English

Application/Administration

Items within each subtest are ordered in such a way that if a subject obtains the maximal score (3) on the first item, the most difficult item, this would predict success with all of the less difficult subscale items. The subject is then credited with having scored 3 on all items of that specific subtest. If the subject does not obtain 3 on the first item, then the easiest item is administered. If a score of zero is obtained, then the subject is not likely to be able to do the remaining items and therefore would be given 0 for all of the items of that specific subtest. If, however, the subject scores less than 3 on the hardest item of a subtest and more than 0 on the easiest item, then all items must be administered. The subject sits on a chair 44 cm above the floor level with the trolley close to the chest. The precise starting location for each task item is set to accommodate for right versus left hemiplegia. A normal performance implies that the subject is able to complete the tasks within the time limit and without losing contact with the back of the chair.[3] To enable the movement to be timed, the subjects are asked to start and finish each task with their hands flat on the table.[4] If someone accomplishes all of the tasks successfully, he/she would obtain a score of 57. De Weerdt and Harrison[6] reported that the test took a mean time of 8 minutes to administer in subacute stroke subjects. It is not specified whether formal training is needed to administer the test.

Typical Reliability Estimates

Internal Consistency
Not available

Interrater[1,3]
- $r = 0.98$
- Spearman's rho: 0.99 (summative score)
- ICC: 0.99 (summative score)
- Weighted kappa: individual items: 0.83 to 1, all items: 0.94 to 1

Test–Retest[4]
- $r = 0.99$
- Spearman's rho: 0.99 (summative score)
- ICC: 0.99 (summative score), 0.95 to 0.98 (individual subscale)
- Weighted kappa: individual items: 0.87 to .0.95, all items: 0.93

Typical Validity Estimates

Content
Not available

Criterion
No gold standard exists for the construct being measured.

Construct—Cross-sectional

Convergent
- Brunnstrom-Fugl-Meyer test: $r = 0.91$ to 0.94[6]
- Motor Assessment scale, upper extremity part: $r = 0.96$[5]
- Motricity index arm subscore: $r = 0.87$[5]
- Modified motor assessment chart upper extremity movement: $r = 0.94$[5]

Known Groups and *Discriminant* are not available.

Construct—Longitudinal/Sensitivity to Change
Not available

Interpretability

General Population Values (Customary or Normative Values)
Mean item performance times of 20 healthy elderly subjects are available.[3,4]

Typical Responsiveness Estimates

Individual Patient. Van der Lee et al[4] estimated the minimal clinically important difference as 5.7. Although the basis for this decision is not apparent, they were able to provide evidence that such a change would likely represent a true change and not only noise owing to measurement error.

Between Group. Not available

References

1. Lyle RC. A performance test for assessment of upper limb function in physical rehabilitation treatment and research. Int J Rehabil Res 1981;4:483–92.

2. Carroll D. A quantitative test of upper extremity function. J Chron Dis 1965;18:479–91.

3. Wagenaar RC, Meijer OG, van Wieringen PC, Kuik DJ, Hazenberg GJ, Lindeboom J, et al. The functional recovery of stroke: a comparison between neuro-developmental treatment and the Brunnstrom method. Scand J Rehabil Med 1990;22:1–8.

4. van der Lee JH, De Groot V, Beckerman H, Wagenaar RC, Lankhorst GJ, Bouter LM. The intra- and interrater reliability of the Action Research Arm Test: a practical test of upper extremity function in patients with stroke. Arch Phys Med Rehabil 2001;82:14–9.

5. Hsieh CL, Hsueh IP, Chiang FM, Lin PH. Inter-rater reliability and validity of the Action Research Arm Test in stroke patients. Age Ageing 1998;27:107–13.

6. De Weerdt WJG, Harrison MA. Measuring recovery of arm-hand function in stroke patients: a comparison of the Brunnstrom-Fugl-Meyer test and the Action Research Arm Test. Physiother Can 1985;37:65–70.

This measure can be found in references 1 and 4.

ACTIVITY SCALE FOR KIDS (ASK)

Developers

Nancy L. Young, The Hospital for Sick Children, Toronto, Ontario, nancy.young@sickkids.ca

Purpose

To measure physical disability in children ages 5 to 15 years who are experiencing limitations in physical activity owing to musculoskeletal disorders.[1] Developed for research and clinical use to assess status at a single point in time or to evaluate change in response to time or therapeutic intervention.[1]

Description

The ASK[1] is a 30-item self-report measure focusing on pediatric physical disability. There are two versions of the scale: (1) performance (ASKp), which assesses what the child "did do" in the previous week, and (2) capability (ASKc), which assesses what the child "could do" during the previous week. There are nine subcategories: personal care (3 items), dressing (4 items), eating and drinking (1 item), miscellaneous (2 items), locomotion (7 items), stairs (1 item), play (2 items), transfers (5 items), and standing skills (5 items).

Response categories range from "all of the time" to "none of the time" on the performance version and from "with no problem" to "I could not do" on the capability version. Individual items are scored on a 5-point ordinal scale (0 to 4). Summary scores are calculated based on the average score of all completed items (0 to 4) multiplied by 25. Summary scores can range from 0 to 100, with high scores indicating greater performance or capability. The ASK was developed in eight stages including review of the literature, interviews, and meetings. Children were assessed throughout the processes of item generation and reduction.

Conceptual/Theoretical Basis of Construct Being Measured

The ASK is based on the 1980 International Classification of Impairment, Disability and Handicap by the World Health Organization.[2] In this model, disability occurs when the performance of activities or behavior of the individual is altered. The ASK focuses on how musculoskeletal disorders impact on everyday physical function at the level of the individual.[1] Capability implies an artificial environment that might serve to reduce apparent disability.[1] Performance implies what the individual is doing in his/her typical environment.[1]

Groups Tested with This Measure

The ASK has been validated in children ages 5 to 15 years with a broad range of musculoskeletal disorders such as muscular dystrophy, juvenile arthritis, fractures, osteogenesis imperfecta, and spina bifida.[1] This measure has also been used with children who are either candidates for or have undergone hemidecorticectomy.[3]

Languages

English, Spanish (translated but not formally validated [unpublished])

Application/Administration

The ASK is an inexpensive self-report questionnaire that can be administered individually or in a group setting. If a child is unable to respond owing to reading ability (usually between the ages of 5 and 9 years), the caregiver can read the questions, but the child is still encouraged to record answers. If the child is unable to respond owing to cognitive limitations, the caregiver can complete the form. Both versions of the ASK are in booklet format. Respondents are asked to check their answer in the corresponding box. Average time to complete is 9 minutes (up to 30 minutes for the first time administered) and rests are allowed, but the respondent is encouraged to complete the questionnaire within 1 day. The booklets and manual are the only equipment needed. The manual provides sample instruction cards and gives meaning to response categories with sample response option cards. The ASK can be mailed or administered in person and should be completed at home, playground, or school to cue children about regular activities. A quiet setting with minimal distractions and adequate lighting is preferred. Summary scores can be calculated quickly with the use of a calculator. Incomplete or not applicable items are not included in the summary score.

Typical Reliability Estimates

Internal Consistency

- Cronbach's alpha = 0.99 in children with physical disabilities[1,4]

Interrater

- ICC (ASKp): 0.96[1,4]
- ICC (ASKc): 0.98[1,4]

Test–Retest

- Children: random effects ICC: ASKp = 0.97, ASKc = 0.98[1,4]
- Parents: random effects ICC: ASKp = 0.94, ASKc = 0.95[1,4]

Typical Validity Estimates

Content

Items were generated using pertinent literature and input from children, caregivers, and clinical experts. Item selection was performed using importance data from parents and children, an expert panel, and a consensus approach.[1] Parents and children were in 85% agreement, kappa = 0.7 on the items generated, confirming content validity.[4] Rasch modeling confirmed that all items measure physical disability.[5]

Criterion

No gold standard exists for the construct being measured.

Construct—Cross-sectional

Convergent

- Clinical observations: Spearman's rho = 0.92, 95% confidence interval = 0.82 to 0.97[6]
- CHAQ (Child Health Assessment Questionnaire): Spearman's correlation = 0.82 to 0.85[5]
- HUI3 (Health Utilities Index) ambulation subscale: Spearman's correlation = 0.71 to 0.74[5]
- HUI3 dexterity subscale: Spearman's correlation = 0.10 to 0.16[5]
- CHQ-PF28 (Child Health Questionnaire-Parent Form 28): $r \geq 0.49$[7]
- PODCI (Pediatrics Outcomes Data Collection Index): $r \geq 0.78$[7]

Known Groups. In 28 children with physical disabilities, those with severe disabilities scored lower on ASKp (one-way ANOVA, $p = 0.0023$).[4] In 200 children with physical disabilities, statistically significant different scores were found on ASKp between children at different levels of disability (ANOVA, $p < 0.0001$).[5]

Discriminant

- HUI3 emotion subscale: Spearman's rho = –0.12 to 0.15[5]
- HUI3 speech subscale: Spearman's rho = 0.08 to 0.09[5]

Construct—Longitudinal/Sensitivity to Change

Convergent

- ASKp showed 16% more change than the CHAQ.[5]
- ASKc showed 2% less change than the CHAQ.[5]

Known Groups and **Discriminant** are not available.

Interpretability

General Population Values (Customary or Normative Values)

Not available

Typical Responsiveness Estimates

Not available

Other

In 200 children, ages 5 to 15 years old[5]: floor effect, 0%; ceiling effect, 4%.

References

1. **Young NL. The Activities Scale for Kids (ASK). Unpublished manual. nancy.young@sickkids.ca.**
2. World Health Organization. International classification of impairments, disabilities and handicaps. Geneva: World Health Organization; 1980.
3. Graveline C, Young NL, Hwang P. Disability evaluation in children with hemidecorticectomy: use of the Activity Scale for Kids and the Pediatric Evaluation Disability Inventory. J Child Neurol 2000;15:7–14.
4. Young NL, Yoshida KK, Williams JI, Bombardier C, Wright JG. The role of children in reporting their physical disability. Arch Phys Med Rehabil 1995;76:913–8.
5. Young NL, Williams JI, Yoshida KK, Wright JG. Measurement properties of the Activities Scale for Kids. J Clin Epidemiol 2000;53:125–37.
6. Young NL, Williams JI, Yoshida KK, Bombardier C, Wright JG. The context of measuring disability. Does it matter whether capability or performance is measured. J Clin Epidemiol 1996;49:1097–101.
7. Pencharz J, Young NL, Owen JL, Wright JG. Comparison of three outcomes instruments in children. J Pediatr Orthop 2001;21:425–32.
8. Young NL. Measurement of capability and performance in pediatric orthopedics: development of a physical function scale [thesis]. Toronto: Univ. of Toronto; 1994.
9. Young NL. Evaluation of pediatric physical disability and exploration of contributing factors [thesis]. Toronto: Univ. of Toronto; 1997.
10. Young NL, Williams JI, Yoshida KK, Wright JG. Exploring determinants of physical disability in paediatric orthopaedics. Orthop Proc J Bone Joint Surg (Br) 1998;80 Suppl I:18–9.

To obtain this measure, contact the developers.

ALBERTA INFANT MOTOR SCALE (AIMS)

Developers

Martha C. Piper and Johanna Darrah, University of Alberta, Edmonton, Alberta, johanna.darrah@ualberta.ca

Purpose

To identify infants who are delayed or deviant in their motor development and to evaluate motor development over time.[1]

Description

The AIMS is a 58-item performance-based, norm-referenced, observational tool for the assessment of motor development in infants from 0 to 18 months of age. Infants are assessed in four positions: supine, prone, sitting, and standing. Items are marked as either "observed" (1 point) or "not observed" (0 points). Any items below the least mature item observed are credited with 1 point. The total AIMS score is a sum of the four positional scores. A graph is provided from which the examiner can determine the infant's percentile rank compared with the normative, age-matched sample.

Conceptual/Theoretical Basis of Construct Being Measured

The AIMS was based on certain aspects of the neuromaturational theory of motor development, as well as certain components of the dynamic systems theory.[1] The AIMS reflects the neuromaturational theory in the sequencing of the individual items on the scale. The AIMS also honors the basic tenets of the dynamic systems theory in the importance that is placed on the testing environment, the task in the assessment context, and the gravitational position of the infant.[1]

Groups Tested with This Measure

Preterm and full-term infants who are developing normally over the first 18 months of life; are considered to be "at risk" owing to prenatal, environmental, genetic, perinatal, or other factors; and display patterns of movement that are normal but exhibit delayed or immature motor development (eg, infants with a diagnosis of Down syndrome) and infants whose development is thought to be "suspect" despite having no predisposing factors in their medical histories.[1] The AIMS has also been used with cocaine-exposed infants.[2,3]

Language

English

Application/Administration

The AIMS can be conducted in a quiet, warm room in the home or clinical environment. Whenever possible, the infant should be completely undressed for the assessment. Parents or caregivers should be present and can comfort the infant during the assessment process if required. The infant should be awake, active, and content during the assessment. Handling of the infant by the examiner is minimal unless positioning or physical prompting is required. The four subscales can be administered in any order. Twenty to 30 minutes are required to administer the AIMS, with an additional 5 to 10 minutes to score the scale. If an infant is particularly irritable or upset and the assessment cannot be completed, the missing items may be administered up to a week after the original assessment. An examining table is required for young infants and a floor mat or carpet for older infants. A stable wooden bench is required for older infants to observe some items in the standing subscale. Toys may be needed to prompt or motivate the infant. The AIMS may be administered by any health professional who has an understanding of the essential components of movement and who has skill in performing observational assessments.

Typical Reliability Estimates

Internal Consistency
Not available

Interrater
- 0.86 to 0.98[1, 4]

Test–Retest
- 0.86 to 0.99[1, 4]

Typical Validity Estimates

Content
Eighty-four items were generated based on published descriptions of early motor performance and were reviewed for appropriateness, clinical impor-

tance, and content by pediatric physical therapists in Alberta, members of the Pediatric Division of the Canadian Physiotherapy Association, and six international experts in infant motor development. Multidimensional scaling indicated that the items fit well into one dimension, with a stress value of 0.04 and an RSQ of 0.995.[1]

Criterion

No gold standard exists for the attribute being measured.

Construct—Cross-sectional

Convergent. Bayley Scales of Motor Development
- $r = 0.84$ to 0.97 (normal infants 0 to < 13 months)[1]
- $r = 0.93$ (abnormal and at-risk infants)[1]
- $r = 0.78$ (assessed at 6 months)[4]
- $r = 0.90$ (assessed at 12 months)[4]

Peabody Developmental Motor Scales (Gross Motor)
- $r = 0.90$ to 0.99 (normal infants 0 to < 13 months)[1]
- $r = 0.95$ (abnormal and at risk infants)[1]

Test of Infant Motor Performance (TIMP)
- $r = 0.60$ to 0.64 (tested at 3 months)[5]

Known Groups. The mean AIMS percentile score in infants exposed to cocaine in utero was significantly different than the mean AIMS percentile score of control infants at 7 months.[2] There were no significant differences in mean raw scores or percentile ranks at 1 and 4 months between exposed and non-exposed infants.[2]

Discriminant. Not available

Construct—Longitudinal/Sensitivity to Change

Convergent Not available

Known Groups. Effect size increases with age in children with in utero cocaine exposure between 1 and 7 months.[3] Cohen's d increased from 0.39 at 1 month to 0.68 at 7 months.[3]

Discriminant. Not available

Other Validity Coefficients
Predictive Validity at 4 Months[6]
- Sensitivity: 30.6 (2nd percentile) to 72.2% (25th percentile)
- Specificity: 96.9 to 69.5%
- Positive predictive value (+PV): 73.3 to 40.0%
- Negative predictive value (–PV): 83.2 to 89.9%

Predictive Validity at 8 Months[6]
- Sensitivity: 52.8 to 86.1%
- Specificity: 96.1 to 66.4%
- +PV: 79.2 to 41.9%
- –PV: 87.9 to 94.4%

Best Combination of Sensitivity and Specificity
- 10th percentile at 4 months and 5th percentile at 8 months

Interpretability

General Population Values (Customary or Normative Values)
The AIMS is a norm-referenced assessment tool, and, as such, an infant's motor performance is interpreted by comparing it with the performance of an age-matched group of Alberta infants.[1] The normative sample was comprised of 2,202 infants, including preterm, full-term, and those with congenital abnormalities. A developmental graph is included with the test score sheet. An infant's raw score can be placed on the graph to determine the percentile rank.

Typical Responsiveness Estimates

Individual Patient. The AIMS has been shown to be responsive to small changes in motor performance over time in infants, as evidenced by the results of the reliability studies.[1] Minimal clinically important difference is not available.

Between Group. Not available

References

1. Piper MC, Darrah J. Motor assessment of the developing infant. Philadelphia: WB Saunders Company; 1994.
2. Fetters L, Tronick EZ. Neuromotor development of cocaine-exposed and control infants from birth through 15 months: poor and poorer performance. Pediatrics 1996;98:938–43.
3. Fetters L, Tronick EZ. Trajectories of motor development: polydrug exposed infants in the first fifteen months. Phys Occup Ther Pediatr 1998;18:1–18.
4. Jeng S, Yau KT, Chen L, Hsaio S. Alberta Infant Motor Scale: reliability and validity when used on preterm infants in Taiwan. Phys Ther 2000;80:168–78.
5. Campbell SK, Kolobe THA. Concurrent validity of the Test of Infant Motor Performance with the Alberta Infant Motor Scale. Pediatr Phys Ther 2000;12:2–9.
6. Darrah J, Piper M, Watt MJ. Assessment of gross motor skills of at-risk infants: predictive validity of the Alberta Infant Motor Scale. Dev Med Child Neurol 1998;40:485–91.

To obtain this measure, contact the developers, or it can be found in reference 1.

ARTHRITIS IMPACT MEASUREMENT SCALES (AIMS)

Developers

Robert Meenan and John Mason,[1–9] Boston University School of Public Health, Boston, Massachusetts, www.dcc2.bumc.bu.edu/rmeenn/, e-mail: rmeenan@bu.edu

Purpose

To measure the health status component of outcome in clients with rheumatic diseases and to compare health status across chronic disease groups.

Description

The AIMS were derived from two health status measures, Bush's Index of Well-being[10] and the Rand Health Insurance Study batteries.[11] They consist of 67 questions, including nine subscales: mobility, physical activity, dexterity, household activity, social activity, activities of daily living (ADL), pain, depression, and anxiety. The subscales can be combined into five health status components: lower extremity function, upper extremity function, affect, symptom, and social interaction.[8] Shortened versions of the AIMS are also available.[12,13] The AIMS have been revised to include three new subscales (arm function, work, and social support), and sections were added to assess satisfaction with function, attribution of problems to arthritis, and self-designation of priority areas for improvement (AIMS2).[6]

Conceptual/Theoretical Basis of Construct Being Measured

The AIMS were developed to measure three dimensions of health (physical, mental, and social) as defined by the World Health Organization.

Groups Tested with This Measure

Adults with rheumatic diseases (osteoarthritis [OA], rheumatoid arthritis [RA], fibromyalgia,[14] psoriatic arthritis),[15] and hip arthroplasty[16] and in a variety of ethnic groups with RA (blacks, Hispanics, whites of Eastern European origin).[17] Testing in children with juvenile arthritis (JA) has shown that the pain and physical activity scales are the most reliable for use with children.[18] In addition, this measure has been used with other chronic diseases, such as diabetes[19] and chronic orthopedic conditions (post-traumatic fracture nonunion, refractory osteomyelitis, lower extremity amputation).[20] The AIMS have been modified for use with patients with ankylosing spondylitis (AS) (AS-AIMS)[21] and with a geriatric population (GERI-AIMS).[22,23]

Languages

English. The AIMS have been translated and validated in a dual-language English-Spanish format,[24] Italian,[25] Dutch (DUTCH-AIMS),[16,26,27] and French.[28] The AIMS have been anglicized and validated in British patients with RA.[29] The AIMS2 have been translated but not formally validated in French.[30]

Application/Administration

Clients are asked to respond based on their status in the previous month. Self-administered, face-to-face, mail-out, and telephone administration is possible. Time to complete AIMS: 15 to 20 minutes, AIMS2: 23 minutes.

Some questions need to be recoded before scoring. Once recoded, the scores in each subscale are added to create raw scores. The raw scores are normalized so that all scores are expressed out of 10 (0 = good health status, 10 = poor health status). The developers will provide support for scoring the data if needed. A one-page computer-generated scoring summary is available.[31] Time to score is not reported.

Typical Reliability Estimates

Internal Consistency
- Cronbach's alpha > 0.6 for AIMS[2,5]
- Cronbach's alpha = 0.72 to 0.91 in RA and 0.74 to 0.96 in OA for AIMS2.[6]

Interrater
Not applicable

Test–Retest
- AIMS2: ICC = 0.78 to 0.94[6]

Typical Validity Estimates

Content

The Total Health Score (function subscales) reflected areas of function perceived as relevant to nursing practice (impaired physical disability and self-care deficit).[32] Pain, anxiety, depression, dexterity, physical activity, household activity (for women only), and ADL (for those with higher disability only) subscales correlated with clients' importance ratings for related aspects of their treatment ($r = 0.22$ to 0.45).[33]

Criterion

Concurrent. No gold standard exists for the construct being measured.

Predictive. In a community-based RA population, the AIMS subscales for lower extremity function and social activity best predicted survival at 5 years.[31]

Construct—Cross-sectional

Convergent. AIMS

- Perceptions of overall health, recent arthritis activity, physician's report of disease activity, functional status, joint count, walking time, grip strength, range of motion: $r = 0.00$ to 0.68[2,35]
- Scores for a variety of clinical variables: $r = 0.17$ to 0.57[35]
- Measures of mobility, pain, and global health preoperatively: $r = 0.21$ to 0.87 and 3 months post joint replacement: $r = 0.25$ to 0.55[36]
- Sickness Impact Profile (SIP): $r = 0.37$ to 0.76[37]
- Self-efficacy (SE) for pain and other symptoms: $r = 0.38$ to 0.57[38]
- Timed Stands Test: $r = 0.31$ to 0.63[39]

AIMS2

- Measures of disease activity: $r > 0.71$[6]

Known Groups. AIMS

In a community-based RA population, those who survived to 5-year follow-up had significantly lower (better) AIMS subscale scores for mobility, physical activity, household activity, social activity, depression, anxiety, and lower extremity function at baseline compared with those who died.[34]

Discriminant AIMS2

No correlations with age, education, income, or duration of RA ($r < 0.32$).[9]

Construct—Longitudinal/Sensitivity to Change

Convergent. In RA, the AIMS change scores for mobility, pain, and emotions correlated with change scores for clinical variables ($r = 0.18$ to 0.41).[35,36] In patients with hip or knee OA, the AIMS total health dimension demonstrated change scores comparable to that of the SIP (ES: AIMS, 0.07 to 0.32; SIP, 0.17 to 0.40).[37]

Known Groups In RA, the AIMS change scores distinguished between the treatment and placebo groups and between the two treatment groups (gold shots and oral gold).[7]

Discriminant. Not available

Interpretability

General Population Values (Customary or Normative Values)

Not available

Typical Responsiveness Estimates

Not available.

References

1. AIMS user guide. Boston: Boston University Multipurpose Arthritis Center; 1985.
2. Meenan RF, Gertman PM, Mason JH. Measuring health status in arthritis: the Arthritis Impact Measurement Scales. Arthritis Rheum 1980;23:146–52.
3. Meenan RF, Gertman PM, Mason JH, Dunaif R. The Arthritis Impact Measurement Scales: further investigations of a health status measure. Arthritis Rheum 1982;25:1048–53.
4. Meenan RF. The AIMS approach to health status measurement: conceptual background and measurement properties. J Rheumatol 1982;9:785–8.
5. Meenan RF. New approaches to outcome assessment: the AIMS questionnaire for arthritis. Adv Intern Med 1986;31:167–85.
6. Meenan RF, Mason JH, Anderson JJ, Guccione AA, Kazis LE. AIMS2: the content and properties of a revised and expanded Arthritis Impact Measurement Scales health status questionnaire. Arthritis Rheum 1992;35:1–10.
7. Meenan RF, Anderson JJ, Kazis LE, Egger MJ, Altz-Smith M, Samuelson CO Jr, et al. Outcome assessment in clinical trials: evidence for the sensitivity of a health status measure. Arthritis Rheum 1984;27:1344–52.
8. Mason JH, Anderson JJ, Meenan RF. A model of health status for rheumatoid arthritis: a factor analysis of the Arthritis Impact Measurement Scales. Arthritis Rheum 1988;31:714–20.
9. Mason JH, Meenan RF, Anderson JJ. Do self-reported arthritis symptom (RADAR) and health status (AIMS2) data provide duplicative or complementary information? Arthritis Care Res 1992;5:163–72.
10. Patrick DL, Bush JW, Chen MM. Toward an operational definition of health. J Health Soc Behav 1973;14:6–23.
11. Brook RH, Ware JE, Davies-Avery A, Stewart AL, Donald CA, Rodgers WH, et al. Overview of adult health status measures fielded in Rand's Health Insurance Study. Med Care 1979;17(9 Suppl):1–131.

12. Lorish CD, Abraham N, Austin JS, Bradley LA, Alarcon GS. A comparison of the full and short versions of the Arthritis Impact Measurement Scales. Arthritis Care Res 1991;4:168–73.

13. Katz JN, Larson MG, Phillips CB, Fossel AH, Liang MH. Comparative measurement sensitivity of short and longer health status instruments. Med Care 1992;30:917–25.

14. Burckhardt CS, Clark SR, Bennett RM. The Fibromylagia Impact Questionnaire: development and validation. J Rheumatol 1991;18:728–33.

15. Duffy CM, Watanabe Duffy KN, Gladman DD, Brubacher BB, Bushkila D, Langevitz P, et al. The utility of the Arthritis Impact Measurement Scales for patients with psoriatic arthritis. J Rheumatol 1992;19:1727–32.

16. Borstlap M, Zant JL, Van Soesbergen RM, Van Der Korst JK. Quality of life assessment: a comparison of four questionnaires: for measuring improvements after total hip replacement. Clin Rheumatol 1995;14:15–20.

17. Coulton CJ, Hyduk CM, Chow JC. An assessment of the Arthritis Impact Measurement Scales in 3 ethnic groups. J Rheumatol 1989;16:1110–5.

18. Coulton CJ, Zborowsky E, Lipton J, Newman AJ. Assessment of the reliability and validity of the Arthritis Impact Measurement Scales for children with juvenile arthritis. Arthritis Rheum 1987;30:819–24.

19. Burckhardt CS, Woods SL, Schultz AA, Ziebarth DM. Quality of life of adults with chronic illness: a psychometric study. Res Nurs Health 1989;12:347–54.

20. Lerner RK, Esterhai JL, Polomono RC, Cheatle MC, Heppenstall RB, Brighton CT. Psychosocial, functional and quality of life assessment of patients with posttraumatic fracture nonunion, chronic refractory osteomyelitis, and lower extremity amputation. Arch Phys Med Rehabil 1991;72:122–6.

21. Guillemin F, Challier B, Urlaacher F, Vancon G, Pourel J. Quality of life in ankylosing spondylitis: validation of the Ankylosing Spondylitis Arthritis Impact Measurement Scales 2, a modified Arthritis Impact Measurement Scales Questionnaire. Arthritis Care Res 1999;12:157–62.

22. Hughes AL, Edelman P, Chang RW, Singer RH, Schuette P. The GERI-AIMS: reliability and validity of the AIMS adapted for elderly respondents. Arthritis Rheum 1991;34:856–65.

23. Falconer J, Hughes SL, Naughton BJ, Singer RH, Chang RW, Sinacore JM. Self-report and performance-based hand function tests as correlates of dependency in the elderly. J Am Geriatr Soc 1991;39:695–9.

24. Hendricson WD, Russell IJ, Prihoda TJ, Jacobson JM, Rogan A, Bishop GD, et al. Development and initial validation of a dual-language English-Spanish format for the Arthritis Impact Measurement Scales. Arthritis Rheum 1989;32:1153–9.

25. Salaffi F, Cavalieri F, Nolli M, Ferraccioli G. Analysis of disability in knee osteoarthritis: relationship with age and psychological variables but not with radiographic score. J Rheumatol 1991;18:1581–6.

26. Taal E, Jacobs JW, Seydel ER, Wiegman O, Rasker JJ. Evaluation of the Dutch Arthritis Impact Measurement Scales (Dutch-AIMS) in patients with rheumatoid arthritis. Br J Rheumatol 1989;28:487–91.

27. Jacobs JWG, Oosterveld FG, Deuxbouts N, Rasker JJ, Taal E, Dequeker J, et al. Opinions of patients with rheumatoid arthritis about their own functional capacity: how valid is it? Ann Rheum Dis 1992;51:765–8.

28. Sampalis JS, Pouchot J, Beaudet F, Carette S, Gutkowske A, Harth M, et al. Arthritis Impact Measurement Scales: reliability of a French version and validity in adult Still's disease. J Rheumatol 1990;17:1657–61.

29. Hill J, Bird HA, Lawton CW, Wright V. The Arthritis Impact Measurement Scales: an anglicized version to assess the outcome of British patients with rheumatoid arthritis. Br J Rheumatol 1990;29:193–6.

30. Poiraudeau S, Dougados M, Ait-Hadad H, Pion-Graff J, Ayral X, Listrat V, et al. [Evaluation of a quality of life scale (AIMS2) in rheumatology]. Rev Rhum Ed Fr 1993;60:561–7.

31. Kazis LE, Anderson JJ, Meenan RF. Health status information in clinical practice: the development and testing of patient profile reports. J Rheumatol 1988;15:338–44.

32. Goeppinger J, Thomas Doyle MA, Charlton SL, Lorig K. A nursing perspective on the assessment of function in persons with arthritis. Res Nurs Health 1988;11:321–31.

33. Potts MK, Brandt KD. Evidence of the validity of the Arthritis Impact Measurement Scales. Arthritis Rheum 1987;30:93–6.

34. Soderlin MK, Nieminen P, Hakala M. Arthritis Impact Measurement Scales in a community-based rheumatoid arthritis population. Clin Rheumatol 2000;19:30–4.

35. Fitzpatrick R, Ziebland S, Jenkinson C, Mowat A, Mowat A. A comparison of the sensitivity to change of several health status instruments in rheumatoid arthritis. J Rheumatol 1993;20:429–36.

36. Liang MH, Larson MG, Cullen KE, Schwartz JA. Comparative measurement efficiency and sensitivity of five health status instruments for arthritis research. Arthritis Rheum 1985;28:542–7.

37. Weinberger M, Samsa GP, Tierney WM, Belyea MJ, Hiner SL. Generic versus disease specific health status measures: comparing the Sickness Impact Profile and the Arthritis Impact Measurement Scales. J Rheumatol 1992;19:543–6.

38. Brekke M, Hjortdahl P, Kvien TK. Self-efficacy and health status in rheumatoid arthritis: a two-year longitudinal observational study. Rheumatology 2001;40:387–92.

39. Newcomer KL, Krug HE, Mahowald ML. Validity and reliability of the Timed-Stands Test for patients with rheumatoid arthritis and other chronic diseases. J Rheumatol 1993;20:21–7.

This measure or ordering information can be found at the Website address included in this review.

ARTHRITIS SELF-EFFICACY SCALE (SES)

Developers

Kate Lorig, R.L. Chastain, E. Ung, S. Shoor, and H.R. Holman,[1-3] Stanford University School of Medicine, California, Lorig@Stanford.edu, Fax: 650-725-9422

Purpose

To measure clients' perceived self-efficacy (SE) to cope with the consequences of chronic arthritis

Description

The Arthritis SES is a self-administered disease-specific questionnaire consisting of 20 questions. There are three subscales: physical function (9 questions), other symptoms (6 questions), and pain (5 questions). Questions are scored on a 9-cm numeric rating scale with anchors (10 = very uncertain, 50 to 60 = moderately uncertain, and 100 = very certain). A higher score indicates higher self-efficacy.

Conceptual/Theoretical Basis of Construct Being Measured

Self-efficacy is defined as the belief in one's capability to do a specific task or achieve a certain result. The theoretical framework of SE was proposed by Bandura in 1986.[4] There is some controversy about whether the measurement of SE is really the measurement of outcome expectations.[3]

Groups Tested with This Measure

Clients with chronic arthritis, including fibromyalgia

Languages

English,[1] Swedish,[5-7] Spanish[8,9]

Application/Administration

Clients are asked to circle a number to indicate their certainty that they can perform each task. Each subscale is scored separately by taking the mean of the subscale items. The Arthritis SES is administered face to face or by mail-out survey. Time to administer is less than 10 minutes. The time to score is not reported. A computer is not needed. If one-fourth or less of the data is missing, the score is a mean of the completed data. If more than one-fourth of the data is missing, no score is calculated.

Typical Reliability Estimates

Internal Consistency

The original SES Subscales[1]
- Physical function: Cronbach's alpha = 0.93
- Other arthritis symptoms: Cronbach's alpha = 0.90.

Revised SES Subscales[1]
- Physical function: Cronbach's alpha = 0.89
- Other symptoms: Cronbach's alpha = 0.87
- Pain: Cronbach's alpha = 0.75

Interrater
Not applicable

Test–Retest
Not available

Typical Validity Estimates

Content
No reference to content validity in the literature

Criterion
No gold standard exists for the construct being measured.

Construct—Cross-sectional

Convergent
- Self-efficacy (mail-out version of original Arthritis SES) correlated with task performance assessed in the clients' homes: $r = 0.61$[1]
- SES pain subscale and ratings of pain threshold: rho = 0.21, and pain tolerance: rho = 0.16[10]
- Higher self-efficacy was related to fewer pain behaviors in clients with rheumatoid arthritis (RA): $r = -0.32$ to -0.39[11]
- Self-efficacy (original version) and health status: $r = 0.35$ to 0.73; revised version: $r = 0.16$ to 0.76[1]
- SES pain subscale and levels of clinical pain reported on the Arthritis Impact Measurement Scales: rho = -0.62[10]
- In RA, self-efficacy and health status: $r = 0.34$ to 0.57[12]
- In RA, self-efficacy and symptoms of depression and less disease activity: $r = -0.25$ to -0.44[11]

Known Groups
- Self-efficacy improved in an experimental group participating in the Arthritis Self-management Course compared to a control group.[1]

- Clients with RA who had greater involvement with their care and those who had higher satisfaction with their care also reported higher self-efficacy than those who had less involvement and those who were less satisfied with their care.[13]
- Clients with osteoarthritis who had high self-efficacy for arthritis pain had higher pain tolerance and higher pain thresholds and rated thermal stimuli as less unpleasant and less intense than subjects in the low self-efficacy group.[10]

Discriminant. Not available

Construct—Longitudinal/Sensitivity to Change
Not available

Other Validity Coefficients
Baseline self-efficacy (original version) correlated with future health status 4 months from baseline ($r = 0.32$ to 0.68). Revised version: 0.21 to 0.71.[1] High self-efficacy (for pain and other symptoms subscales) has been associated with improved health status 2 years from baseline in clients with RA ($r = 0.12$ to 0.22).[12]

Interpretability

General Population Values
(Customary or Normative Values)
Not available

Typical Responsiveness Estimates
Not available.

Comments

There are no data to support this measure's ability to detect change in individuals or groups; therefore, it needs to be used as an outcome measure with caution until this measurement property has been tested.

A shortened eight-item version of the Arthritis Self-efficacy Scale is now available by contacting the developer (see above). The reliability and validity of this measure have not been reported in the literature.

References

1. Lorig K, Chastain RL, Ung E, Shoor S, Holman HR. Development and evaluation of a scale to measure perceived self-efficacy in people with arthritis. Arthritis Rheum 1989;32:37–44.
2. Lorig K, Stewart A, Ritter P, Gonzalez V, Laurent D, Lynch J. Outcome measures for health education and other health care interventions. Thousand Oaks (CA): Sage Publications; 1996.
3. Lorig K, Holman H. Arthritis self-efficacy scales measure self-efficacy. Arthritis Care Res 1998;11:155–7.
4. Bandura A. Social foundations of thought and action. Englewood Cliffs (NJ): Prentice Hall; 1986.
5. Lomi C, Burckhardt C, Norholm L, Bjelle A, Ekdahl C. Evaluation of a Swedish version of the Arthritis Self-Efficacy Scale in people with fibromyalgia. Scand J Rheumatol 1995;24:282–7.
6. Lomi C, Nordholm LA. Validation of a Swedish version of the Arthritis Self-Efficacy Scale. Scand J Rheumatol 1992;21:231–7.
7. Lomi C. Evaluation of a Swedish version of the Arthritis Self-Efficacy Scale. Scand J Caring Sci 1992;6:131–8.
8. Lorig K, Gonzalez VM, Ritter P. Community-based Spanish language arthritis education program: a randomized controlled trial. Med Care 1999;37:957–63.
9. Gonzalez VM, Stewart A, Ritter PL, Lorig K. Translation and validation of arthritis outcome measures into Spanish. Arthritis Rheum 1995;38:1429–46.
10. Keefe FJ, Lefebvre JC, Maixner W, Salley AN Jr, Caldwell DS. Self-efficacy for arthritis pain: relationship to perception of thermal laboratory pain stimuli. Arthritis Care Res 1997;10:177–84.
11. Buescher KL, Johnston JA, Parker JC, Smarr KL, Buckelew SP, Anderson SK, et al. Relationship of self-efficacy to pain behavior. J Rheumatol 1991;18:968–72.
12. Brekke M, Hjortdahl P, Kvien TK. Self-efficacy and health status in rheumatoid arthritis: a two-year longitudinal observational study. Rheumatology (Oxford) 2001;40:387–92.
13. Brekke M, Hjortdahl P, Kvien TK. Involvement and satisfaction: a Norwegian study of health care among 1,204 patients with rheumatoid arthritis and 1,509 patients with chronic noninflammatory musculoskeletal pain. Arthritis Care Res 2001;45:8–15.

To obtain this measure, contact the developers, or it can be found in reference 1 and a shorter version in reference 9.

BACK PAIN FUNCTIONAL SCALE (BPFS)

Developers

P. W. Stratford and J. M. Binkley, McMaster University, Hamilton, Ontario, stratfor@mcmaster.ca

Purpose

To assess functional status and pain-related disability status in clients with low back pain.

Description

The BPFS[1,2] consists of 12 items, each scored on a 6-point scale (0 to 5). Adjectives with approximately equal interval properties define the scale points. The total BPFS scores can vary from 0, the lowest functional level, to 60, the highest functional level.

Conceptual/Theoretical Basis of Construct Being Measured

The BPFS was conceived as a self-report functional status measure appropriate for clinical practice and clinical research. Guiding principles were that the measure should (1) be based on the World Health Organization's model of impairment, disability (activity), and handicap (participation); (2) have sound psychometric properties; (3) be able to be completed in less than 5 minutes; and (4) be able to be scored in less than 30 seconds.

Groups Tested with This Measure

Outpatients seen in physical therapy settings with acute, subacute, and chronic low back pain. Most clients received conservative interventions; however, some clients were postsurgical cases.

Language

English

Application/Administration

This is a self-report measure in which clients respond by circling the appropriate score associated with each item. Most clients can complete the questionnaire in 3 to 5 minutes. The score is obtained by summing the circled responses. Clinicians can score this measure without the use of computational aids in less than 15 seconds.

Typical Reliability Estimates

Internal Consistency

Coefficient alpha value 0.93[1,2]

Interrater

Not applicable

Test–Retest

Type 2,1 intraclass correlation coefficient values 0.82 to 0.88[1,2]

Typical Validity Estimates

Content

Existing questionnaires, clients, and clinical experts surveyed to achieve content validity.

Criterion

No gold standard exists for the attribute being assessed.

Construct—Cross-sectional

Convergent. Correlation with Roland-Morris Questionnaire: 0.79.[1] Correlation with duration of symptoms: 0.26.[2]

Known Groups. Capable of discriminating among persons with different levels of impairment ($F_{1,136} = 75.4$), work status ($F_{2,146} = 20.18$), location of pain ($F_{2,148} = 10.32$), and education level ($F_{1,149} = 4.29$)

Discriminant. Not available

Construct—Longitudinal/Sensitivity to Change

Convergent. Correlation with Roland-Morris Questionnaire change scores: 0.82.[1] Correlation with prognostic rating of change: 0.17 to 0.56.[1,2] Correlation with duration of symptoms: –0.56.[1]

Known Groups. Capable of discriminating amount of change between a dichotomized duration of symptom standard ($F_{1,113} = 10.80$).[2]

Discriminant. Not available

Interpretability

General Population Values (Customary or Normative Values)

Not available

Typical Responsiveness Estimates

Individual Patient. Confidence in a measured score: $SEM_{internal\ consistency} = 3.2$ BPFS.[2] True change estimate: $SEM_{test-retest} = 3.9$ to 4.8 BPFS.[1,2]

Between Group. Not available

References

1. Stratford PW, Binkley JM, Riddle DL. Development and initial validation of the Back Pain Functional Scale. Spine 2000;25:2095–102.
2. Stratford PW, Binkley JM. A comparison study of the Back Pain Functional Scale and Roland-Morris Questionnaire. North American Orthopaedic Rehabilitation Research Network. J Rheumatol 2000;27:1928–36.

This measure can be found on the accompanying CD-ROM. Prior to using the measure, you are strongly advised to contact the developers for administration and scoring guidelines and revisions to the measure not available at time of publication.

BARTHEL INDEX (BI)

Developers

Florence I. Mahoney and Dorothea W. Barthel[1]

Purpose

The index was developed to measure functional independence in personal care and mobility.

Description

This is a 10-item performance-based instrument that evaluates activities of daily living (ADL). Scores range between 0 and 100, with a score of 100 representing the highest level of independence. A perfect score does not mean that the individual is able to live alone or perform instrumental ADL (such as cooking and house cleaning). Each item is assigned a score of 0, 5, 10, or 15; each item is weighted differently and hence reflects the relative importance of each type of disability in terms of assistance required.[1] The items assessed are feeding, transferring from wheelchair to bed and back, personal hygiene, getting on and off toilet, bathing self, walking on a level surface/propelling wheelchair, ascending/descending surface, dressing, controlling bowels, and controlling bladder.

An adapted version consists of 15 items scored on a 4-point scale.[2] The original 10 items are expanded; for example, feeding was expanded to "drinking from a cup" and "eating." Another adaptation proposed making the BI more sensitive to change by increasing the number of categories in the rating scale.[3]

Conceptual/Theoretical Basis of Construct Being Measured

This is an index of independence that scores the ability of a client with a neuromuscular or musculoskeletal disorder to care for himself/herself.[1]

Groups Tested with This Measure

Individuals with stroke, spinal cord injuries, neurologic conditions (such as multiple sclerosis), burns, cardiac problems, rheumatoid arthritis, amputations, and elderly people.

Language

English

Application/Administration

It can be administered in 20 minutes if performance is observed or in 5 minutes if information is obtained verbally from the client. A health care professional, a trained interviewer, a proxy respondent, or the client may complete it. It may be performed in clinic or community settings.

Typical Reliability Estimates

Internal Consistency

Cronbach's alpha = 0.87 at admission and 0.92 at discharge for a sample of 258 stroke clients undergoing rehabilitation.[3]

Interrater

A Pearson product-moment correlation coefficient on a sample of 25 inpatients in a neurorehabilitation unit, with mixed diagnoses was 0.99 ($p < 0.001$).[4] Kappa scores among five therapists using the total score to rate seven inpatients with stroke for each patient ranged from 0.70 to 0.88.[5]

Test–Retest

Repeatability of testing among 50 clients with stroke who were interviewed by two of three research nurses on two occasions, 2 to 3 weeks apart: kappa score of 0.98.[6]

Other

When scores on interview were compared with those obtained from observation of 25 inpatients with various neurologic conditions,[4] a Pearson product-moment correlation coefficient of 0.88 ($p < 0.001$) was reported.

When telephone interview responses were compared with those during a home interview among 366 rehabilitation inpatients with stroke or orthopedic conditions, an ICC of 0.89 was reported. Kappa scores for agreement between these modes of interview according to type of interviewers were laypersons, 0.75, versus health professionals, 0.76, and according to type of respondents were self, 0.71, versus proxy, 0.75.[7]

Intrarater reliability of five therapists using the total score to rate seven inpatients with stroke: kappa scores ranged from 0.84 to 0.97 and the Spearman rank-order correlation coefficients ranged from 0.95 to 1.00.[5]

Typical Validity Estimates

Content

In a study designed to compare three popular ADL scales, the BI was the only scale among the three that included all 11 of the most commonly used variables.[8]

Criterion

Concurrent. The BI has been used many times as the gold standard for the concurrent validation of other scales, but it has not been validated in this way. When the BI was developed, there were no gold standards to use for validation purposes. Over time, the BI seems to have been generally accepted by the rehabilitation community and continues to be used as a disability outcome measure.

Predictive. The BI predicted living arrangements, productivity outcomes, and overall independent living in 84 stroke clients.[9]

Another study compared the number of deaths within 6 months following admission among four groups of stroke clients (defined according to BI admission scores); clients with higher BI admission scores were less likely to die than clients with lower scores.[10] Although *p* values were not reported, a statistical test was conducted for the purpose of this review, resulting in a *p* value of $p < 0.005$.

In a study of 110 clients in stroke rehabilitation, a greater proportion of clients with initial BI scores above 40 were discharged home, compared with clients with scores under 40. Clients with initial scores above 60 had shorter lengths of stay than clients with scores below 60. All clients who returned to an acute care facility had BI admission scores below 40.[11] Although *p* values were not reported, a chi-square test was conducted for the purpose of this review, and a *p* value of $p < 0.001$ was obtained, indicating that it is highly unlikely that these results are attributable to chance alone.

Construct—Cross-sectional

Convergent. Correlations between 0.73 and 0.77 were reported between the BI and the Motricity Index in a study of 976 stroke clients ($p < 0.001$).[12] The BI achieved a significant positive agreement with the Katz Index of ADL (0.77; $p < 0.0001$) and with the Kenny Self-Care Evaluation (0.42, $p < 0.0001$; Spearman's rank-order correlation rho = 0.73, $p < 0.001$).[8]

In a study with 204 stroke clients, BI scores were compared to Functional Independence Measure (FIM) scores by creating ordered categories

that placed the scores on the same scale. The results indicate a high concordance between FIM and Barthel ordered categories. Crude agreement on individual item scores between the FIM and Barthel scale ranged from 62 to 97%.[13]

Known Groups. Patterns of recovery in 459 stroke clients with varying degrees of severity were described using five different instruments and varying cutoff points for each.[14] Using a BI score of > 90 (out of 100) to indicate full functional recovery after stroke, 16% of the group of clients who had suffered major strokes reached full recovery, whereas 52% and 89% of clients recovered in the moderate and minor stroke severity groups, respectively.[14]

The proportion of clients considered to have recovered by 6 months post-stroke differed according to the definition used for recovery; 57.3% of clients recovered when recovery was defined by a BI score > 90 (Table 1).[14]

TABLE 1

Definition of Recovery	% of Cohort (n = 459) Fully Recovered
Barthel > 90	57.3
NIH Stroke Scale ≤ 1	44.9
Fugl-Meyer > 90	36.8
Women SF-36 > 66	24.0
Men SF-36 > 75	28.5
Rankin Scale ≤ 1	24.4
Rankin Scale ≤ 2	53.8

NIH = National Institutes of Health; SF-36 = 36-Item Short-Form Health Survey.

BI scores varied in magnitude in the same direction as changes observed using the Rankin scale. However, BI scores were better able to discriminate between patients who obtained lower Rankin scores than between those with higher scores.[14] Rankin scores 0, 1, 2, 3, 4, and 5 corresponded to BI scores of 99, 99, 96, 83, 43, and 6, respectively.

Discriminant. Not available

Construct—Longitudinal/Sensitivity to Change

Convergent. Not available

Known Groups. Patterns of recovery in a group of 459 stroke clients illustrated that changes in BI scores changed over time and that these changes differed across three severity groups.[14] The figures in Table 2 have been approximated from a chart provided by the authors.[14]

TABLE 2

Severity Group	N*	Barthel Scores			
		Baseline	1 Mo	3 Mo	6 Mo
Minor	179	80	90	95	95
Moderate	230	40	65	75	75
Major	50	10	20	35	45

*459 clients total; 39% had a minor stroke, 50% had a moderate stroke, and 11% had a major stroke.

These results indicate that the BI measured more change early on in the group with moderate stroke than in the other groups; the BI measured less change after 3 months among clients with minor or moderate strokes. BI scores continued to change over the entire study period for clients with severe strokes.

These findings were consistent with those of an earlier study[12] that classified 531 stroke clients into one of four severity categories (Table 3).

Using the Wilcoxon signed rank test for repeat measures, all changes were significant ($p < 0.01$) except for deterioration in scores between 3 weeks and 6 months for the mildly disabled group.

Discriminant. Not available

Interpretability

General Population Values
(Customary or Normative Values)
Guidelines have been proposed for interpreting the scores obtained on the BI. Shah et al[3] proposed that a total BI score of 0 to 20 suggests total dependency, 21 to 60 severe dependency, 61 to 90 moderate dependence, and 91 to 99 slight dependence, and 100 indicates that a patient is independent of assistance from others. Granger et al[2,15] proposed a score of 60 as the cut point between independence and more marked dependence; 40 or less is said to be indicative of severe dependence, whereas 20 or below indicates total dependence.

Sensitivity. *Single-Group Indexes*
An effect size of 0.37 ($p < 0.0001$) in a group of 201 clients with multiple sclerosis and an effect size of 0.95 ($p < 0.0001$) in a group of 82 clients with stroke.[16]

Multigroup Indexes
A study comparing five different outcome measures (representing 10 different measurement strategies) in stroke reported a standardized response mean (SRM) of 0.99 for the BI. The Barthel SRM ranked fourth highest among the 10 strategies (with a higher SRM representing greater sensitivity to change).[17] When grouped by severity of stroke, the BI scores of the more severely disabled group were very sensitive to change (surpassed only by one other scale). Among the moderately or mildly disabled groups, the BI performed as well as other instruments.

Typical Responsiveness Estimates
Not available

Comments

Websites of interest:
- Scale and calculator: www.info.med.yale.edu/neurol/Residency/barthel.htm
- Printable copy of scale: www.neuro.mcg.edu/mcgstrok/Indices/Barthel_Ind.htm
- or www.strokecenter.org/trials/scales/barthel.pdf

TABLE 3

Severity Group	N	Barthel Scores*		
		Baseline	3 Wk	6 Mo
Mild	69	85	95	90
Moderate	61	60	85	90
Severe	79	35	60	70
Very severe	67	10	40	60

*Scores were estimated from figure and were converted from the 20-point scale to the 100-point scale.

References

1. Mahoney FI, Barthel DW. Functional evaluation: the Barthel Index. Md State Med J 1965;14:61–5.

2. Granger CV, Albrecht GL, Hamilton BB. Outcome of comprehensive medical rehabilitation: measurement by PULSES profile and the Barthel Index. Arch Phys Med Rehabil 1979;60:145–54.

3. Shah S, Vanclay F, Cooper B. Improving the sensitivity of the Barthel Index for stroke rehabilitation. J Clin Epidemiol 1989; 42:703–9.

4. Roy CW, Togneri J, Hay E, Pentland B. An inter-rater reliability study of the Barthel Index. Int J Rehabil Res 1988;11:67–70.

5. Loewen SC, Anderson BA. Reliability of the Modified Motor Assessment Scale and the Barthel Index. Phys Ther 1988; 68:1077–81.

6. Wolfe CD, Taub NA, Woodrow EJ, Burney PG. Assessment of scales of disability and handicap for stroke patients. Stroke 1991; 22:1242–4.

7. Korner-Bitensky N, Wood-Dauphinee S. Barthel Index information elicited over the telephone: is it reliable? Am J Phys Med Rehabil 1995;74:9–18.

8. Gresham GE, Phillips TF, Labi ML. ADL status in stroke: relative merits of three standard indexes. Arch Phys Med Rehabil 1980;61:355–8.

9. DeJong G, Branch LG. Predicting the stroke patient's ability to live independently. Stroke 1982;13:648–55.

10. Wylie CM. Measuring end results of rehabilitation of patients with stroke. Public Health Rep 1967;82:893–8.

11. Granger CV, Dewis LS, Peters NC, Sherwood CC, Barrett JE. Stroke rehabilitation: analysis of repeated Barthel Index measures. Arch Phys Med Rehabil 1979;60:14–7.

12. Wade DT, Hewer RL. Functional abilities after stroke: measurement, natural history and prognosis. J Neurol Neurosurg Psychiatry 1987;50:177–82.

13. Gosman H, Svensson E. Parallel reliability of the Functional Independence Measure and the Barthel ADL Index. Disabil Rehabil 2000;22:702–15.

14. Duncan PW, Lai SM, Keighley J. Defining post-stroke recovery: implications for design and interpretation of drug trials. Neuropharmacology 2000;39:835–41.

15. Granger CV, Sherwood CC, Greer DS. Functional status measures in a comprehensive stroke care program. Arch Phys Med Rehabil 1977;58:555–61.

16. van der Putten JJ, Hobart JC, Freeman JA, Thompson AJ. Measuring change in disability after inpatient rehabilitation: comparison of the responsiveness of the Barthel Index and the Functional Independence Measure. J Neurol Neurosurg Psychiatry 1999;66:480–4.

17. Salbach NM, Mayo NE, Higgins J, Ahmed S, Finch LE, Richards CL. Responsiveness and predictability of gait speed and other disability measures in acute stroke. Arch Phys Med Rehabil 2001;82:1204–12.

This measure or ordering information can be found at the Website address included in this review.

BATH ANKYLOSING SPONDYLITIS FUNCTIONAL INDEX (BASFI)

Developers

A. Calin, S. Garrett, H. Whitelock, L. G. Kennedy, J. O'Hea, P. Mallorie, and T. Jenkinson

Purpose

To assess functional ability in patients with ankylosing spondylitis (AS).[1] This index is intended to be used either in a clinical setting (eg, monitoring functional status) or in research studies (eg, clinical trials).[1–3]

Description

The BASFI is a 10-item, self-completed instrument used to measure the functional ability of clients with AS.[1] Eight questions relate to functional ability and two additional questions assess the client's ability to cope with everyday life. Each question is scored on a 10-cm visual analogue scale (VAS), with anchors of easy (score = 0) to impossible (score = 10). The mean of the 10 scales gives the BASFI score (range: 0 to 10).

Conceptual/Theoretical Basis of Construct Being Measured

None reported

Groups Tested with This Measure

Clients with AS,[1–4] clients receiving physiotherapy treatment,[4,5] and clients in clinical trials comparing nonsteroidal anti-inflammatory drugs (NSAIDs) to placebo.[2,6,7]

Languages

English,[1] Swedish,[5] German,[6] Finnish[4]

Application/Administration

This is a self-completed measure, whereby clients place a vertical mark on the 10-cm VAS for each item. The questionnaire takes an average of less than 2 minutes to complete.[1] The score for each item is determined by measuring the distance (in cm) from the lower anchor (ie, easy). The total index score is the arithmetic mean of the 10 item scores. No advice for missing values is provided.

Typical Reliability Estimates

Internal Consistency
0.81^6 to $0.94^{1,4}$

Interrater
Not applicable

Test–Retest:
- $r = 0.89^1$
- ICC = 0.89^6 to 0.99^4

Typical Validity Estimates

Content
Items were selected from a preliminary list of 20 potential questions, through consultations with rheumatologists, physiotherapists, research associates, and clients with AS.[1]

Criterion
No gold standard exists for the attribute being assessed.

Construct—Cross-sectional

Convergent
- Correlation with other functional status measures: 0.85^4
- Correlation with physiotherapist rating of functional status: 0.78^5 to 0.87^1
- Correlation with disease activity measures: 0.68^5 to 0.74^4

Known Groups. Not available

Discriminant
- Correlation with global well-being measure: 0.54^8 to 0.67^5
- Correlation with impairment measures: 0.47^4 to 0.55^5

Construct—Longitudinal/Sensitivity to Change

Convergent. Not available

Known Groups. Significant difference in standardized response mean (SRM) ($p < 0.0001$) between NSAID-treated and placebo clients[2]

Discriminant. Not available

Other. Significant improvement ($p = 0.004$) during 3-week intensive physiotherapy course[1]

Interpretability

General Population Values (Customary or Normative Values)

Reference centile charts available by gender and disease duration.[9]

Typical Responsiveness Estimates

Individual Patient. Not available

Between Group

- Expected improvement group's responsiveness statistics in NSAID versus placebo trial: SRM = 0.46, effect size (ES) = 0.36, Guyatt's Change Index (GCI) = 0.70, Norman's S coefficient = 0.59[7]
- Expected deterioration group's responsiveness statistics in NSAID versus placebo trial: SRM = 0.72, ES = 0.70[7]

References

1. Calin A, Garrett S, Whitelock H, Kennedy LG, O'Hea J, Mallorie P, et al. A new approach to defining functional ability in ankylosing spondylitis: the development of the Bath Ankylosing Spondylitis Functional Index. J Rheumatol 1994;21:2281–5.

2. Calin A, Nakache JP, Gueguen A, Zeidler H, Mielants H, Dougados M. Outcome variables in ankylosing spondylitis: evaluation of their relevance and discriminant capacity. J Rheumatol 1999;26:975–9.

3. Ruof J, Stucki G. Comparison of the Dougados Functional Index and the Bath Ankylosing Spondylitis Functional Index. A literature review. J Rheumatol 1999;26:955–60.

4. Heikkila S, Viitanen JV, Kautianen H, Kauppi M. Evaluation of the Finnish versions of the functional indices BASFI and DFI in spondylarthropathy. Clin Rheumatol 2000;19:464–9.

5. Cronstedt H, Waldner A, Stenstrom CH. The Swedish version of the Bath Ankylosing Spondylitis Functional Index. Reliability and validity. Scand J Rheumatol Suppl 1999;111:1–9.

6. Ruof J, Sangha O, Stucki G. [Evaluation of a German version of the Bath Ankylosing Spondylitis Functional Index (BASFI) and Dougados Functional Index (D-FI)]. Rheumatol 1999;58:218–25.

7. Ruof J, Sangha O, Stucki G. Comparative responsiveness of 3 functional indices in ankylosing spondylitis. J Rheumatology 1999;26:1959–63.

8. Jones SD, Steiner A, Garrett SL, Calin A. The Bath Ankylosing Spondylitis Patient Global Score (BAS-G). Br J Rheumatol 1996; 35:66–71.

9. Taylor AL, Balakrishnan C, Calin A. Reference centile charts for measures of disease activity, functional impairment, and metrology in ankylosing spondylitis. Arthritis Rheum 1998;41:1119–25.

This measure can be found in reference 1.

Berg Balance Scale (BBS)

Developers

K. Berg, S. Wood-Dauphinee, J. I. Williams, and D. Gayton[1]

For information, contact Katherine.Berg@mcgill.ca. For copies of the scale and full instructions, go to www.chcr.brown.edu/BALANCE.HTM.

Purpose

To monitor functional balance over time and to evaluate clients' response to treatment. It has also been used for screening and as a prognostic indicator.

Description

The BBS is a 14-item performance-based instrument intended for individuals with some degree of balance impairment. Each item is scored on a 5-point scale, 0 to 4. Higher scores are awarded for independent performance that meets specific time or distance requirements. The maximum score is 56.

Conceptual/Theoretical Basis of Construct Being Measured

The BBS addresses two dimensions of balance: the ability of subjects to maintain upright posture and to make appropriate adjustments for voluntary movement. Degree of difficulty is manipulated by narrowing the base of support, asking subjects to lean toward the edges of the base of support, and altering sensory input. Timing of movements is considered a marker for the efficiency of postural adjustments for voluntary movements.

Groups Tested with This Measure

Older adults and clients undergoing rehabilitation with varying diagnoses.

Languages

English, French Canadian, Danish, Icelandic, Swedish, Norwegian, Finnish, Italian, German, Portuguese, Portuguese-Brazilian, Korean, Japanese, Dutch, and Spanish. No formal list of publications for cultural adaptations is available.

Application/Administration

Subjects are graded as to their performance on 14 tasks. Instructions should be clearly stated and/or demonstrated because the subject's first effort is scored. Required equipment is a stopwatch, ruler, chair, and step stool 7 to 8" in height or the lower step of a staircase. Time to complete averages 10 to 20 minutes, depending on the ability of the subject.

Typical Reliability Estimates

Internal Consistency

Cronbach's alpha was 0.83 for 113 older adults and 0.97 for 70 patients with stroke.[1,2] Cronbach's alpha was 0.96 based on scores of 14 clients with varying diagnoses.[1]

Interrater

ICC for older adults was 0.91 and 0.99 for clients with stroke.[2]

Test–Retest

ICCs were 0.92 for older adults and 0.98 for clients with stroke.[2] Assessments were made by two raters independently at two different points in time.

Typical Validity Estimates

Content

Content was developed in three phases, each including a different panel of clients and professionals. A total of 38 clients and 32 professionals participated.[1]

Criterion

Concurrent. See Construct-Cross-Sectional

Predictive. Higher BBS scores were associated with lower odds of falling within 1 year.[4] The relationship between a 1-point lower score and the odds of falling has been described as a 3 to 4% increase in odds if BBS scores are between 54 and 56 and a 6 to 8% increase if scores are between 46 and 54.[5] Subjects with BBS scores of 36 and below are at extremely high risk of falling.[5] BBS scores and a history of falls have been suggested as having utility and good sensitivity and specificity for predicting falls.[5]

Admission BBS scores of clients with stroke were correlated with length of stay in rehabilitation (0.60) and were predictive of discharge location from inpatient rehabilitation post stroke.[6] The mean admission BBS scores by place of eventual discharge were 28.5 (SD 1.7) (home), 21.8 (SD 5.7) (residential), 7.9 (SD 4.8) (nursing home), and 1.4 (SD 6.1) for rehospitalized clients. BBS scores accounted for 22% of variation in Functional Independence Measure efficiency score across all impairment groups.[7]

Construct—Cross-Sectional

Convergent. BBS scores showed an average correlation of 0.55 with laboratory measures assessing spontaneous sway[3] and a multiple R of 0.81 for measures representing postural adjustments for voluntary movements.[8] BBS scores showed a correlation of 0.91 with Tinetti Performance Oriented Mobility Assessment (POMA) (balance subscale).[3] BBS scores of older adults showed a correlation of 0.67 with the Barthel Mobility subscale and 0.76 with Timed Up and Go scores.[3]

Known Groups. BBS scores discriminated among persons using different types of walking aids ($F_{3,109} = 29.61$).[4] Moreover, the BBS showed a larger effect size (1.044) when differentiating among older individuals who use a walker, cane, or no walking aids than did the Tinetti POMA (0.89), Barthel Index (0.53), Timed Up and Go (1.02), or spontaneous platform measures (0.51).[3] Admission and discharge BBS scores differed between patients with stroke who did and did not require an ankle-foot orthosis. On admission to inpatient rehabilitation, BBS scores were 17.0 (SD 15.2) for orthosis users versus 31.8 (SD 16.1) for nonusers ($p < 0.005$), whereas at discharge, the BBS scores were 32.1 (SD 12.7) for orthosis users versus 41.7 (SD 14.6) for nonusers, $p < 0.013$.[10]

Discriminant. Not available

Construct—Longitudinal/Sensitivity to Change

Convergent. BBS scores showed correlations of > 0.80 with the Barthel Index and between 0.62 and 0.94 with the Fugl-Meyer index at 2, 6, and 12 weeks post stroke.[4] Both the Barthel Index and the BBS showed linear improvements over time and a similar magnitude of change.[11] The standardized response means (SRM) for a 12-week period were 1.20 (CI 0.95 to 1.44) for the Barthel Index, 1.08 (CI 0.89 to 1.26) for the BBS, and 0.87 (CI 0.69 to 1.02) for the Fugl-Meyer.

A similar SRM for the BBS, 1.0 (CI 0.77 to 1.29), was reported during a 4-week period following commencement of walking post stroke.[12] When comparing five measures (5-m walk, 10-m walk, Barthel Index, STREAM, Timed Up and Go), the 5-m walk was most responsive to change 1.22 (CI 0.93 to 1.50). However, the BBS was most responsive for the group with slow walking speeds on entry to the study.

Additional evidence for sensitivity to change in response to treatment is suggested based on a systematic increase in scores reported for patients with stroke when comparing scores before and after a treatment session.[13]

Known Groups and *Discriminant* are not available.

Other Validity Coefficients

A BBS score below 48 or a gait speed of less than 0.57 m/sec demonstrated a sensitivity of 91% and a specificity of 70% for identifying older adults living in residential care who needed referral to physical therapy evaluation.[9]

Interpretability

General Population Values (Customary or Normative Values)

Based on assessments of 247 older community-dwelling residents of an inner city, the most common value on the BBS (mode) was 53 (range = 29 to 56).

Typical Responsiveness Estimates

Individual Patient. Minimal detectable change score has been reported at ±6 points to be 90% confident of genuine change in patients with stroke.[13] Differences in the minimal detectable change are acknowledged, depending on the level of ability of the subject. However, anecdotal reports from clinicians to the author have suggested that as little as 2 points represents clinically meaningful change for individuals with scores above 50, 3 points in the high forties and progressively more points, possibly 6 or 7, below 40.

Between Group. Not available

Other. The BBS has a ceiling effect for very active individuals living in the community.

References

1. Berg K, Wood-Dauphinee S, Williams JI, Gayton D. Measuring balance in the elderly: preliminary development of an instrument. Physiother Can 1989;41:304–311.

2. Berg K, Wood-Dauphinee S, Williams JI. The Balance Scale. Reliability assessment for elderly residents and patients with an acute stroke. Scand J Rehabil Med 1995;27:27–36.

3. Berg K, Maki B, Williams JI, Holliday P, Wood-Dauphinee S. A comparison of clinical and laboratory measures of postural balance in an elderly population. Arch Phys Med Rehabil 1992; 73:1073–83.

4. Berg K, Wood-Dauphinee S, Williams JI, Maki B. Measuring balance in the elderly: validation of an instrument. Can J Public Health 1992;2:S7–11.

5. Shumway-Cook A, Baldwin M, Polissar NL, Gruber W. Predicting the probability for falls in community-dwelling older adults. Phys Ther 1997;77:812–9.

6. Wee JY, Bagg SD, Palepu A. The Berg Balance Scale as a predictor of length of stay and discharge destination in an acute stroke rehabilitation setting. Arch Phys Med Rehabil 1999;80:448–52.

7. Juneja G, Czyrny JJ, Linn RT. Admisson balance and outcomes of patients admitted for acute inpatient rehabilitation. Am J Phys Med Rehabil 1998;77:388–93.

8. Stevenson TJ, Garland J. Standing balance during internally produced perturbations in subjects with hemiplegia: validation of the Balance Scale. Arch Phys Med Rehabil 1996;77:656–62.

9. Harada N, Chiu V, Damron-Rodriques J, Fowler E, Siu A, Reuben DB. Screening for balance and mobility impairment in elderly individuals living in residential care facilities. Phys Ther 1995;75:462–9.

10. Teasall RW, McRae MP, Foley N, Bhardwaj A. Physical and functional correlations of ankle-foot orthosis use in the rehabilitation of stroke patients. Arch Phys Med Rehabil 2001;82:1047–9.

11. Wood-Dauphinee S, Berg K, Brave G, Williams JI. The Balance Scale: responding to clinically meaningful changes in patients with stroke. Can J Rehabil 1997;10:35–50.

12. Salbach NM, Mayo NE, Higgins J, Ahmed S, Finch LE, Richards CI. Responsiveness and predictability of gait speed and other disability measures in acute stroke. Arch Phys Med Rehabil 2001;82:1204–211.

13. Stevenson TJ. Detecting change in patients with stroke using the Berg Balance Scale. Aust J Physiother 2001;47:29–38.

14. Baer HR, Wolf SL. Modified Emory Functional Ambulation Profile. An outcome measure for the rehabilitation of poststroke gait dysfunction. Stroke 2001;32:973–9.

15. Newton R. Balance screening of an inner city older adult population. Arch Phys Med Rehabil 1997;78:587–91.

This measure or ordering information can be found at the Website address included in this review.

BORG'S RATING SCALE OF PERCEIVED EXERTION (RPE)

Developers

Gunnar Borg, Department of Psychology, Stockholm University, Stockholm, Sweden; Fax: +46-8-159342; e-mail: gbg@psychology.su.se

Purpose

Borg's 15-grade rating scale of perceived exertion provides an index of the person's perception of physical effort or strain during work or leisure-time activities, diagnostic situations, and exercise prescriptions. The modified Borg's 12-grade scale is recommended for use to measure symptoms such as dyspnea, aches, and pain.

Description

The 15-grade RPE or Borg's scale is an ordinal category scale that can be used to measure the client's perceived exertion. Grades 6 to 20 are associated with heart rate (HR) ranging from 60 to 200 beats/min in some people, although the relationship between HR and RPE can vary depending on age, fitness, health status, environment, and type of exercise. This scale does not have interval properties. Subsequently, Borg developed a newer 12-grade scale, also known as the modified Borg scale, that has ratio properties (ie, each grade is equivalent in the amount of perceived exertion). For example, a measure of 10 is described as being five times the intensity of 2.[1]

Conceptual/Theoretical Basis of Construct Being Measured

The Borg's scale was initially developed to estimate the sensation of effort. Later, it was used as an indicator of exercise production. In other words, individuals who had received RPE values during an exercise test were later asked to produce an equivalent exercise intensity based on the RPE.[2-6]

Groups Tested With This Measure

Borg's scales have been used in many diverse populations but have been validated for the following:

- measures of RPE in both genders[6]; healthy children[7] and younger and older adults[2,6]; parasympathetic and sympathetic blocking agents[2]; hot environments[2]; lean and obese individuals[2]; and trained and untrained individuals, including elite athletes[2]
- measures of RPE or dyspnea in respiratory conditions including cystic fibrosis[8]; cardiovascular disease including coronary artery disease, arterial hypertension, vasoregulatory asthenia syndrome, and angina pectoris[6]; in children[6]; and in psychiatric clients[6]
- measures of back muscle fatigue in healthy individuals[9]

Languages

The 15-grade RPE scale has been translated into many different languages, including French, German, Japanese, Hebrew, and Russian.[10]

Application/Administration

Method and instructions for administration of the 15-grade and 12-grade Borg's scales during an exercise test recommended by the American College of Sports Medicine[11] are as follows: "During the exercise test we want you to pay close attention to how hard you feel the exercise work rate is. This feeling should reflect your total amount of exertion and fatigue, combining all sensations and feelings of physical stress, effort, and fatigue. Don't concern yourself with any one factor such as leg pain, shortness of breath or exercise intensity, but try to concentrate on your total, inner feeling of exertion. Try not to underestimate or overestimate your feeling of exertion; be as accurate as you can." Asking clients to rate their perceived exertion using Borg's scale may take a couple of minutes during the first trial. Thereafter, administering the test may take several seconds. The Borg scale is usually presented to the client on a small poster board (~30 × 60 cm). No other special equipment is required. The test administrator should have an appreciation of the development of the test and the importance of standardized instructions.

6	
7	Very, very light
8	
9	Very light
10	
11	Fairly light
12	
13	Somewhat hard
14	
15	Hard
16	
17	Very hard
18	
19	Very, very hard
20	

FIGURE 1 The 15-grade scale for ratings of perceived exertion, the RPE scale.

0	Nothing at all	
0.5	Very, very weak	(just noticeable)
1	Very weak	
2	Weak	(light)
3	Moderate	
4	Somewhat strong	
5	Strong	(heavy)
6		
7	Very strong	
8		
9		
10	Very, very strong	(almost max)
•	Maximal	

FIGURE 2 The newer rating scale, also known as the modified Borg's scale, is constructed as a category scale with ratio properties.

Typical Reliability Estimates

Internal Consistency
Not applicable

Interrater
Not applicable

Test–Retest
- ICC = 0.97 to measure dyspnea in 28 patients on mechanical ventilation[16]
- ICC = 0.84 to measure back fatigue in healthy subjects on three occasions[9]

Typical Validity Estimates

Content
Not reported

Criterion

Concurrent
- Spearman's rho of 0.84 and 0.76 between Borg's 12-grade scale and dyspnea visual analogue scale at two test times 30 minutes apart[16]

Predictive. Not available

Construct —Cross-sectional

Convergent
- Heart rate over a wide range of workloads from moderate to heavy intensity in healthy adults[2,17] and children[7]; $r = 0.80$ to 0.90
- Heart rate has low correlations (0.20 to 0.50) at constant intensities and low workloads[6]
- When HR is manipulated by a β-adrenergic receptor blocking agent to lower it or by envi-

ronmental heat to increase it, RPE remains related to workload intensity and not HR. This lends credence to the postulate that HR is not a major central sensory cue for RPE.[6]

- Oxygen consumption (VO_2); $r = 0.76$ to 0.97[2,6]
- Ventilatory function and respiratory rate; $r = 0.46$ to 0.94[2,6]
- Distance on modified shuttle test by adults with cystic fibrosis; $r = 0.99$[8]

Known Groups. Not available

Discriminant
- Poor correlation with angina[12]

Construct—Longitudinal/Sensitivity to Change
Not available

Interpretability

General Population Values (Customary or Normative Values)
Not available

Typical Responsiveness Estimates
Not available

Comments

The Borg scale was initially developed to estimate the sensation of effort but was later used as an indicator of exercise production. The data to support criterion validity would depend on the construct being measured.

References

1. Borg GAV. Psychophysical bases of perceived exertion. Med Sci Sports Exerc 1982;4:377–81.

2. Mihevic PM. Sensory cues for perceived exertion: a review. Med Sci Sports Exerc 1981;13:150–63.

3. Pandolf KB, Noble BJ. The effect of pedaling speed and resistance changes on perceived exertion of equivalent power outputs on the bicycle ergometer. Med Sci Sports Exerc 1973;5:132–6.

4. Pandolf KB. Advances in the study and application of perceived exertion. Exerc Sport Sci Rev 1983;11:118–58.

5. Robertson RJ. Central signals of perceived exertion during dynamic exercise. Med Sci Sports Exerc 1982;14:390–6.

6. Sullivan SB. Perceived exertion. A review. Phys Ther 1984; 64:343–6.

7. Eakin BL, Finta KM, Serwer GA, Beekman RH. Perceived exertion and exercise intensity in children with or without structural heart defects. J Pediatr 1992;120:90–3.

8. Bradley J, Howard J, Wallace E, Elborn S. Reliability, repeatability, and sensitivity of the modified shuttle test in adult cystic fibrosis. Chest 2000;117:1666–71.

9. Elfving B, Németh G, Arvidsson I, Lamontagne M. Reliability of EMG spectral parameters in repeated measurements of back muscle fatigue. J Electromyogr Kinesiol 1999;9:235–43.

10. Borg GAV, Noble BJ. Perceived exertion. In: Wilmore JH, editor. Exercise sport sciences review. New York: Academic Press; 1974. p. 131–53.

11. American College of Sports Medicine. Guidelines for exercise testing and prescription. 5th ed. Philadelphia: Lea & Febiger; 1995. p. 77.

12. Noble BJ. Clinical applications of perceived exertion. Med Sci Sports Exerc 1982;14:406–11.

13. Whaley MH, Brubaker PH, Kaminsky LA, Miller CR. Validity of rating perceived exertion during graded exercise testing in apparently healthy adults and cardiac patients. J Cardiopulm Rehabil 1997;17:261–7.

14. Mahon AD, March ML. Reliability of the rating of perceived exertion at ventilatory threshold in children. Int J Sports Med 1992;13:567–71.

15. Eston RG, Williams JG. Reliability of ratings of perceived effort regulation of exercise intensity. Br J Sports Med 1988; 22:153–5.

16. Powers J, Bennett SJ. Measurement of dyspnea in patients treated with mechanical ventilation. Am J Crit Care 1999;8: 254–61.

17. Borg GAV. Perceived exertion as an indicator of somatic stress. Scand J Rehabil Med 1970;2–3:92–8.

18. Dunbar CC, Roberson RJ, Baun R, Blandin MF, Metz K, Burdett R, et al. The validity of regulating exercise intensity by ratings of perceived exertion. Med Sci Sports Exerc 1992;24:94–9.

This measure can be found on the accompanying CD-ROM and in references 1 and 11.

BOX AND BLOCK TEST (BBT)

Developers

Initially developed by Jean A. Ayres and Patricia Holser Buehler and modified by the latter and Elisabeth Fucks.[1] Mathiowetz, Volland, Kasman, and Weber standardized its measurement procedure.[2]

Purpose

To measure unilateral gross manual dexterity.

Description

The BBT is a short performance-based test that consists of moving, one by one, the maximum number of blocks from one compartment of a box to another of equal size, within 60 seconds.

Conceptual/Theoretical Basis of Construct Being Measured

None reported

Groups Tested with This Measure

People of different ages with various upper extremity disabilities.

Languages

English and French[3]

Application/Administration

Time to administer is 5 minutes. A 15-second trial period precedes the testing.[2] The evaluator must be sure that the fingertips cross the partition before releasing the block. The score is the number of blocks moved during the allowed 60-second period.

Typical Reliability Estimates

Internal Consistency
Not applicable

Interrater
Spearman's rho = 1 for both hands[2] with occupational therapy students without upper extremity impairments.

Test–Retest
Spearman's rho = 0.98 for the right hand and 0.94 for the left.[1] Spearman's rho = 0.98 for the right hand and 0.94 for the left[2] with occupational therapy

students. ICCs of 0.97 (right hand) and 0.96 (left hand) for people with impairments and 0.90 and 0.89 for those without (with people $\geq$ 60 years).[3]

Typical Validity Estimates

Content
Not reported in the literature

Criterion
No gold standard exists for the construct being measured.

Construct—Cross-sectional

Convergent. The BBT was found to be highly correlated ($r = 0.91$)[2] to the Minnesota Rate Manipulative Test.[4] The BBT is also correlated with the Action Research Arm test[5] (r: 0.80 and 0.82, depending on the hand) as studied with 35 older people with upper extremity disabilities.[3] The BBT is moderately correlated with a measure of functional independence (the SMAF[6]) ($r = 0.42$ to 0.54).[3]

Known Groups. In a community-based sample of 360 elderly persons,[3] the number of blocks transferred decreased linearly across groups defined by age, 60 to 64 years, 65 to 69, 70 to 74 years, 75 to 79, 80 to 84, and 85 years and older, but there was no difference between men and women. Differences were also observed for the right and left hands, although these differences were quite small.[3]

Discriminant. Not available

Construct—Longitudinal/Sensitivity to Change
Not available

Interpretability

General Population Values
(Customary or Normative Values)
Mathiowetz et al[2] developed norms for adults using 628 volunteer subjects aged 20 to 94 who were recruited in shopping centers, universities, fairs, and day centers. Normative data were also developed with a random sample of 360 healthy community-living individuals aged 60 and over.[3] The mean number of blocks transferred in 1 minute, for the right hand in persons aged 60 to 64 years, was 74.0, and in persons 85 years of age and older, the

mean was 57.9; the corresponding values for the left hand were 74.8 and 57.1, for the youngest and the oldest group, respectively.

Typical Responsiveness Estimates
Not available

Comments

There are no data to support this measure's ability to detect change in individuals or groups; therefore, it needs to be used with caution as an outcome measure until sensitivity to change and responsiveness are tested.

References

1. Cromwell FS. Occupational therapists manual for basic skills assessment: primary prevocational evaluation. Pasadena, (CA): Fair Oaks Printing; 1965: p. 29–31.

2. Mathiowetz V, Volland G, Kashman N, Weber K. Adult norms for the Box and Block Test of manual dexterity. Am J Occup Ther 1985;39:386–91.

3. Desrosiers J, Bravo G, Hébert R, Dutil É, Mercier L. Validation of the Box and Block Test as a measure of dexterity of elderly people: reliability, validity and norms studies. Arch Phys Med Rehabil 1994;75:751–5.

4. American Guidance Service. The Minnesota Rate Manipulative Tests. Examiner's manual. Circle Pines, (MN): Author; 1969.

5. Lyle RC. A performance test for assessment of upper limb function in physical rehabilitation treatment and research. Int J Rehabil Res 1981;4:483–92.

6. Hébert R, Carrier R, Bilodeau A. The functional autonomy measurement system (SMAF): description and validation of an instrument for the measurement of handicaps. Age Ageing 1988; 17:293–302.

This measure can be found in reference 2.

CANADIAN OCCUPATIONAL PERFORMANCE MEASURE (COPM)

Developers

Mary Law, Sue Baptiste, Mary Ann McColl, Ann Carswell, Helene Polatajko, and Nancy Pollock.[1] For more information, www.caot.ca/COPM

Purpose

To detect change in a client's self-perception of performance and satisfaction in self-care, productivity, and leisure occupations over time.

Description

The COPM is an outcome measure with a semi-structured interview format and structured scoring method. It is a standardized instrument as it has specific instructions and methods for administration and scoring. Change scores between assessment and reassessment using the COPM are collected in identified problem areas. The COPM is also used to establish performance goals based on the client's perceptions of need in the areas of self-care, productivity, and leisure.

Conceptual/Theoretical Basis of Construct Being Measured

The COPM is a measure of occupational performance developed for use by occupational therapists. The Canadian Model of Occupational Performance defines occupational performance as the product of the interactions between the person, his/her environment, and the occupation being performed.[1]

Groups Tested with This Measure

Adults in rehabilitation,[2] young children with disabilities (COPM was completed with the parents),[3] individuals on intrathecal baclofen therapy,[4] individuals attending a pain management program,[5] and individuals with depressive disorder.[6]

Languages

French, Hebrew, Icelandic, Japanese, German, Danish, Swedish, Greek, Spanish, Mandarin Chinese, Korean, Norwegian, Russian, Slavic, and Portuguese

Application/Administration

The individual respondent identifies activities or tasks within each area of self-care, productivity, and/or leisure that are perceived to be difficult to perform. The individual also rates each task in terms of importance on a scale of 1 to 10 (not important at all to extremely important). The five activities that are ranked the highest by the individual are then rated on two additional scales of 1 to 10. One scale is for the individual's perception of his/her performance of the activity (not able to do it to able to do it extremely well). The other scale is to rank the individual's satisfaction with his/her performance (not satisfied at all to extremely satisfied). On reassessment at appropriate intervals, the individual reports the rating of his/her performance and satisfaction for the five targeted activities.

The assessment takes 20 to 40 minutes to administer, is not diagnosis specific, and can be used across all developmental ages and with caregivers as well as individuals. No formal training is required to administer the COPM. Administration and scoring instructions are available in the COPM manual.[1]

Typical Reliability Estimates

Internal Consistency[7]
- Performance: 0.41 to 0.56
- Satisfaction: 0.71

There is a high degree of correlation between the COPM performance and satisfaction scores (0.68, $p < .01$).

Interrater
Not applicable

Test–Retest
- ICC: performance, 0.63; satisfaction, 0.84
- In a sample of young children with disabilities whose COPM was completed by their parents: performance, 0.79; satisfaction, 0.75
- In an adult rehabilitation setting: performance, 0.80; satisfaction, 0.89

Typical Validity Estimates

Content

"Good" rating on the overall relevance of COPM's test content to the evaluation of occupational performance.[8]

Criterion

Concurrent. The COPM problems were similar in a majority of cases to the criterion of the spontaneous reporting of problems by individuals. Fifty-three percent of respondents named at least one identical problem spontaneously. Respondents named more problems when offered the structured approach of the COPM.[9] "Adequate to good" at reflecting clients' problems in occupational performance.[8]

Predictive. Sixty-five percent accurate predictions of discharge status when combining the COPM and Functional Independence Measure (FIM) (compared with 29% accurate predictions of discharge status when using the FIM alone).[10]

Construct—Cross-sectional

Convergent. There is a high degree of correlation between the COPM performance and satisfaction scores (0.68, $p < .01$). The COPM satisfaction score correlates with (1) the Satisfaction with Performance Scaled Questionnaire (0.39, $p < .01$), (2) the Reintegration to Normal Living Index (0.38, $p < .01$), and (3) the Life Satisfaction Scale (0.46, $p < .01$).[9]

Known Groups. Not available

Discriminant. Predischarge COPM performance subscale and the FIM cognitive subscale ($r = 0.20$).[8]

Construct—Longitudinal/Sensitivity to Change

Convergent. COPM change scores reflected changes in global function (ranked on a 7-point Likert scale) as perceived by clients (0.62, 0.53), families (0.55, 0.56), and therapists (0.30, 0.33).

Correlations in changes in hand function were 0.32 with changes in COPM performance and 0.28 with changes in COPM satisfaction.[11] Correlations in changes in movement were 0.29 with COPM performance and 0.21 with COPM satisfaction.[11] The correlation of predischarge COPM performance subscale scores and FIM motor subscale scores was 0.32, $p < 0.05$.[8]

Known Groups and *Discriminant* are not available.

Interpretability

General Population Values (Customary or Normative Values)

Not applicable

Typical Responsiveness Estimates

Supported through investigations,[2,12–14] initial and final scores for performance and satisfaction for the COPM show significant changes over time ($p < 0.0001$ to 0.001).

Individual Patient and *Between Group* are not available.

References

1. **Law M, Baptiste S, Carswell-Opzoomer A, McColl M, Polatajko H, Pollock N. Canadian Occupational Performance Measure. 3rd ed. Ottawa (ON): CAOT Publications; 1998.**
2. Law M, Polatajko H, Pollock N, McColl MA, Carswell A, Baptiste S. The Canadian Occupational Performance Measure: results of pilot testing. Can J Occup Ther 1994;61:191–7.
3. Pollock N, Stewart D. Occupational performance needs of school-aged children with physical disabilities in the community. Phys Occup Ther Pediatr 1998;18:55–68.
4. Steeden B. Occupational therapy guidelines for client-centred practice and Canadian Occupational Performance Measure [review]. Br J Occup Ther 1994;57:23.
5. Carpenter L, Baker GA, Tyldesley B. The use of the Canadian Occupational Performance Measure as an outcome of a pain management program. Can J Occup Ther 2001;68:16–22.
6. Waters D. Recovering from a depressive episode using the Canadian Occupational Performance Measure. Can J Occup Ther 1995;62:278–82.
7. Bosch J. The reliability and validity of the Canadian Occupational Performance Measure [thesis]. Hamilton, (ON): McMaster Univ; 1995.
8. Chan CCH, Lee TMC. Validity of the Canadian Occupational Performance Measure. Occup Ther Int 1997;4:229–47.
9. McColl M, Paterson M, Davies D, Doubt L, Law M. Validity and community utility of the Canadian Occupational Performance Measure. Can J Occup Ther 1999;67:22–30.
10. Simmons DC, Blesedell Crepeau E, Prudhomme White B. The predictive power of narrative data in occupational therapy evaluation. Am J Occup Ther 2000;54:471–6.
11. Law M, Russell D, Pollock N, Rosenbaum P, Walter S, King G. A comparison of intensive neurodevelopmental therapy plus casting and a regular occupational therapy program for children with cerebral palsy. Dev Med Child Neurol 1997;39:664–70.
12. Mirkopolous C, Butler K. Quality assurance: Clients' perceptions of goal performance and satisfaction. 11th World Congress of Occupational Therapy, London; 1994.
13. Sanford J, Law M, Swanson L, Guyatt G. Assessing clinically important change an outcome of rehabilitation in older adults. Conference of the American Society of Aging, San Francisco (CA), 1994.
14. Wilcox A. A study of verbal guidance for children with development coordination disorder [thesis]. London (ON): Univ. of Western Ontario; 1994.

This measure or ordering information can be found at the Website address included in this review.

CHEDOKE-MCMASTER STROKE ASSESSMENT

Developers

Carolyn (Kelley) Gowland, McMaster University; Hamilton, Ontario; Sandra VanHullenaar, Hamilton Health Sciences Corporation; Hamilton, Ontario; Wendy Torresin, Hamilton Health Sciences Corporation and McMaster University; Julie Moreland, St. Joseph's Hospital, Hamilton, Ontario, and McMaster University; Bernadette Vanspall; Susan Barecca, Hamilton Health Sciences Corporation and McMaster University; Maureen Ward; Maria Huijbregts, Baycrest Hospital and University of Toronto, Toronto, Ontario; Paul Stratford, McMaster University; Ruth Barclay-Goddard, University of Manitoba, Winnipeg, Manitoba.

Purpose

The Chedoke-McMaster Stroke Assessment (Chedoke Assessment) is a two-part measure designed for use with clients with stroke.[1,2] It consists of a Physical Impairment and an Activity Inventory. The purpose of the Impairment Inventory is to determine the presence and severity of common physical impairments. This provides guidance for the selection of appropriate interventions and the evaluation of their effectiveness and is used in outcome prediction within 6 months of onset of stroke. The principal purpose of the Activity Inventory is to measure functional outcome (clinically important change in physical function). It is designed for use in program evaluation and the determination of the effectiveness of therapeutic interventions.

Description

The Chedoke Assessment is a performance-based measure. The Impairment Inventory has six dimensions, each measured on a 7-point scale (1 = low, 7 = high). The dimensions include shoulder pain, postural control, the arm, the hand, the leg, and the foot. The 7-point scale corresponds to seven stages of motor recovery (with the exception of shoulder pain, which has a unique scale based on severity). The Activity Inventory is made up of two indices: gross motor function and walking. The gross motor function index consists of 10 items and the walking index consists of 5 items. The inventory has a max-

imum total score of 100, with 100 representing normal function.

Conceptual/Theoretical Basis of Construct Being Measured

Four conceptual domains provide the theoretical basis for the measure: physical performance following stroke, measurement theory, the World Health Organization classification of disease consequences, and client-centered practice. The theoretical basis related to these conceptual domains is described in detail in Chapter 3 of the development manual[2] and in an independent publication.[3]

Groups Tested with This Measure

Subjects were from the inpatient stroke unit of Chedoke-McMaster Rehabilitation Centre, a regional tertiary care institution,[1,2,4–6] stroke survivors, and caregivers in the community; survivors were discharged from the inpatient or day hospital stroke population 6 to 24 months prior to this study.[7] Two additional studies examined the suitability of the Chedoke Assessment for use on a population of individuals with acute neurologic disorders and acquired brain injury.[8,9]

Language

English

Application/Administration

Detailed administration guidelines are contained in the development manual.[2] Approximately 45 to 60 minutes is required to complete the assessment, depending on the client's level of endurance and concentration. Equipment needed includes a footstool, pillows, stopwatch, 2-m line marked on the floor, floor mat, chair with armrests, pitcher with water, measuring cup, ball 2.5 inches in diameter, and an adjustable table. Clinical use of the measure over time provides adequate training for most clinicians; however, in a recently completed study, it was determined that reliability in administration was improved significantly by attendance at a training workshop.[10]

Typical Reliability Estimates

Internal Consistency
Not applicable.

Interrater

To evaluate the interrater reliability of the Impairment Inventory, clients were assessed concurrently by both a treating and a research physical therapist during the first week of admission. To estimate intrarater reliability, the initial assessment was videotaped, and the treating therapist scored the videotape after a minimum interval of 2 weeks (see Table 1).

Test–Retest

To examine the test–retest reliability of the Impairment Inventory, both the treating and research therapists assessed clients separately on admission and again within 5 days. Because the Activity Inventory is designed to assess change in a client's function, it was important to assess the amount of variability that a client would demonstrate in a "stable" state. Test–retest reliability was therefore estimated in addition to interrater reliability (see Table 1).[1,2]

Typical Validity Estimates

Content

A survey was carried out to test the assumption that the content in the Activity Inventory is representative of skills that are important to clients (clients with stroke and caregivers; n = 34).[7] On a scale where 1 = not at all important and 7 = extremely important, all items received a 7 from at least one person in each group.

Criterion

Concurrent. Not available

Predictive. A study of 182 clients consecutively admitted to a rehabilitation center was carried out.[2,6] Regression analysis was performed on outcomes of interest and prognostic variables to identify those variables that were the most statistically significant in predicting outcomes. The prognostic variables analyzed were selected following a systematic literature review. The resulting equations for predicting clinical outcomes following rehabilitation are contained in Chapter 8 of the development manual.[2] Two previous studies also reported on similar work on a previous version of the measure.[5,6]

Construct—Cross-sectional

Convergent. Table 2 shows the relationships established between the Chedoke Assessment and two other measures. The Fugl-Meyer is a measure of impairment and the Functional Independence Measure is a measure of activity.[1,2]

Known Groups and *Discriminant* are not available.

Construct—Longitudinal/Sensitivity to Change

There is a correlation ($r = 0.749$) between important change as perceived by clients and the change score of the measure. Also, there is a relationship between the severity of the disability and the value clients place on change in function and a correla-

TABLE 1 Reliability of the Chedoke Assessment

Inventory	Intrarater		Interrater		Test–Retest	
	ICC	95% CI	ICC	95% CI	ICC	95% CI
Impairment						
Shoulder pain	0.96	0.92–0.98	0.95	0.91–0.98	0.75	0.55–0.87
Postural control	0.96	0.93–0.98	0.92	0.84–0.96	0.80	0.63–0.90
Arm	0.95	0.89–0.97	0.88	0.76–0.94	0.84	0.72–0.92
Hand	0.93	0.85–0.96	0.93	0.84–0.96	0.85	0.72–0.92
Leg	0.98	0.96–0.99	0.85	0.73–0.93	0.92	0.85–0.96
Foot	0.94	0.87–0.97	0.96	0.91–0.98	0.85	0.71–0.92
Total score	0.98	0.95–0.99	0.97	0.94–0.98	0.94	0.89–0.97
Activity						
Gross motor function	—	—	0.98	0.97–0.99	0.96	0.93–0.98
Walking	—	—	0.98	0.95–0.99	0.98	0.96–0.99
Total score	—	—	0.99	0.98–1.00	0.98	0.95–0.99

TABLE 2 Construct and Concurrent Validities of the Chedoke Assessment by Comparing It to the Fugl-Meyer Measure and Functional Independence Measure (n = 32)[1,2]

Chedoke Assessment	Fugl-Meyer Measure					Functional Independence Measure		
	Balance	Shoulder, Elbow, Forearm, Wrist, and Hand	Hip, Knee, Foot, and Ankle	Upper Limb Joint Pain	Total Score	Mobility Subscore	Locomotion Subscore	Total Score
Impairment Inventory								
Postural control	0.84*	0.53	0.65	0.46	0.69	0.74	0.66	0.73
Arm and hand	0.46	0.95†	0.76	0.49	0.89	0.40	0.46	0.36
Leg and foot	0.68	0.79	0.93†	0.56	0.87	0.58	0.53	0.58
Shoulder pain	0.38	0.49	0.59	0.76*	0.66	0.40	0.36	0.36
Total score	0.67	0.88	0.90	0.65	0.95†	0.59	0.57	0.57
Activity Inventory								
Gross Motor Function	0.88	0.49	0.67	0.40	0.65	0.90†	0.85	0.81
Walking	0.68	0.40	0.41	0.31	0.49	0.83	0.85*	0.64
Total score	0.85	0.46	0.61	0.38	0.62	0.91	0.89	0.79†

$p > 0.60$ (one-tailed) of numbers on diagonal based on Fisher's Z transformation; *$p < 0.05$; †$p < 0.01$; ‡$p < 0.001$.

tion ($r = 0.62$) between total score on the Activity Inventory and living arrangements.[7]

Interpretability

General Population Values (Customary or Normative Values)
Not available

Typical Responsiveness Estimates
Mean change scores for the gross motor function index, walking index, and Activity Inventory were determined. For the Activity Inventory, a score of 0 equated with no change, 8 with small change, and 20 with large change. Details for subgroups and the importance of the change to individuals and their caregivers are contained in a recent publication.[2,7]

References

1. Gowland C, Stratford P, Ward M, Moreland J, Torresin W, VanHullenaar S, et al. Measuring physical impairment and disability with the Chedoke-McMaster Stroke Assessment. Stroke 1993;24:58–63.

2. Gowland C, VanHullenaar S, Torresin W, et al. Chedoke-McMaster Stroke Assessment: development, validation, and administration manual. Hamilton (ON): School of Rehabilitation Science, McMaster University; 1995.

3. Moreland J, Gowland C, VanHullenaar S, Huijbregts M. Theoretical basis of the Chedoke-McMaster Stroke Assessment. Physiother Can 1993;45:231–8.

4. Gowland C. Predicting physical outcomes in stroke: implications for clinical decision making. In: Proceedings of the 6th Annual Stroke Rehabilitation Conference. Cambridge; 1994.

5. Gowland C. Recovery of motor function following stroke: profile and predictors. Physiother Can 1982;34:77–84.

6. Gowland C. Predicting sensorimotor recovery following stroke rehabilitation. Physiother Can 1984;36:313–20.

7. Huijbregts MP, Gowland C, Gruber R. Measuring clinically important change with the Activity Inventory of the Chedoke McMaster Stroke Assessment. Physiother Can 2000;52:295–304.

8. Barclay-Goddard R. Physical function outcome measures suitable for use in acute neurology. Synapse 1996;16:2–5.

9. Crowe J, Harmer D, Sharpe D. Reliability of the Chedoke-McMaster Disability Inventory in acquired brain injury [abstracts]. Physiother Can 1996;48 Suppl:25.

10. Miller P, Stratford P, Gowland C, VanHullenaar S, Torresin W. Comparing two methods to train therapists to use the Chedoke-McMaster Stroke Assessment. In: Proceedings of the 13th International Congress of WCPT. Yokohama (Japan): WCPT; 1999.

This measure can be found on the accompanying CD-ROM. Prior to using the measure, you are strongly advised to contact the developers for administration and scoring guidelines and revisions to the measure not available at time of publication.

CHILD HEALTH QUESTIONNAIRE (CHQ)

Developers

Jeanne M. Landgraf, Linda Abetz, and John E. Ware Jr, Child Health Assessment Project, The Health Institute, New England Medical Center, Boston, Massachusetts, Fax: 617-636-8077

Purpose

To measure the physical and psychosocial well-being of children ages 5 years and older.[1]

Description

The CHQ[1] is designed for completion by children or their caregivers. The three CHQ parent forms, the CHQ-PF28, CHQ-PF50, and CHQ-PF98, are for use with caregivers of children older than 5 years. The numbers added to each parent form correspond to the number of items in each questionnaire. The child form, the CHQ-CF87, has 87 items and is intended for self-completion by children ages 10 years and older. The questionnaires encompass 14 concepts related to global health. Item responses are based on 4- to 6-point scales. Transformed total scores range from 0 to 100, with higher scores reflecting better overall health.

Conceptual/Theoretical Basis of Construct Being Measured

The CHQ was based on the World Health Organization's definition of health as "a state of complete physical, mental and social well-being and not merely the absence of disease or infirmity."[2]

Groups Tested with This Measure

- CHQ-PF50 psychometric testing[1]: US sample of children, children with asthma, attention-deficit hyperactivity disorder, cystic fibrosis, epilepsy, juvenile rheumatoid arthritis, and psychiatric disorders
- CHQ-PF28 psychometric testing[1]: US sample of children
- CHQ-CF87 psychometric testing[1]: African-American middle-school–aged children, children with attention-deficit hyperactivity disorder, cystic fibrosis, and end-stage renal failure

Languages

At the time of writing the manual, translation, feasibility testing, cultural validation, and psychometric testing had been initiated in Australia, Britain, Canada, France, Germany, Ireland, Scotland, Sweden, and The Netherlands.[1] In 2001, the Pediatric Rheumatology International Trials Organisation (PRINTO) published an introductory paper on the cross-cultural and psychometric evaluation of the CHQ in 32 countries.[3]

Application/Administration

The CHQ can be administered in a variety of settings. If done in a clinic setting, questionnaires should be completed prior to interacting with the health care professional. Telephone and in-person interview scripts have also been developed. Suggested equipment is a firm writing surface and a number 2 pencil (if the scannable response form is used). Respondents are asked to answer questions in relation to the past 4 weeks except for a change in health that is related to the past year. The manual also provides specific instructions for item recoding, calculating raw scale scores, and transforming scores. Raw scores equal the algebraic mean of all completed items. The administrator is instructed to ask respondents about incomplete items, but these are not included in the calculations. Specific scoring algorithms are provided in each chapter related to which form is used. Scoring codes are available for SAS programs. The CHQ-PF28 and CHQ-PF50 can be used to calculate Physical (PhS) and Psychosocial (PsS) summary measures. Summary measures can then be standardized using a linear T-score transformation and are normalized to the general pediatric population.

Typical Reliability Estimates

Internal Consistency

- CHQ-PF50: Cronbach's alpha = 0.46 to 0.98
- CHQ-PF28: Cronbach's alpha = 0.35 to 0.95
- CHQ-CF87: Cronbach's alpha = 0.62 to 0.97
- CHQ-PF50 summary measures: PhS = 0.84 to 0.97, PsS = 0.88 to 0.97
- CHQ-PF28 summary scores: PhS = 0.79 to 0.93, PsS = 0.87 to 0.92

Interrater

Not available and not applicable for CHQ-CF87

Test–Retest

- CHQ-PF50: ICC = 0.49 to 0.82[4]

Typical Validity Estimates

Content
Concepts were included based on comparisons with other health status measures, expert review, and consensus approach.[1]

Criterion
No gold standard exists for many of the health domains included in the CHQ.[4]

Construct—Cross-sectional

Convergent
- CHQ-PF28[5]: ASK (Activity Scale for Kids): $r \geq 0.49$
- PODCI (Pediatrics Outcomes Data Collection Index): $r \geq 0.60$
- Clinician global rating: $r = 0.5$ for physical summary score, $r = 0.4$ for pain subscale
- Parent global rating: $r = 0.6$ for physical summary score; $r = 0.4$ for pain subscale
- CHQ-PF50[6]: bodily pain: HUI2 (Health Utilities Index) = 0.58, HUI3 = 0.60
- CHQ Physical with HUI2 mobility and HUI3 ambulation, both = 0.45
- CHQ mental health with HUI2 emotional – 0.64, HUI3 emotional = 0.54
- CHQ general health scale with HUI2 global utility = 0.43, HUI3 global utility = 0.44

Known Groups. US normative sample and clinical samples[1,5]: all scales statistically significant at $p < 0.001$

Discriminant. Not available

Construct—Longitudinal/Sensitivity to Change
Not available

Interpretability

General Population Values
(Customary or Normative Values)
- Normative data for CHQ-PF50 and CHQ-PF28[1] are available.

Typical Responsiveness Estimates
Not available

Other
- CHQ-CF80 (modified from 87)[7]: floor effects = 0.0 to 3.6%, ceiling effects = 1.1 to 81.6%
- CHQ-PF28[5]: potential floor effects = 17%; potential ceiling effects = 37%

Comment

There are no data to support this measure's ability to detect change in individuals or groups; therefore, it needs to be used with caution as an outcome measure until sensitivity to change and responsiveness are tested.

References

1. **Landgraf JM, Abetz L, Ware JEJ. The Child Health Questionnaire (CHQ): a user's manual. 1st ed. Boston: The Health Institute, New England Medical Center; 1996.**
2. World Health Organization. World Health Organization constitution. In: Basic documents. Geneva: WHO; 1948.
3. Pratsidou-Gertsi P, Vougiouka O, Tsitsami E, Ruperto N, Siamopoulou-Mavridou A, Dracou C, et al. Paediatric International Trials Organisation. The Greek version of the Childhood Health Assessment Questionnaire (CHAQ) and the Child Health Questionnaire (CHQ). Clin Exp Rheumatol 2001;19(4 Suppl 23):S76–80.
4. Waters EB, Salmon LA, Wake M. The parent-form Child Health Questionnaire in Australia: comparison of reliability, validity, structure and norms. J Pediatr Psychol 2000;25:381–91.
5. Pencharz J, Young NL, Owen JL, Wright JG. Comparison of three outcomes instruments in children. J Pediatr Orthopaed 2001;21:425-32.
6. Nixon Speechley KN, Maunsell F, Desmeules M, Schanzer D, Landgraf JM, Feeny DH, et al. Mutual concurrent validity of the Child Health Questionnaire and the Health Utilities Index: an exploratory analysis using survivors of childhood cancer. Int J Cancer 1999;125.95–105.
7. Waters EB, Salmon LA, Wake M, Wright M, Hesketh KD. The health and well-being of adolescents: a school-based population study of the self-report Child Health Questionnaire. J Adolesc Health 2001;29:140–9.
8. Landgraf JM, Abetz L. Influences of sociodemographic characteristics on parental reports of children's physical and psychosocial well-being: early experiences with the Child Health Questionnaire. In: Drokar D, editor. Measuring health-related quality of life in children and adolescents. Mahwah (NJ): Lawrence Erlbaum; 1998.
9. Waters EB, Wright E, Wake M, Landgraf J, Salmon L. Measuring the well-being of children and adolescents: a preliminary comparative evaluation of the Child Health Questionnaire. Ambul Child Health 1999;5:131–41.
10. Waters EB, Salmon LA, Wake M, Hesketh K, Wright M. The Child Health Questionnaire in Australia: reliability, validity and population means. Aust N Z J Public Health 2000;24:207–10.
11. Landgraf JM, Maunsell E, Speechley KN, Bullinger M, Campbell S, Abetz L, et al. Canadian-French, German and UK versions of the Child Health Questionnaire: methodology and preliminary item scaling results. Qual Life Res 1998;7:433–45.
12. Wake M, Hesketh K, Cameron F. The Child Health Questionnaire in children with diabetes: cross-sectional survey of parent and adolescent-reported functional health status. Diabet Med 2000;17:700–7.
13. Asmussen L, Olson LM, Grant EN, Landgraf JM, Fagan J, Weiss KB. Use of the Child Health Questionnaire in a sample of moderate and low-income inner-city children with asthma. Am J Respir Crit Care Med 2000;162(4 Pt 1):1215–21.
14. Landgraf JM, Abetz LN. Functional status and well-being of children representing three cultural groups: initial self-reports using the CHQ-CF87. Psychol Health 1997;12:839–54.

To obtain this measure, contact the developers.

CHRONIC RESPIRATORY DISEASE QUESTIONNAIRE (CRQ)

Developers

Gordon H. Guyatt, McMaster University, Hamilton, Ontario

Purpose

To assess the physical and emotional aspects of quality of life in patients with chronic airflow limitation.

Description

The CRQ is a disease-specific interviewer-administered health-related quality of life instrument. Patients respond on a numeric 7-point modified Likert scale to 20 items or questions asked by the interviewer. The 20 items have been derived from a large set of items identified by clients with chronic airflow limitation as the most important problems in their emotional and physical functioning. There are four domains: dyspnea, fatigue, emotional function, and mastery. The dyspnea domain is individualized, that is, patients identify activities important to their health. A standardized version is being tested.[1]

Conceptual/Theoretical Basis of Construct Being Measured

The CRQ is designed to evaluate change in a client's health-related quality of life over time focusing on the two constructs of physical and emotional functioning.

Groups Tested with This Measure

Clients with chronic airflow limitation (primarily those with chronic obstructive pulmonary disease, but also cystic fibrosis); in addition, this instrument has been used in clients with allergic rhinitis.

Languages

English.[1] The measure has been translated, culturally adapted, and validated in Dutch,[2] Japanese,[3] and Spanish.[4] It has been translated and culturally adapted but not formally validated in Danish,[5] French,[6] German,[7] Italian,[8] and Chinese.

Application/Administration

Clients receive a brief introduction to the questionnaire from the interviewer, who then elicits the five most important activities that limit physical functioning. The severity of shortness of breath with each of these activities is recorded using colored cards shown to the patients. Thereafter, 15 questions are asked and answered by the patient using the colored response cards provided with the original questionnaire. Most clients complete the interviewer-administered version in approximately 15 to 20 minutes. Repeat administration takes approximately 10 to 15 minutes. Currently, a self-administered version is under testing. Total score and subscores in the two physical and two emotional domains are reported; higher scores correspond to better health-related quality of life. The scores for each question of each dimension are added together and divided by the number of questions asked. Thus, using a 7-point scale for the responses, the minimum and maximum scores for each dimension are the same: 1 is the worst (if the patient answered each question by choosing option 1) and 7 is the best (if the patient answered each question by choosing 7). Missing data will occur only in the dyspnea domain.

Typical Reliability Estimates

Internal Consistency

- Dyspnea domain: 0.51 to 0.82, fatigue domain: 0.71 to 0.94, emotional function domain: 0.81 to 0.90, mastery domain: 0.83 to 0.85[2–4,9,10]
- Cronbach's alpha: dyspnea domain: 0.53 to 0.90, fatigue domain: 0.20 to 0.87, emotional function domain: 0.84 to 0.87, mastery domain: 0.68 to 0.88[2,10–12]

Test–Retest

- Spearman Brown reliability coefficient: > 0.7 for all four domains[2]

Typical Validity Estimates

Content

No reference to content validity in the literature

Criterion

No gold standard exists for the construct being measured

Construct—Cross-Sectional

Convergent

- VO_{2max}: $r = 0.48$[3] (dyspnea domain)

- Forced expiratory volume in 1 second (FEV$_1$): $r = 0.34$[3] (dyspnea domain)
- St. George's Respiratory Questionnaire: $r = 0.47$ to 0.70[13] (all domains)

Known Groups and ***Discriminant*** are not available.

Construct—Longitudinal/Sensitivity to Change

Convergent

- Kappa between predicted and observed correlations for changes in different measures (6-minute walk distance and global ratings of change) = 0.51[1]
- FEV$_1$: $r = 0.55$ to 0.66[14,15]
- 6-minute walk: $r = 0.26$ to 0.52[14,16]
- Global rating dyspnea: $r = 0.46$ to 0.61[16] (for all four domains)
- Oxygen cost diagram: $r = 0.30$ (with dyspnea domain)[16]
- Transitional dyspnea index: $r = 0.34$ to 0.59[16]
- 36-Item Short-Form Health Survey (SF-36) physical domains: $r = 0.43$ to 0.66 (with CRQ physical domains)[17]
- SF-36 emotional domains: $r = 0.57$ to 0.71 (with CRQ emotional domains)[17]
- St. George's Respiratory Questionnaire: $r = 0.32$ to 0.53[13]

Known Groups and ***Discriminant*** are not available.

Interpretability

General Population Values
(Customary or Normative Values)
Not available

Typical Responsiveness Estimates
A change in the score of 0.5 on the 7-point scale reflects a clinically significant small change. A change of 1.0 reflects a moderate change, and a difference of 1.5 represents a large change.[18,19]

References

1. Guyatt GH, Berman LB, Townsend M, Pugsley SO, Chambers LW. A measure of quality of life for clinical trials in chronic lung disease. Thorax 1987;42:773–8.

2. Wijkstra PJ, Tenvergert EM, VanAltena R, Otten V, Postma D, Kraan J, et al. Reliability and validity of the Chronic Respiratory Questionnaire (CRQ). Thorax 1994;49:465–7.

3. Hajiro T, Nishimura K, Tsukino M, Ikeda A, Koyama H, Izumi T. Comparison of discriminative properties among disease-specific questionnaires for measuring health-related quality of life in patients with chronic obstructive pulmonary disease. Am J Respir Crit Care Med 1998;157:785–90.

4. Guell R, Casan P, Sangenis M, Morante F, Belda J, Guyatt GH. Quality of life in patients with chronic respiratory disease: the Spanish version of the Chronic Respiratory Questionnaire (CRQ). Eur Respir J 1998;11:55–60.

5. Hansen NC, Evald T, Ibsen TB. Terbutaline inhalations by the Turbuhaler as replacement for domiciliary nebulizer therapy in severe chronic obstructive pulmonary disease. Respir Med 1994; 88:267–71.

6. Bourbeau J, Rouleau MY, Boucher S. Randomised controlled trial of inhaled corticosteroids in patients with chronic obstructive pulmonary disease. Thorax 1998;53:477–82.

7. Kirsten DK, Wegner RE, Jorres RA, Magnussen H. Effects of theophylline withdrawal in severe chronic obstructive pulmonary disease. Chest 1993;104:1101–7.

8. Clini EM, Scalvini S, Simoni P, Foglio K, Rocchi S, Bruletti G. Cycloergometer effort test evaluation and quality of life in chronic obstructive lung disease. Ital J Chest Dis 1993;47:71–6.

9. Larson JL, Covey MK, Berry JK, Wirtz S, Kim MJ. Reliability and validity of the Chronic Respiratory Disease Questionnaire. Am J Crit Care Med 1993;147:A350.

10. Martin LL. Validity and reliability of a quality-of-life instrument. The Chronic Respiratory Disease Questionnaire. Clin Nurs Res 1994;3:146–56.

11. Harper R, Brazier JE, Waterhouse JC, Walters SJ, Jones NMB, Howard P. Comparison of outcome measures for patients with chronic obstructive pulmonary disease in an outpatient setting. Thorax 1997;52:879–87.

12. Lacasse Y, Wong E, Guyatt G. A systematic overview of the measurement properties of the Chronic Respiratory Questionnaire. Can Respir J 1997;4:131–9.

13. Rutten-van Molken M, Roos B, Van Noord J. An empirical comparison of the St. George's Respiratory Questionnaire (SGRQ) and the Chronic Respiratory Disease Questionnaire (CRQ) in a clinical trial setting. Thorax 1999;54:995–1003.

14. Guyatt GH, Townsend M, Keller JL, Singer J, Nogradi S. Measuring functional status in chronic lung disease: conclusions from a randomized controlled trial. Respir Med 1989;83:293–7

15. Guimont C, Bourbeau J. Dyspnea by the Chronic Respiratory Disease Questionnaire in patients with chronic obstructive pulmonary disease. Am J Crit Care Med 1995;151:A466.

16. Guyatt GH, King DR, Feeny DH, Stubbing D, Goldstein RS. Generic and specific measurement of health-related quality of life in a clinical trial of respiratory rehabilitation. J Clin Epidemiol 1999;52:187–92.

17. Schünemann HJ, Guyatt GH, Griffith L, Stubbing D, Goldstein RS. A randomized controlled trial to evaluate the effect of informing patients about their pretreatment responses to two respiratory questionnaires. Submitted.

18. Jaeschke R, Singer J, Guyatt GH. Measurement of health status ascertaining the minimal clinically important difference. Controlled Clin Trials 1989;10:407–15.

19. Redelmeier DA, Guyatt GH, Goldstein RS. Assessing the minimal important difference in symptoms: a comparison of two techniques. J Clin Epidemiol 1996;49:1215–9.

This measure or ordering information can be found at the Website address of the American Thoracic Society: www.atsqol.org

Continuing Care Activity Measure (CCAM)

Developers

Maria P. J. Huijbregts, Baycrest Centre for Geriatric Care, University of Toronto, Toronto, Ontario, Theresa M. Kay, Sunnybrook and Women's College Health Sciences Centre, University of Toronto[1,2]; and Staff of the Physiotherapy Department at Baycrest Centre for Geriatric Care. To obtain the measure and guidelines or videotape, e-mail physiotherapy@baycrest.org. Fax: 416-785-4227

Purpose

To measure gross motor function and mobility and screen upper extremity function in the adult population ($\geq$ 19 years) residing in long-term care (complex continuing care or nursing home). The measure is developed to assist in (1) determining the need for physiotherapy intervention, (2) setting client-centered goals, and (3) evaluating change in client performance.[1-4]

Description

The CCAM is a performance-based measure. It consists of 16 items that relate to gross motor function and mobility: 6 items pertain to bed mobility, 3 to seating, 2 to transfers, 2 to ambulation, and 1 to wheelchair mobility. Two items assess left and right upper extremity functioning, respectively. Scoring is on a 1 to 7 scale. The total score ranges from 16 to 112. A higher score reflects a higher level of function.[1-4] The measure was developed from the Clinical Outcome Variables Scale (COVS). For clients who are independently ambulatory, it is recommended that the 2-minute walk test be used in combination with the CCAM.[2]

Conceptual/Theoretical Basis of Construct Being Measured

Gross motor function and mobility are related to the concept of activity in the World Health Organization model of disease consequences.[2,3] The CCAM assesses activities that are of particular importance to long-term care clients and scores these on a grading scale that distinguishes between relatively small changes in function. In some of the activities, clients do not have to be independent to achieve the maximum score.

Groups Tested with This Measure

Clients residing in complex continuing care[1-4] and in a nursing home[2,4]

Language

English

Application/Administration

Administered in the client's own living space, using the client's own bed, ambulation device, and/or wheelchair. The full guidelines must be used for test administration. The abbreviated guidelines are designed to inform staff reviewing the chart on clients' performance. Total score is obtained by summing the scores for the different items. The measure takes about 20 minutes to administer and < 1 minute to score. No computer is required. Equipment needs include the client's bed, ambulation aids, and wheelchair as applicable, a cup with water, a comb, and a timer or watch. A training videotape is available and recommended.[5]

Typical Reliability Estimates

Internal Consistency
- 0.75 to 0.95[1]

Interrater
- ICC: 0.9[1]

Test–Retest
- ICC: 0.9[1]

Typical Validity Estimates

Content
Professional physiotherapy, occupational therapy, and nursing staff, as well as family members, were involved in the development (item generation and reduction) of the measure.[1]

Criterion
No gold standard exists for the construct being measured.

Construct—Cross-sectional

Convergent

- Correlation with the COVS: $r = 0.9$[1,3,4]
- Correlation with physiotherapists' perception of function: $r = 0.8$[1,3,4]

Known Groups and *Discriminant* are not available.

Construct—Longitudinal/Sensitivity to Change

Convergent

- Correlation between change in CCAM score and the therapist's perception of change: $r = 0.84$[4]
- Correlation between change in CCAM score and the importance of that change to the therapist: $r = 0.81$[4]

Known Groups and *Discriminant* are not available.

Interpretability

General Population Values (Customary or Normative Values)
Not applicable

Typical Responsiveness Estimates

Individual Patient and *Between Group* are not available.

Comments

Results from a multicenter standardization study will be available in spring 2002.

References

1. Huijbregts M, Kay T. The Continuing Care Disability Measure (CCDM): a gross motor function and mobility outcome measure for continuing care clients. In: Congress of the World Confederation of Physical Therapy. Washington (DC); 1995.

2. Huijbregts M, McCullough C, Kay T. The Continuing Care Activity Measure (CCAM): a gross motor function and mobility measure for long term care clients. Pinnacles, CPA Gerontology Division Newletter 2000;54:2–4.

3. Huijbregts M, Gurber R. Functional outcome measurement in the elderly. Phys Ther Clin North Am 1997;6:383–401.

4. Huijbregts M. The CCAM: a gross motor function and mobility outcome measure for the long term care client. Can J Rehabil 1997;40:18–9.

5. McCullough C, Huijbregts MPJ. The Continuing Care Activity Measure (CCAM) training video. Gerontology 2001;47:553–4.

This measure can be found on the accompanying CD-ROM. Prior to using the measure, you are strongly advised to contact the developers for administration and scoring guidelines and revisions to the measure not available at time of publication.

COPD SELF-EFFICACY SCALE (CSES)

Developers

Joan K. Wigal, Thomas L. Creer, and Harry Kotses, Department of Psychology, Ohio University, Athens, Ohio, 45701, USA

Purpose

To assess self-efficacy in adults with chronic obstructive pulmonary disease (COPD). Intended for use in both clinical and research environments.[1]

Description

The CSES is a self-report, condition-specific measure intended for people with chronic bronchitis and/or emphysema. It contains 34 items that describe situations or activities that tend to provoke shortness of breath in people with COPD. Items can be divided into five subscales including negative affect, intense emotional arousal, physical exertion, weather/environment, and behavioral risk factors. Respondents are asked to rate how confident they are, on a 5-point Likert scale, that they could manage breathing difficulty or avoid breathing difficulty in each of the 34 situations.[1] Items are scored as follows: 1 = not at all confident, 2 = not very confident, 3 = somewhat confident, 4 = pretty confident, and 5 = very confident. Total and subscale scores are obtained by first adding responses and then dividing by the number of items answered to obtain a mean score. Mean scores can range from 1 to 5, with higher scores indicating higher self-efficacy.[2]

Conceptual/Theoretical Basis of Construct Being Measured

The CSES is based on Self-Efficacy Theory,[3] which suggests that the degree of confidence an individual has in his/her ability to bring about a certain outcome determines how much effort an individual will put into coping with a difficult situation. Specifically, "self-efficacy refers to the personal convictions people have regarding whether or not they feel they can successfully execute particular behaviours in order to produce certain outcomes."[1]

Groups Tested with This Measure

This measure has been used, but not formally validated, in adults aged 35 to 85 years with chronic bronchitis and/or emphysema.[1,2,4]

Language

English[1]

Application/Administration

A self-administered questionnaire in which respondents circle the relevant response. Most clients can complete the questionnaire in less than 10 minutes. This measure can be scored in less than 5 minutes with the use of a calculator.

Typical Reliability Estimates

Internal Consistency
- Cronbach's alpha (total score) = 0.95[1]

Interrater
Not applicable

Test–Retest
Measures taken approximately 2 weeks apart: $r = 0.77$[1]

Typical Validity Estimates

Content
No reference to content validity in the literature.

Criterion
No gold standard exists for the attribute being assessed (self-efficacy).

Construct—Cross-sectional

Convergent
- Human Activity Profile Dyspnea Scale: $r = -0.56$[2]
- 12-Minute Walk Test: $r = 0.43$[2]

Known Groups and *Divergent* are not available.

Construct—Longitudinal/Sensitivity to Change
Not available

Interpretability

General Population Values (Customary or Normative Values)
Not available

Typical Responsiveness Estimates
Not available

Comments

There are no data to support this measure's ability to detect change in individuals or groups; therefore, some caution is needed when using this as an outcome measure until sensitivity to change and responsiveness are tested. Some items on the questionnaire are of a sensitive nature (eg, "When I feel sexually inadequate or impotent").

References

1. Wigal JK, Creer TL, Kostes H. The COPD Self-Efficacy Scale. Chest 1991;99:1193–6.
2. Scherer YK, Schmieder LE. The effect of a pulmonary rehabilitation program on self-efficacy, perception of dyspnea and physical endurance. Heart Lung 1997;26:15–22.
3. Bandura A. Self-efficacy: toward a unifying theory of behavioural change. Psychol Rev 1977;84:191–215.
4. Scherer YK, Schmieder LE, Shimmel S. The effects of education alone and in combination with pulmonary rehabilitation on self-efficacy in patients with COPD. Rehabil Nurs 1998;23:71–7.

To obtain this measure, contact the developers, or it can be found in reference 1.

COVS (PHYSIOTHERAPY CLINICAL OUTCOME VARIABLES SCALE)

Developers

Louise Seaby and George Torrance, The Rehabilitation Centre, Ottawa, Ontario. Copyright is held by and detailed rating guidelines, a training videotape, and database software are available through The Institute for Rehabilitation Research and Development, 505 Smyth Road, Ottawa, ON K1H 8M2. Contact information: www.rehab.on.ca/irrd/covs/index.html

Purpose

To measure mobility in an active rehabilitation population of individuals with spinal cord injury, stroke, other neurologic conditions, amputation, multiple trauma, and postsurgical hip or knee replacement.[1,2] This clinical tool also assists therapists with treatment goal setting.

Description

The COVS is a performance-based measure comprised of 13 items (tasks). The seven-level ordinal scale is based on the Patient Evaluation Conference System (PECS)[3] 0 to 7 scale, with some scale categories modified to facilitate rating precision. The composite score ranges from 13 to 91. A higher score denotes greater mobility and function. The COVS includes four items adopted from the PECS,[3] four from the CPA Health Status Form,[4] and five items identified by physiotherapy staff. Using COVS items, treatment goals (predicted outcomes) are formulated and quantified on admission. Predicted and discharge scores can be compared. Grouping clients into diagnostic categories facilitates outcome prediction.

Conceptual/Theoretical Basis of Construct Being Measured

The COVS is related to Nagi's model of the process of disablement and is intended to measure dysfunction in the mobility functional domain. Mobility is defined as "movement from one postural position to another or from one location to another within walking or wheeling distance."[2] Item inclusion criteria were that items contribute to the mobility construct, are believed to be a primary physiotherapy treatment focus in an active rehabilitation setting and are an important factor in determining overall functional ability.

Groups Tested with This Measure

Those individuals with spinal cord injury,[1,2] stroke,[1,2,5,6] amputation,[1,2] multiple trauma,[1,2] postsurgical total hip or knee replacements,[1,2] other neurologic conditions,[1,2] traumatic brain injury (TBI),[5] acute adult neurologic conditions,[7] and a general geriatric population.[8]

Languages

English and French. The French version has not been formally validated.

Application/Administration

Each item represents a functional task (eg, Gets to a sitting position from supine lying in bed. Patient is asked to "sit up"). There is no demonstration by the tester, and the first trial is rated. Administration time is 15 to 45 minutes. Scoring time is < 5 minutes, obtained by summing the ratings for the individual items. Equipment needed includes a stopwatch, plastic hospital mug, penny and slotted can, or pincushion and straight pins. To simulate an outdoor environment requires an exercise mat, a ramp (1 to 12-inch rise), and a 6-inch platform. Training consists of a review of the 34-page written guidelines including the data collection form (available in English and French), observation of a physiotherapist experienced in the application of COVS ratings, and viewing the COVS videotape. The authorized data collection software prompts during data entry if data are missing; cases with missing data are not saved.

Typical Reliability Estimates

Internal Consistency
Not available

Interrater
- Cronbach's alpha = 0.93[1,2]
- Weighted kappas = 0.66 to 0.97 ($p < 0.001$)[1,2]
- Spearman's rho = 0.74 to 0.94[1,2]
- Composite scale ICC = 0.97[1,2,7]

Test–Retest
- Weighted kappas: 0.87 to 0.98[1,2]
- Spearman's rho: all > 0.90[1,2]

Other
Rasch analysis. It was found that the COVS items form adequate Rasch Scales for admission and discharge assessments as indicated by item fit and item separation.[9]

Typical Validity Estimates

Content
A panel of experienced physiotherapists determined the item content and scaling. As a result of reliability testing, one item was removed to form the final COVS.[1,2]

Criterion
No gold standard available.

Construct—Cross-sectional

Convergent
- Kenny Self Care evaluation and CPA Health Status Rating Form. Spearman's rho = 0.52 to 0.95[2]
- Functional Independence Measure: Spearman's rho = 0.82
- Bartel Index: Spearman's rho = 0.71[6]
- Chedoke Disability Index (Chedoke DI): $r = 0.97$[7]

Known Groups
- Admission scores for stroke and TBI were significantly different from discharge scores ($p < 0.001$).[5]
- Admission and discharge scores for the 21 diagnostic groups were significantly different from each other and the size of the difference was in the expected direction (eg, paraplegic mobility ratings > quadriplegic ratings).[10]

Discriminant. Not available

Construct—Longitudinal/Sensitivity to Change

Convergent
- COVS and Chedoke DI change scores: $r = 0.89$[7]

Known Groups
- Change scores for 21 diagnostic groupings were significantly different: $F = 7.3$ ($p < 0.001$).[10]
- In a nursing home with a general geriatric population, a comparison of COVS scores between 2 groups of patients, assigned according to PT/OT staffing levels, using stratified random allocation by severity of condition, demonstrated a trend in favour of the higher staffing level at the 6, 12, 18 and 24 month intervals.[8]

Discriminant. Not available

Interpretability

General Population Values (Customary or Normative Values)
Not applicable

Typical Responsiveness Estimates

Individual Patient. Minimal clinically important difference for neurology patient is COVS 5.[7]

Between Group. Not available

References

1. Seaby L, Torrance G. Reliability of a physiotherapy functional assessment used in a rehabilitation setting. Physiother Can 1989;41:264–71.
2. Seaby L. Mobility: a functional domain for clinical assessment and program evaluation in physiotherapy [thesis]. 1987.
3. Harvey RF, Jellinek HM. Functional performance assessment: a program approach. Arch Phys Med Rehabil 1981;62:456–61.
4. Tapping C. Instruments to measure health status of patients receiving physiotherapy. Towards assessment in quality of care, vol 2. Ottawa (ON): Institutional and Professional Services Division, Health Services Directorate, Health Services Promotion Branch, Health and Welfare Canada; 1981.
5. Eng JJ, Rowe SJ, McLaren L. Mobility status during inpatient rehabilitation: a comparison of patients with stroke and traumatic brain injury. Arch Phys Med Rehabil. In press.
6. Hajek VE, Gagnon S, Ruderman JE. Cognitive and functional assessments of stroke patients: an analysis of their relation. Arch Phys Med Rehabil 1997;78:1331–7.
7. Barkley-Goddard R. Physical function outcome measurement in acute neurology. Physiother Can 2000;52:138–45.
8. Przybylski BR, Dumont D, Watkins ME, Warren SA, Beaulne PA, Lier DA. Outcomes of enhanced physical and occupational therapy service in a nursing home. Arch Phys Med Rehabil 1996;77:554–61.
9. Torrance GM, Seaby LS. Rasch analysis of the physiotherapy clinical outcome variables scale (COVS) [abstract]. Physiother Can 1994;46 Suppl PO-004-T:4.
10. Seaby LS, Torrance GM. Measurement properties of the physiotherapy clinical outcomes variables scale (COVS): a mobility functional assessment [abstract]. Physiother Can 1994;46 Suppl PL-220-M:76.

This measure or ordering information can be found at the Website address included in this review, or contact the developers.

CYSTIC FIBROSIS QUESTIONNAIRE (CFQ)

Developers

Alexandra L. Quittner, Anne Buu, Marc Watrous, and Melissa Davis.[1] Contact information: Alexandra L. Quittner, PhD, Department of Clinical and Health Psychology, University of Florida, 1600 SW Archer Road, DG-136, Gainsville, Florida 32610-0165, USA, e-mail: aquittne@ hp.ufl.edu

Purpose

The CFQ comprises disease-specific, developmentally appropriate, health-related quality of life (HRQL) questionnaires designed to measure the multidimensional impact (physical, emotional, and social) of cystic fibrosis (CF) on individuals and their families.[1]

Description

The CFQ contains five domains of HRQL[1]: physical symptoms, role functioning, energy/fatigue, psychological and emotional functioning, and social functioning.[1] Four domains specific to CF are also measured: body image, eating disturbances, social marginalization, and treatment burden.[1] The three versions are as follows[1,2]:

1. CFQ Teen/Adult Version (CFQ-14+). The CFQ-14+ is filled out by adolescents/adults who are 14 years of age and older. It is a self-report measure that consists of 48 items. Items are rated on a 4-point scale to measure frequency (always to never), difficulty (a lot of difficulty to no difficulty), and true-false ratings (very true to very false) or weighted statements (on a 4- or 5-point scale).

2. CFQ Parent Version (CFQ-P). The parent or primary caregiver (parent report) completes the 44-item CFQ-P on the basis of the child's HRQL. It is used in conjunction with the child questionnaire. Items are rated in terms of frequency, difficulty, true-false categories, or weighted statements using the same response choices described for the Teen/Adult Version.

3. CFQ Child Version (CFQ-C). The CFQ-C is for children ages 6 to 13 years. It is provided in two different formats: interviewer administered for children ages 6 to 11 or self-administered (self-report) for children who are 12 or 13 years old. Thirty-five items are answered on a 4-point scale

with a frequency response ranging from always to never. Fifteen items require a true-false rating on a 4-point scale (very true to not at all true).

Conceptual/Theoretical Basis of Construct Being Measured

Quittner states that HRQL is a multidimensional construct, including several core dimensions such as physical functioning and symptoms, emotional and psychological state, social relationships, and activities of daily living.[1–3]

Groups Tested with This Measure

Children with CF (6 to 13 years of age) and their parents and adolescents and adults with CF (14 years of age and older).

Languages

French,[4,5] English,[2,6,7] German, and Spanish[2,4,8]

Application/Administration

Each measure takes 15 to 20 minutes to complete.[2] The questionnaire should be administered before the child undergoes a physical examination or completes other clinic procedures so that the respondent is not influenced by the person administering the clinical procedures. Respondents should be able to read at a 5th grade level. In some cases (eg, visual impairment), the questionnaire may be read to the child/parent. Children who are 12 or 13 years old can self-administer the questionnaire (self-report).[1] An interviewer administers the version for children ages 6 to 11.[1] The primary caregiver should be the one who is asked to complete the CFQ-P questionnaire at the first and subsequent visits as he/she should be aware of the child's normal behaviors, schedule, and symptoms.[1] Two practice questions are used with colored rating cards to train the child on the two types of response choices.[2] Items in the CFQ are written either positively or negatively[1]; therefore, some items must be recoded before the scores for the dimensions are calculated. There are scoring programs written for SAS and SPSS (for all three questionnaires). The score is calculated by adding the score obtained for each item of a dimension (scale) after any necessary recoding. Scores for a dimension can be computed only if at least two-thirds of the items have been completed.

If less than two-thirds of the items have been completed, the dimension should be considered missing for that particular individual.

Typical Reliability Estimates

Internal Consistency
- CFQ-14+: Cronbach's alpha = 0.63 to 0.94[7]
- CFQ-P: Cronbach's alpha = 0.63 to 0.90[6]
- CFQ-C: not available

Interrater
Not applicable

Test–Retest
Not available

Typical Validity Estimates

Content
The original French version was developed through extensive review of literature, interviews with experts and CF associations, and qualitative interviews with children with CF, their parents, and adolescents and adults with CF.[2]

Criterion
No gold standard exists for the construct being measured.

Construct—Cross-sectional

Convergent
CFQ-14+
- Age: $r = -0.23$ to -0.35 in teens and adults with CF ages 14 to 53[7]
- Percentage of forced expiratory volume in 1 second: $r = 0.22$ to 0.42[7]
- 36-Item Short-Form Health Survey: $r = 0.43$[7]

CFQ-P
- PedsQL-Parent: $r = 0.32$ to 0.72[6]
- CFQ-C, physical, respiratory, and eating/digestive disorders scales: $r = 0.30$ to 0.53[6]
- CFQ-C, school/social functioning scales: $r = 0.28$[6]

CFQ-C
As reported above

Known Groups. Significant difference on several CFQ scales for three age groups (7 to 13 years, 14 to 17 years, 18 years of age and older) including treatment burden, social functioning, and respiratory functioning.[9]

Discriminant. Not available

Construct—Longitudinal/Sensitivity to Change
Not available

Interpretability

General Population Values (Customary or Normative Values)
Not published, but some can be found in the manual[1]

Typical Responsiveness Estimates
Not available

Comments
There are no data to support this measure's ability to detect change in individuals or groups; therefore, it needs to be used as an outcome measure with caution until this measurement property has been tested.

References

1. Quittner AL, Buu A, Watrous M, Davis MA. CFQ Cystic Fibrosis Questionnaire: a health-related quality of life measure. User manual. English version 1.0. 2000.
2. Quittner AL, Sweeny S, Watrous M, Munzenberger P, Bearss K, Nitza AG, et al. Translation and linguistic validation of a disease-specific quality of life measure for cystic fibrosis. J Pediatr Psychol 2000;25:403–14.
3. Quittner AL. Measurement of quality of life in cystic fibrosis. Curr Opin Pulm Med 1998;4:326–31.
4. Henry B, Aussage P, Grosskopf C, Goehrs J-M. Evaluating quality of life (QOL) in children with cystic fibrosis (CF): should we believe the child or the parent? Pediatr Pulmonol 1998; 26 Suppl.
5. Henry B, Grosskopf C, Aussage P, Goehr J-M, Launois R, and the French CFQoL Study Group. Construction of a disease-specific quality of life questionnaire for cystic fibrosis. Pediatr Pulmonol 1997; 13 Suppl;337–8.
6. Quittner AL, Espelage DL, Davis MA, Watrous M. National validation of a health-related quality of life measure [abstract]. Pediatr Pulmonol 2000; Suppl 20:334.
7. Quittner AL, Espelage DL, Watrous M, Davis MA. National validation of a health-related quality of life measure for adolescents and adults with cystic fibrosis [abstract]. Pediatr Pulmonol 2000; Suppl 20:335.
8. Henry B, Staab D, Prados C, Aussage P, DeFontbrune S, Grosskopf C, et al. How to measure quality of life in cystic fibrosis (CF) patients across countries and cultures: the Cystic Fibrosis Questionnaire (CFQ) [abstract]. Pediatr Pulmonol [CD-ROM edition]. 1998.
9. Modi AC, Davis MA, Quittner AL, Accurso F, Koenig J. The relationship between demographic and health status variables and health-related quality of life in individuals with cystic fibrosis [abstract]. Pediatr Pulmonol 2001; Suppl 22:349.

This measure can be found on the accompanying CD-ROM. Prior to using the measure, you are strongly advised to contact the developers for administration and scoring guidelines and revisions to the measure not available at time of publication. It can also be found in reference 2.

DASH (Disabilities of the Arm, Shoulder and Hand)

Developers

The Institute for Work & Health, Toronto, Ontario, DASH@iwh.on.ca; http://www.iwh.on.ca and the American Academy of Orthopaedic Surgeons, Rosemont, Illinois[1]

Purpose

To quantify symptoms and disability among individuals with upper extremity musculoskeletal disorders[1] and to evaluate changes over time.[1,2]

Description

The DASH is a 30-item self-report condition-specific disability measure. The questionnaire includes 21 physical function items, 6 symptom items, and 3 social/role function items. There are also two optional 4-item modules: one is intended for athletes/performing artists and the other is for working populations. Each item of the DASH is scored on a 5-point scale (1 to 5). Lower scores reflect less disability and higher scores reflect more disability.

Conceptual/Theoretical Basis of Construct Being Measured

The DASH is intended to measure physical function at the level of disability.[1] The disablement process[3,4] was used to define the concept of physical function; therefore, the DASH evaluates a client's ability to perform an activity, regardless of how it is done (eg, using an assistive device).[1] During development, the upper extremity was conceptualized as a single functional unit, and, as such, the DASH is intended to have broad applicability to any or all joints of the upper extremity.[1]

Groups Tested with This Measure

Adults with wrist/hand,[1,5–8] elbow,[1,9] and shoulder disorders[1,5,10–13]; with psoriatic arthritis[14]; and cumulative trauma disorder.[15]

Languages

English and official translations of Swedish[16] and French

Application/Administration

Clients circle the appropriate response to each question based on their condition in the last week. If clients did not perform a specific activity in the past week, they are asked to make their best estimate of which response would be most accurate. Most clients can complete the questionnaire in 10 minutes.[1] To calculate the overall DASH score, responses to the 30-item DASH are summed. The sum is then transformed so that it falls between 0 and 100 by subtracting 30 and dividing by 1.2 (ie, DASH score = [raw score − 30]/1.2). If less than three items are left blank, the mean score of the other items may be substituted for the missing scores. If four or more items are left blank, a DASH score cannot be calculated. The optional modules are scored separately from the 30-item DASH by transforming them to a 0 to 100 scale (ie, optional module score = [raw score − 4]/1.6). Optional module scores cannot be calculated if any of the items are missing.[1]

Typical Reliability Estimates

Internal Consistency
- Cronbach's alpha: 0.96 to 0.97[1,5]

Interrater
Not applicable

Test–Retest
- $ICC_{2,1}$: 0.96 among individuals with upper extremity disorders[5]
- $ICC_{2,1}$: 0.92 among individuals with elbow disorders[9]

Typical Validity Estimates

Content
During development, experts in upper extremity pathology were consulted and the literature was reviewed.[1,17]

Criterion
No gold standard exists for the attribute being assessed.

Construct—Cross-sectional

Convergent:

- Other upper extremity functional outcome measures: $r = 0.77$ to 0.89[5,6,9,10]
- Visual analogue scale ratings of pain: $r = 0.65$ to 0.72[5,9]; of problem severity, $r = 0.69$[5]; of function, $r = 0.79$ to 0.80[5,9]; and of ability to work: $r = 0.77$[5]
- 36-Item Short-Form Health Survey (SF-36) physical function and pain indices: $r = 0.65$ to 0.73[1,6] and $r = 0.56$ to 0.70,[1,6] respectively
- Clinical and impairment measures (eg, strength, ROM, Constant-Murley Shoulder Score): $r = 0.47$ to 0.93[11–15]

Known Groups

- Individuals who are able to cope and perform all of their activities of daily living/those not able to do so ($p < 0.0001$)[5]
- Individuals not able to work owing to their upper extremity disorder/those able to work ($p < 0.0001$)[1,5]
- Individuals working without restrictions/those working with restrictions ($p < 0.0001$)[6]
- Individuals with severe versus mild self-rated conditions ($F_{4,61} = 16.08$, $p < 0.0001$)[6,9]; between individuals with severe versus mild clinician-rated conditions ($F_{3,54} = 7.69$, $p < 0.0002$)[9]; ($F = 19.85$, $p < 0.0001$)[1]

Discriminant

- SF-36 mental health indices: $r = 0.29$ to 0.38[1,6]
- Damaged joint count in those with psoriatic arthritis[14]: $r = 0.09$

Construct—Longitudinal/Sensitivity to Change

Convergent

- Change in index of self-rated change: $r = 0.76$[10]
- Change in rating of pain intensity: $r = 0.65$[5]
- Change in rating of function: $r = 0.69$[5]
- Change in rating of problem severity: $r = 0.66$[5]

Known Groups. Sensitivity and specificity of various change scores in terms of being able to distinguish individuals shifting to being able to cope with their problem over time from those unable or always able to cope are available.[5]

Discriminant. Not available

Other

- Change in groups expected to improve: standardized response mean (SRM) = 0.71 to 2.52[2]
- Change in groups estimated to have improved by an external marker: SRM = 0.91 to 1.44[2,18]
- Change in groups estimated to have an important improvement by an external marker: SRM = 1.06 to 1.27[2,18]

Interpretability

General Population Values (Customary or Normative Values)

Not available

Typical Responsiveness Estimates

Individual Patient. A change in DASH score of 15 points has been found to be the most accurate change score in terms of distinguishing individuals who become able to cope with their problem over time from those who do not.[5] MDC$_{95}$: 12.7 among individuals with various disorders of the upper extremity[2,5] and 17.2 among individuals with elbow disorders.[2,9] MDC$_{90}$: 10.7 among individuals with various disorders of the upper extremity[5] and 14.5 among individuals with elbow disorders.[9]

Between Group. Not available

Other. The DASH is able to describe a range of disability experiences without running out of descriptive space at the top or bottom of the scale (ie, no ceiling or floor effects).[2]

References

1. McConnell S, Beaton DE, Bombardier C. The DASH outcome measure user's manual. Toronto: Institute for Work & Health; 1999.

2. Beaton DE, Davis AM, Hudak P, McConnell S. The DASH (Disabilities of the Arm, Shoulder and Hand) outcome measure: what do we know about it now? Br J Hand Ther 2001;6:109–18.

3. Jette AM. Physical disablement concepts for physical therapy research and practice. Phys Ther 1994;74:380–6.

4. Verbrugge LM, Jette AM. The disablement process. Soc Sci Med 1994;38:114.

5. Beaton DE, Katz JN, Fossell AH, Wright JG, Tarasuk V, Bombardier C. Measuring the whole or the parts? Validity, reliability and responsiveness of the Disabilities of the Arm, Shoulder and Hand outcome measure in different regions of the upper extremity. J Hand Ther 2001;14:128–46.

6. Jain R, Hudak PL, Bowen CV. Validity of health status measures in patients with ulnar wrist disorders. J Hand Ther 2001; 14:147–53.

7. Hannah SD, Hudak PL. Splinting and radial nerve palsy: a single-subject experiment. J Hand Ther 2001;14:195–201.

8. MacDermid JC, Richards RS, Donner A, Bellamy N, Roth JH. Responsiveness of the Short-Form 36, disability of the arm, shoulder and hand questionnaire, patient-rated wrist evaluation and physical impairment measurements in evaluating recovery after a distal radius fracture. J Hand Surg [Am] 2000;25:330–40.

9. Turchin DC, Beaton DE, Richards RR. Validity of observer-based aggregate scoring systems as descriptors of elbow pain, function, and disability. J Bone Joint Surg Am 1998;80:154–62.

10. Kirkley A, Griffin S, McLintock H, Ng L. The development and evaluation of a disease-specific quality of life measurement tool for shoulder instability. The Western Ontario Shoulder Instability Index. Am J Sports Med 1998;26:764–72.

11. Ring D, Perey BH, Jupiter JB. The functional outcome of operative treatment of ununited fractures of the humeral diaphysis in older patients. J Bone Joint Surg Am 1999;81:177–90.

12. McKee MD, Wilson TL, Winston L, Schemitsch EH, Richards RR. Functional outcome following surgical treatment of intra-articular distal humeral fractures through a posterior approach. J Bone Joint Surg Am 2000;82:1701–7.

13. Skutek M, Fremerey RW, Zeichen J, Bosch U. Outcome analysis following open rotator cuff repair. Early effectiveness validated using four different shoulder assessment scales. Arch Orthopaed Trauma Surg 2000;120:432–6.

14. Navsarikar A, Gladmann DD, Husted JA, Cook RJ. Validity assessment of the Disabilities of Arm, Shoulder and Hand questionnaire (DASH) for patients with psoriatic arthritis. J Rheumatol 1999;26:2191–4.

15. Brouwer B, Mazzoni C, Pearce GW. Tracking ability in subjects symptomatic of cumulative trauma disorder: does it relate to disability? Ergonomics 2001;44:443–56.

16. Atroshi I, Gummesson C, Anderson B, Dahlgren E, Johansson A. The Disabilities of the Arm, Shoulder and Hand (DASH) outcome questionnaire. Reliability and validity of the Swedish version evaluated in 176 patients. Acta Orthop Scand 2000; 71:613–8.

17. Davis AM, Beaton DE, Hudak P, Amadio P, Bombardier C, Cole D, et al. Measuring disability of the upper extremity: a rationale supporting the use of a regional outcome measure. J Hand Ther 1999;12:269–74.

18. Beaton DE. Are you better? Describing and explaining changes in health status in persons with upper limb musculoskeletal disorders [thesis]. Toronto: Univ. of Toronto; 2000.

This measure or ordering information can be found at the Website address included in this review.

BASELINE/TRANSITIONAL DYSPNEA INDEX

Developers

D. A. Mahler, D. H. Weinberg, C. K. Wells, and A. R. Feinstein,[1] Section of Pulmonary and Critical Care Medicine, Dartmouth Hitchcock Medical Centre, Lebanon, NH 03756-0001. Contact information to request permission for use: Donald.A.Mahler@Hitchcock.org.

Purpose

The Baseline Dyspnea Index (BDI) is used to rate the severity of dyspnea at a single point in time. Its follow-up scale is the Transitional Dyspnea Index (TDI), which is used to denote changes from the baseline condition.[1]

Description

Both the BDI and TDI are interviewer-administered scales consisting of ratings or grades in each of three categories: functional impairment, magnitude of task needed to evoke dyspnea, and magnitude of effort needed to evoke dyspnea. At the initial evaluation, the BDI is used to rate the client's condition from 0 (severe) to 4 (unimpaired) for each category. The ratings are added to form a baseline focal score (range from 0 to 12), with a lower focal score representing a greater severity of dyspnea. Changes in dyspnea are rated using the TDI, which compares the current condition to the baseline state. There are seven grades for each category ranging from –3 (major deterioration) to 0 (unchanged) to +3 (major improvement). The ratings on each of the three categories are added to form a transitional focal score (range –9 to +9).[1]

Conceptual/Theoretical Basis of Construct Being Measured

Dyspnea is defined as "an uncomfortable awareness of breathing or an increased respiratory effort that is unpleasant and regarded as inappropriate by the patient."[1]

Groups Tested with This Measure

The BDI/TDI has been validated in chronic obstructive pulmonary disease (COPD),[1,2] asthma,[1] interstitial fibrosis,[1] and cystic fibrosis.[3] In addition, the measure has been used in people with congestive heart failure.[4]

Languages

English.[1] The measure has been translated but not formally evaluated in Japanese.[2]

Application/Administration

The client is asked open-ended questions about his/her breathlessness focusing on the criteria indicated on the scale during a subjective examination. The interviewer scores the client on each of the three categories based on the client's responses. The interview takes 5 to 10 minutes to complete. The focal score is obtained by simply adding the ratings from each of the three categories.[1]

Typical Reliability Estimates

Internal Consistency
Not available

Interrater
BDI focal score: κ_w = 0.70 to 0.72, functional impairment: κ_w = 0.53 to 0.73, magnitude of task: κ_w = 0.68 to 0.72, magnitude of effort: κ_w = 0.66 to 0.73.[1–5]

TDI focal score: κ_w = 0.63, functional impairment: κ_w = 0.66; magnitude of task: κ_w = 0.57, magnitude of effort: κ_w = 0.65.[1]

Test–Retest
Not available

Typical Validity Estimates

Content
No reference to content validity in the literature.

Criterion
No gold standard exists for the criterion being assessed.

Construct—Cross-sectional

Convergent. BDI focal score
- Forced expiratory volume in 1 second (FEV$_1$): r = 0.31 to 0.56 in COPD[1,2,6,7]
- Forced vital capacity (FVC): r = 0.41 to 0.76 in COPD[1,6,7]
- FEV$_1$: r = 0.77 and FVC: r = 0.78 in asthma[5]
- Maximal inspiratory pressure (PImax): r = 0.34 to 0.41 in COPD[5,6] and r = 0.89 in heart failure[4]
- Maximal expiratory pressure (PEmax): r = 0.35 to 0.36 in COPD[5,6] and r = 0.67 in heart failure[4]

- Medical Research Council Dyspnea Scale: $r = -0.70$ to -0.83[5,8]
- Oxygen Cost Diagram (OCD): $r = 0.54$[5,8]
- 12-minute walk distance: $r = 0.60$[1]
- VO_{2max}: $r = 0.46$ to 0.50[2,3]
- 36-Item Short-Form Health Survey (SF-36): $r = 0.91$ in COPD[7]

Known Groups. BDI focal score discriminates between patients with COPD limited by breathlessness (BDI = 5.4 ± 2.3) versus leg fatigue (BDI = 8.3 ± 2.9) on the cycle ergometer exercise test.[3]

Discriminant
- SF-36, role functioning: $r = 0.24$ in COPD[7]
- SF-36, social functioning: $r = 0.42$ in COPD[7]
- SF-36, health perceptions $r = 0.28$ in COPD[7]

Construct—Longitudinal/Sensitivity to Change

Convergent. TDI focal score: changes in FEV_1, $r = -0.04$, and in FVC, $r = -0.01$[1]; change in 12-minute walk distance: $r = 0.33$[1]

Known Groups and **Discriminant** are not available.

Interpretability

General Population Values (Customary or Normative Values)
Not available

Typical Responsiveness Estimates
Not available

Comments

The transitional version of the measure that indicates change in dyspnea is not a true outcome measure as it does not provide an absolute rating of dyspnea.

References

1. **Mahler DA, Weinberg DH, Wells CK, Feinstein AR. The measurement of dyspnea: contents, interobserver agreement, and physiologic correlates of two new clinical indexes. Chest 1984;85:751–8.**
2. Hajiro T, Nishimura K, Tsukino M, Ikeda A, Koyama H, Izumi T. Analysis of clinical methods used to evaluate dyspnea in patients with chronic obstructive pulmonary disease. Am J Respir Crit Care Med 1998;158:1185–9.
3. Mahler DA, Harver A. Prediction of peak oxygen consumption in obstructive airway disease. Med Sci Sports Exerc 1988; 20:574–8.
4. McParland C, Krishnan B, Wang Y, Gallagher CG. Respiratory muscle weakness and dyspnea in chronic heart failure. Am Rev Respir Dis 1992;146:467–72.
5. Mahler DA, Wells CK. Evaluation of clinical methods for rating dyspnea. Chest 1988;93:580–6.
6. Mahler DA, Harver A. A factor analysis of dyspnea ratings, respiratory muscle strength, and lung function in patients with chronic obstructive pulmonary disease. Am Rev Respir Dis 1992;145:467–70.
7. Mahler DA, Mackowiak JI. Evaluation of the short-form 36-item questionnaire to measure health-related quality of life in patients with COPD. Chest 1995;107:1585–9.
8. Mahler DA, Rosiello RA, Harver A, Lentine T, McGovern DF, Daubenspeck JA. Comparison of clinical dyspnea ratings and psychophysical measurements of respiratory sensation in obstructive airway disease. Am Rev Respir Dis 1987;135:1229–33.

To obtain this measure, contact the developers.

MODIFIED MEDICAL RESEARCH COUNCIL (MRC) DYSPNEA SCALE

Developers

Developed by the Medical Research Council (MRC) of Great Britain (1960)[1,2] and adopted by the American Thoracic Society[3]

Purpose

The modified MRC Dyspnea Scale is part of a larger measure, the MRC Respiratory Questionnaire, developed to standardize the assessment of patients with occupational respiratory diseases for epidemiologic studies.[1,4] The Dyspnea Scale assesses the level of physical activity necessary to precipitate breathlessness.

Description

The modified MRC Dyspnea Scale is a self-administered scale consisting of five descriptive statements regarding levels of physical activity that precipitate shortness of breath. The client is asked to read the descriptive statements and select the grade (0 to 4) that best describes his/her shortness of breath, with 0 representing the least severe shortness of breath and 4 the most severe shortness of breath.[3]

Conceptual/Theoretical Basis of Construct Being Measured

No conceptual basis for dyspnea was included by the original authors.

Groups Tested with This Measure

The measure has been validated in the following groups: individuals with occupational respiratory ailments,[1,3] chronic obstructive pulmonary disease (COPD),[1,5,6] interstitial lung disease,[6] and asthma.[6] The measure has also been used in patients following lung transplant[7] and lung volume reduction surgery.[8]

Language

English

Application/Administration

The scale is self-administered and takes less than 5 minutes to complete. The client reads each of the statements and chooses the one that best applies to his/her condition. Each statement is associated with a grade and degree of breathlessness from 0 (none) to 4 (very severe).

Typical Reliability Estimates

Internal Consistency
Not applicable

Interrater
- $\kappa_w = 0.92$[6]

Test–Retest
Not available

Typical Validity Estimates

Criterion
No gold standard exists for the construct being measured.

Construct—Cross-sectional

Convergent. In COPD
- Baseline Dyspnea Index: $r = -0.70$ to -0.83[6,9]
- Oxygen Cost Diagram: $r = -0.53$ to -0.71[6,9]
- Forced expiratory volume in 1 second: $r = -0.39$ to -0.54 [6,8] and forced vital capacity: $r = -0.41$[6]
- Maximal inspiratory pressure (PImax): $r = -0.38$[9]
- Maximal expiratory pressure (PEmax): $r = -0.29$[9]
- Airway resistance: $r = -0.25$[9]
- VO_{2max}: $r = 0.60$[10]

Known Groups and *Discriminant* are not available.

Construct—Longitudinal/Sensitivity to Change

Convergent. Effect size (ES) = 0.31 for clients with COPD taking theophylline over a 2-week period and 0.35 for clients taking salbutamol (n = 24).[5]

Known Groups and *Discriminant* are not available.

Interpretability

General Population Values (Customary or Normative Values)
Not available for healthy populations, but a MRC dyspnea score of 0 (none) in healthy individuals is to be expected.

Typical Responsiveness Estimates

Not available

References

1. Medical Research Council. Standardized questionnaire on respiratory symptoms. Br J Med 1960;2:1665.

2. Medical Research Council. Instructions for use of the questionnaire on respiratory symptoms. Dawlish: WJ Holman; 1966.

3. American Thoracic Society. Surveillance for respiratory hazards in the occupational setting. Am Rev Respir Dis 1982;126: 952–7.

4. Samet JM. Historical and epidemiologic perspective on respiratory symptoms questionnaires. Am J Epidemiol 1978;108:435–47.

5. Guyatt GH, Townsend M, Keller J, Singer J, Norgradi S. Measuring functional status in chronic lung disease: conclusions from a randomized control trial. Respir Med 1989;83:293–7.

6. Mahler DA, Wells CK. Evaluation of clinical methods for rating dyspnea. Chest 1988;93:580–6.

7. Speich R, Boehler A, Russi EW, Weder W. A case report of a double-blind, randomized trial of inhaled steroids in a patient with lung transplant bronchiolitis obliterans. Respiration 1997; 64:375–80.

8. O'Donnell DE, Webb KA, Bertley JC, Chau LK, Conlan AA. Mechanisms of relief of exertional breathlessness following unilateral bullectomy and lung volume reduction surgery in emphysema. Chest 1996;110:18–27.

9. Mahler DA, Rosiello RA, Harver A, Lentine T, McGovern DF, Daubenspeck JA. Comparison of clinical dyspnea ratings and psychophysical measurements of respiratory sensation in obstructive airway disease. Am Rev Respir Dis 1987;135:1229–33.

10. Hajiro T, Nishimura K, Tsukino M, Ikeda A, Koyama H, Izumi T. Analysis of clinical methods used to evaluate dyspnea in patients with chronic obstructive pulmonary disease. Am J Respir Crit Care Med 1998;158:1185–9.

This measure can be found in reference 3.

EuroQoL-5D
(European Quality of Life Scale)

Developers

The EuroQoL Group, a network of interdisciplinary researchers from Europe; www.euroqol.org

Purpose

The EuroQoL-5D (EQ-5D) provides a descriptive profile and a single index value of health status for use in clinical and economic evaluation of health care and population surveys. It has been specifically designed to complement other health-related quality of life (HRQL) measures such as the 36-Item Short-Form Health Survey, Nottingham Health Profile, Sickness Impact Profile, or disease-specific instruments.

Description

The EuroQoL comprises two sections, the EQ-5D index and the EQ-5D visual analogue scale (VAS). The EQ-5D index is a 5-item standardized generic measure of HRQL. Domains of mobility, self-care, usual activities, pain/discomfort, and anxiety/depression are assessed using a 3-point response scale. Each possible combination of response choice describes a health state. The EQ-5D index describes 243 unique health states. Each health state may be converted to a 0 (worst possible health state) to 1.0 (best possible health state) utility value using a scoring formula. The scoring formulae integrate preference weights obtained from the general population using the time trade-off technique. The EQ-5D VAS is a 0 to 100 thermometer scale that assesses self-perceived health status. Anchors on the thermometer are 0 (worst possible health state) and 100 (best possible health state). Both the EQ-5D index and EQ-5D VAS assess health on that day.

Conceptual/Theoretical Basis of Construct Being Measured

The EuroQoL group recognizes that its instrument is not a comprehensive measure of HRQL, yet they believe that the domains frequently assessed in this area,[1] physical, mental, and social functioning, need to be covered.[1,2] Simplicity was prioritized over the multidimensionality of the instrument. Ease of completion also influenced developmental strategies of the group. The EQ-5D index is based on the concept of utilities. The EuroQoL group strongly believes that attributes of health must be weighted to determine which, on balance, seems best.[1] Using appropriate investigatory methods, a single index value can then be generated for each health state, taking into account each attribute's weight.[1]

Groups Tested with This Measure

Individuals with rheumatic disorders,[3,4] stroke,[5,6] osteoarthritis,[7] Parkinson's disease,[8] low back pain,[9] intermittent claudication,[10] and acute care elderly clients[11] (refer to Website for a complete list of references: www.euroqol.org).

Languages

The EuroQoL was simultaneously developed in Dutch, English (United Kingdom), Finnish, Norwegian, and Swedish. It has been translated into Spanish, Catalan, French (Canadian), English (Canadian), German, Italian, Japanese, and Greek (refer to the Website for a complete list of languages). Preference weights are culture (population) based and are available for the following countries: United Kingdom, Spain, Japan, Germany, and Zimbabwe.

Application/Administration

The EQ-5D was developed to be a self-completed questionnaire. Age and cognition have been reported to affect the ability to self-complete both the index and VAS in an elderly acute care population.[11] It can be completed in 2 to 3 minutes. It can be done over the telephone, and completion by proxies has been assessed in the stroke population group.[6] Values from the EQ-5D index typically range from 0 to 1, where 0 represents the worst possible health state and 1 the best possible one. The EQ-5D VAS possible values range from 0 to 100, in which case a high value expresses a better health state.

Typical Reliability Estimates

Internal Consistency
Not available

Interrater

TABLE 1 Estimates of Interrater Agreement for EQ-5D

Population	EQ-5D Index	EQ-5D VAS
Stroke[6]	Kappa: 0.38 to 0.62 between patient and proxy when self-completed (mobility, 0.57; self-care, 0.62; usual activities, 0.57; pain, 0.54; anxiety/depression, 0.38) Kappa: 0.05 to 0.64 between patient and proxy when interview based (mobility, 0.48; self-care, 0.62; usual activities, 0.37; pain, 0.30; anxiety/depression, 0.05)	ICC: 0.53 between patient and proxy when self-completed by patient, 0.32 between patient and proxy when interview-based

Test–Retest

TABLE 2 Estimates of Test Retest Reliability for EQ-5D

Population	EQ-5D Index	EQ-5D VAS
Rheumatic diseases[4,7]	ICC: 0.70 at 1 wk 0.78 at 2 wk 0.73 at 3 mo	ICC: 0.73 at 1 wk 0.85 at 2 wk 0.70 at 3 mo
Stroke[12]	ICC: 0.83 at 3 wk (0.81 by proxy)	ICC: 0.86 at 3 wk (0.74 by proxy)
General population[2]	ICC: 0.73 at 10 wk	ICC: 0.78 at 10 wk

Typical Validity Estimates

Content
No reference to content validity in the literature

Criterion
No gold standard measure available

Construct—Cross-sectional

Convergent. Pearson product-moment correlations in Table 3 provide good indications of the convergence (high correlations) between the EQ-5D Index or VAS and other frequently used outcome measures in rehabilitation.

TABLE 3 Pearson Correlation Coefficients of EQ-5D with Other Measures

Population	EQ-5D Index	EQ-5D VAS
Rheumatic diseases [3,4,7]	0.67, 0.78 with health (HAQ); 0.74 with functional class; 0.62, 0.65, 0.73 with pain; 0.56 with HADS-mood; 0.48 and 0.55 with AIMS anxiety and depression	0.47, 0.61 with health (HAQ); 0.55 with functional class; 0.52, 0.63 with pain-VAS; 0.59 with HADS-mood; 0.48 and 0.52 with AIMS anxiety and depression
Parkinson's disease[8]	0.63 with depression; 0.66 to 0.68 with disease severity, 0.75 with PDQ, 0.61 with physical score of SF-36, NS for mental score of SF-36	0.63 with depression, NS for disease severity, 0.60 with PDQ, 0.55 with physical score of SF-36, NS for mental score of SF-36

TABLE 3 *Continued*

Population	EQ-5D Index	EQ-5D VAS
Elderly acute care[11]	NS with age at baseline, $p = 0.01$ at 4 wk, NS with self-reported disability 0.35 to 0.59 with COOP-Wonca (physical feelings, ADL [0.59], social activities, change in health [0.35], overall health, pain)	$p = 0.03$ with age at baseline, $p = 0.004$ at 4 wk, NS with self-reported disability, $p = 0.003$ at 4 wk 0.29 to 0.65 with COOP-Wonca (physical [0.29] feelings, ADL [0.59], social activities [0.29], change in health [0.35], overall health [0.65], pain)
Chronic fatigue syndrome[13]	0.08 to 0.83 with SF-36 subscales (PF: 0.80, RP: 0.08,* SF: 0.69, BP: 0.83, MH: 0.50, RE: 0.43, VT: 0.70, GH: 0.57), *NS	0.08 to 0.66 with SF-36 subscales (PF: 0.74, RP:0.0,* SF: 0.70, BP: 0.72, MH: 0.46, RE: 0.40, VT: 0.74, GH: 0.73), *NS
Stroke[5,14]	0.17 to 0.64 with SF-36 subscales	0.08 to 0.66 with SF-36 subscales 0.25 to 0.49 with standard instruments of domains of EQ-5D index (OPCS locomotion subscale: −0.42, Barthel Index: 0.26, Frenchay Activities Index: 0.49, HADS anxiety/depression: −0.25/−0.54

COOP-Wonca = Dartmouth Primary Care Cooperative Information Project—World Organization of Family Doctors, HAQ = Health Assessment Questionnaire; HADS – Health Anxiety and Depression Scale; AIMS = Arthritis Impact Measurement Scales; SF-36 = 36-Item Short-Form Health Survey; ADL = activities of daily living; NS = not significant; OPCS = Office of Population Census and Surveys; PDQ = Parkinson Disease Questionnairre

Known Groups

TABLE 4

Population	EQ-5D Index	EQ-5D VAS
Rheumatoid arthritis[4]	Discriminates between functional classes; lower mean values (0.02 ± 0.31) reported for functional class 4 compared with class 1 clients (0.73 ± 0.14)	Does not discriminate between class 3 (43.6 ± 17.5) and class 4 (45.0 ± 23.2) but discriminates between class 1 (76.8 ± 14.7), 2 (58.3 ± 19.2), and 3
Parkinson's disease[8]	Discriminates between patients presenting clinical features from those who did not: depression (mean: 0.4 vs 0.7), MMS (mean: 0.2 vs 0.7), falls (0.4 vs 0.8), postural instability (mean: 0.4 vs 0.8).	Discriminates between patients presenting clinical features from those who did not: depression (mean: 54.9 vs 76.7), MMS (mean: 51.1 vs 69.0), falls (58.6 vs 71.7), postural instability (57.2 vs 77.6)

Discriminant. Not available

Construct—Longitudinal/Sensitivity to Change

Although no studies have assessed this directly, many have reported potential weakness of the EQ-5D index in its ability to be sensitive to change because of a bimodal distribution of scores[3,7,13] that transposes in a ceiling or floor effect.

Convergent. Not available

Known Groups.

TABLE 5

Population	EQ-5D Index	EQ-5D VAS
Elderly acute care[11]	Mean differences following expected change in patients [stroke: almost no difference in score (–0.05 at 4 wk and –0.005 at 3 mo) compared to total knee replacement (+0.31 at 4 wk and 0.28 at 3 mo)]	Mean differences following expected change in patients [stroke: almost no difference in score (+2.1 at 4 wk and –0.09 at 3 mo) compared to total knee replacement (+11.9 at 4 wk and 15.1 at 3 mo)]

Discriminant. Not available

Interpretability

General Population Values

The EQ-5D index has population-based utility weights from different countries. These weights provide a standard set of utility values for EQ-5D–generated health states. Values for the EQ-5D VAS were reported to be 87.2 and 88.3 among subjects with no health problems compared with 0.76 among those with a chronic condition.[15]

Typical Responsiveness Estimates

TABLE 6

Population	EQ-5D Index	EQ-5D VAS
Rheumatoid arthritis[4]	SRM: 0.70 over 3 mo	SRM: 0.71 over 3 mo
Low back pain[9]	SRM: 0.12 at 6 wk and 0.51 at 6 mo	

SRM = standardized response mean.

Comments

The domains of the EuroQoL are weighted, but the estimation of a utility (index) value requires a computerized program and may therefore not be readily accessible to clinicians. The EQ-5D VAS may be of interest to clinicians as this simple and brief question has been shown to be a valid measure of self-perceived health on a day in several population groups.

References

1. Anonymous. EuroQol—a new facility for the measurement of health-related quality of life. The EuroQol Group. Health Policy 1990;16:199–208.
2. Brooks R. EuroQol: the current state of play. Health Policy 1996;37:53–72.
3. Wolfe F, Hawley DJ. Measurement of the quality of life in rheumatic disorders using the EuroQol. Br J Rheumatol 1997;36:786–93.
4. Hurst NP, Kind P, Ruta D, Hunter M, Stubbings A. Measuring health-related quality of life in rheumatoid arthritis: validity, responsiveness and reliability of EuroQol (EQ-5D). Br J Rheumatol 1997;36:551–9.
5. Dorman PJ, Dennis M, Sandercock P. How do scores on the EuroQol relate to scores on the SF-36 after stroke? Stroke 1999;30:2146–51.
6. Dorman PJ, Waddell F, Slattery J, Dennis M, Sandercock P. Are proxy assessments of health status after stroke with the EuroQol questionnaire feasible, accurate, and unbiased? Stroke 1997;28:1883–7.
7. Fransen M, Edmonds J. Reliability and validity of the EuroQol in patients with osteoarthritis of the knee. Rheumatology (Oxf) 1999;38:807–13.
8. Shrag A, Selai C, Jahanshahi M, Quinn NP. The EQ-5D a generic quality of life measure is a useful instrument to measure quality of life in patients with Parkinson's disease. J Neurol Neurosurg Psychiatry 2000;69:67–73.
9. Garratt AM, Klaber Moffett J, Farrin AJ. Responsiveness of generic and specific measures of health outcome in low back pain. Spine 2001;26:71–7.

10. Bosch JL, Hunink MGM. Comparison of the Health Utilities Index Mark 3 (HUI3) and the EuroQol EQ-5D in patients treated for intermittent claudication. Qual Life Res 2000;9:591–601.

11. Coast J, Peters TJ, Richards SH, Gunnell DJ. Use of the Euro-Qol among elderly acute care patients. Qual Life Res 1998;7:1–10.

12. Dorman P, Slattery J, Farrell B, Dennis M, Sandercock P. Qualitative comparison of the reliability of health status assessments with the EuroQol and SF-36 questionnaires after stroke. United Kingdom Collaborators in the International Stroke Trial. Stroke 1998;29:63–8.

13. Myers C, Wilks D. Comparison of EuroQol EQ-5D and SF-36 in patients with chronic fatigue syndrome. Qual Life Res 1999;8:9–16.

14. Dorman PJ, Waddell F, Slattery J, Dennis M, Sandercock P. Is the EuroQol a valid measure of health-related quality of life after stroke? Stroke 1997;28:1876–82.

15. Mayo E, Goldberg MS, Kind P. Performance of the Euroquol EQ-5D in a Canadian population. Presented at the EuroQol Business Meeting, Rotterdam, 1997.

This measure or ordering information can be found at the Website address included in this review.

FACIAL DISABILITY INDEX

Developers

Jessie M. VanSwearingen and Jennifer S. Brach[1]

Purpose

To provide the clinician with information about the disability and related social and emotional well-being of clients with facial nerve disorders.

Description

The Facial Disability Index (FDI) was developed to provide an account of the client's daily experience of living with a facial nerve disorder. The FDI is intended to assess disability and the outcome of intervention in terms of meaningful change in the client's physical disability and psychosocial status. The FDI is a 10-item self-report questionnaire that consists of two sections: physical function and social/well-being function. Scores on each section range from 0 to 100, with a score of 100 indicating no disability. Questionnaires with unanswered items can still be scored.

Conceptual/Theoretical Basis of Construct Being Measured

The FDI was designed to measure the construct of "disability" as defined in the World Health Organization's International Classification of Impairment, Disease, and Handicap original version, briefly meaning person-level problems or difficulty doing tasks considered typical for humans. Specifically, the FDI physical disability is intended to measure physical disabilities associated with facial function, and the FDI social is intended to measure emotional and social well-being associated with facial function.

Groups Tested with This Measure

People with acute and chronic facial nerve disorders.

Language

English[1]

Application/Administration

This is a self-report measure in which clients check the relevant responses. Most clients can complete the questionnaire in less than 5 minutes. Separate scores are obtained for each section of the FDI. The clinician can calculate a score in 3 to 5 minutes using a simple formula and a calculator.

Typical Reliability Estimates

Internal Consistency

- (theta) 0.88 for FDI physical function and 0.83 for FDI social/well-being function[1]

Interrater

Not applicable

Test–Retest

Not available

Typical Validity Estimates

Content

The items were selected from the disability component of other instruments designed to measure person-level problems and adapted based on the recorded comments of clients with facial nerve disorders describing problems they experienced in their usual human functions and roles living with a facial movement disorder.[1]

Criterion

No gold standard available for the attribute being measured

Construct—Cross-sectional

Convergent. FDI physical function correlates with a clinical scale of facial movement (0.51) and FDI social/well-being function correlates with psychosocial status, 36-Item Short-Form Health Survey (0.69). Using a principal components factor analysis to identify factors describing persons with facial paralysis, the FDI physical and social scores contributed about 25% to the description of persons with facial nerve disorders, with 28% explained by facial impairment measures and about 18% by the temporal characteristics of the disorder.[2] Disability was related to the psychological distress experienced by persons with a facial nerve disorder as indicated by correlation with the Beck Anxiety Inventory and the Beck Depression Inventory, FDI physical, $r = 0.60$, 0.50, and FDI social, $r = 0.50$, 0.48, respectively.[3]

Known Groups. Individuals with facial nerve disorders and individuals without facial nerve disorders:

FDI physical 73.0 and 99.3, respectively, $p < 0.001$; FDI social/well-being 70.7 and 83.9, respectively, $p = 0.002$.[4] The mean scores for the FDI physical and social subscales demonstrated expected differences between groups of clients classified into four treatment-based categories: multivariate analysis of variance, Wilks's lambda 0.81, $F_{1,6218} = 3.97$, $p = 0.00$.[5]

Discriminant. FDI physical did not correlate with psychosocial status, SF-36 (0.23) and the FDI social/well-being function did not correlate with a clinical scale of facial movement (0.07).[1]

Construct—Longitudinal/Sensitivity to Change

Convergent. Correlation coefficients for the relation between change in facial impairment and change in disability for all clients was $r = 0.40$ for the FDI physical disability and $r = 0.30$ for the FDI social disability measures.

Known Groups. The standardized response mean (SRM) for facial impairment for stable and improved clients was 0.35 and 1.61, respectively. Moreover, the change in disability in FDI physical function was 0.12 and 0.61, respectively, and 0.11 and 0.46 for FDI social function for stable and improved clients, respectively. For clients who improved, an effect size (ES) for change in impairment of 1.44 was associated with moderate ES changes in disability, FDI physical, 0.63, and FDI social, 0.47. The receiver operating characteristic curve plot of sensitivity (y-axis) versus 1-specificity (x-axis) was to the left and above the diagonal indicating some degree of discriminative ability of the disability measures.[6]

Discriminant. Not available

Interpretability

General Population Values (Customary or Normative Values)
Not available

Typical Responsiveness Estimates
Not available

References

1. VanSwearingen JM, Brach JS. The Facial Disability Index: reliability and validity of a disability assessment instrument for disorders of the facial neuromuscular system. Phys Ther 1996; 76:1288–300.
2. Brach JS, VanSwearingen J, Delitto A, Johnson PC. Impairment and disability inpatients with facial neuromuscular dysfunction. Otolaryngol Head Neck Surg 1997;117:315–21.
3. VanSwearingen JM, Cohn JF, Turnbull J, Mrzai T, Johnson P. Psychological distress: linking impairment with disability in facial neuromotor disorders. Otolaryngol Head Neck Surg 1998; 118:790–6.
4. Kahn JB, Gliklich RE, Boyev KP, Stewart MG, Metson RB, McKenna MJ. Validation of a patient-graded instrument for facial nerve paralysis: the FaCE scale. Laryngoscope 2001;111:387–98.
5. VanSwearingen JM, Brach JS. Validation of a treatment-based classification system for individuals with facial neuromotor disorders. Phys Ther 1998;78:678–89.
6. VanSwearingen JM, Berry MJ, Brach JS. Assessing the responsiveness of the facial Disability Index to clinical change: is the patient better? Presented at the Combined Sections Meeting, American Physical Therapy Association, Seattle (WA), February 1999.

This measure can be found in reference 1.

FIBROMYALGIA IMPACT QUESTIONNAIRE (FIQ)

Developers

C. S. Burckhardt, S. R. Clark, and R. M. Bennett,[1] Division of Arthritis and Rheumatic Diseases, Oregon Health Sciences University, Portland, Oregon

Purpose

To assess the current health status of women with fibromyalgia syndrome.[1] The measure has since been used for men as well as women to evaluate the effects of treatment and to compare the health status of persons with fibromyalgia to other groups.

Description

The FIQ is a 10-item self-report condition-specific questionnaire for persons with fibromyalgia. The first item (physical function component) has 10 questions on how frequently the respondent performs specific activities. The remaining items pertain to the severity of symptoms and how they affect work. All item scores are standardized to a range of 0 to 10 and are added to obtain a total FIQ score (range 0 to 100, or 0 to 80 if the work questions are omitted). A higher score indicates a poorer health status. The physical function component can be reported as a separate subscale.

Conceptual/Theoretical Basis of Construct Being Measured

The developers began with the premise that a health status instrument for fibromyalgia should contain physical, psychosocial, social, and global well-being components. Items were derived from clients, the literature on fibromyalgia characteristics, and existing health status instruments.[1]

Groups Tested with This Measure

Persons with fibromyalgia (mainly women), post–Lyme disease syndrome,[2] rheumatoid arthritis,[3] and Gulf War syndrome.

Languages

English. The FIQ has been translated into 12 languages and has been culturally adapted and validated in German,[4] Hebrew,[5] and Swedish.[6]

Application/Administration

For the 10 questions of the physical function component, respondents check the best answer from 0 (always perform task) to 3 (never perform task); in the next 2 questions, they circle the appropriate frequency, and in the last 7 items, they mark a 10-cm visual analogue scale. It takes 5 to 10 minutes to complete. To score the FIQ, the clinician must reverse score one item, standardize scores by appropriate multiplication on 3 items, measure 7 visual analog scales, and total the results. It should take less than 5 minutes. Complete scoring instructions are available from Dr. Bennett (see above) on request.

Typical Reliability Estimates

Internal Consistency
0.92 for the German version[4]

Interrater
Not applicable

Test–Retest
$r = 0.56$ for a pain item to 0.95 for physical function over a 1-week period.[1]

Typical Validity Estimates

Content
Assessed by calculating the percentage of missing data (because the item was not relevant to the subject). Eleven percent of the subjects did not do dishes, 20% did not do yard work, and 38% did not work outside the home. Factor analysis yielded five factors. All items of the physical function scale loaded on one factor. Three factors had only one item each: anxiety, depression, and days of work missed. The remaining items loaded on one factor.[1]

Criterion
No gold standard for the attribute being measured.

Construct—Cross-sectional

Convergent. The FIQ physical function scale correlated ($r = 0.67$) with the Arthritis Impact Measurement Scale (AIMS) lower extremity physical function scale. The correlations of the pain, depression, and anxiety items with their respective AIMS scales were 0.69, 0.73, and 0.76 respectively. All items on the FIQ correlated significantly ($r = 0.28$ to 0.83, $p < 0.05$) with the syndrome activity scale of the AIMS.[1]

Known Groups. There were significant differences between healthy women and women with fibromyalgia (*t* values not provided).[7]
Scores below 60 (only 9% work disabled) and above 79 (83% work disabled) were reasonably accurate at predicting work disability.[8]

Discriminant. Not available

Construct—Longitudinal/Sensitivity to Change

Convergent. FIQ change scores were significantly correlated (Spearman's rho = 0.51) with patients' global ratings of symptom change.[9]

Known Groups. FIQ change scores (after 6 months of treatment) were significantly different between groups with global ratings of improved, unchanged, or worsened (analysis of variance summary not provided).[9]

Discriminant. Not available

Other Validity Coefficients
FIQ item scores were not significantly correlated with age, time since diagnosis, education, or income (coefficients not provided).[1] Comparable values for patients with global ratings of "improved" or "worsened" were effect size = −1.38 and 0.13, standardized response mean = −1.04 and 0.19, and Guyatt's statistic = −1.44 and 0.18, respectively.[9]

Interpretability

General Population Values
(Customary or Normative Values)
A total of 124 healthy control subjects had mean scores on the 10 items ranging from 0 to 0.2.[8]

Typical Responsiveness Estimates
Not available

Comments

Rasch analysis revealed a problem with missing (or not applicable) items that resulted in underestima-

tion of the severity of the disability in the physical function component. The physical function component of the FIQ was determined to be nonlinear.[10] Several studies only included women or noted differences in the FIQ properties when used by men compared to women. A modified version of the FIQ has been used with children with fibromyalgia.[11]

References

1. Burckhardt CS, Clark SR, Bennett RM. The Fibromyalgia Impact Questionnaire: development and validation. J Rheumatol 1991;18:728–33.
2. Fallon J, Bujak DI, Guardino S, Weinstein A. The Fibromyalgia Impact Questionnaire: a useful tool in evaluating patients with post-Lyme disease syndrome. Arthritis Care Res 1999;12:42–7.
3. Martinez JE, Ferraz MB, Sato EI, Atra E. Fibromyalgia versus rheumatoid arthritis: a longitudinal comparison of the quality of life. J Rheumatol 1995;22:270–4.
4. Offenbaecher M, Waltz M, Schoeps P. Validation of a German version of the fibromyalgia impact questionnaire (FIQ-G). J Rheumatol 2000;27:1984–8.
5. Buskila D, Neumann L. Assessing functional disability and health status of women with fibromyalgia: validation of a Hebrew version of the Fibromyalgia Impact Questionnaire. J Rheumatol 1996;23:903–6.
6. Hedin PJ, Hamne M, Burckhardt CS, Engstrom-Laurent A. The Fibromyalgia Impact Questionnaire, a Swedish translation of a new tool for evaluation of the fibromyalgia patient. Scand J Rheumatol 1995;24:69–75.
7. Neumann L, Buskila D. Quality of life and physical functioning of relatives of fibromyalgia patients. Semin Arthritis Rheum 1997;26:834–9.
8. White KP, Speechley M, Harth M, Østbye T. Comparing self-reported function and work disability in 100 community cases of fibromyalgia syndrome versus controls in London, Ontario. Arthritis Rheum 1999;42:76–83.
9. Dunkl PR, Taylor AG, McConnell CG, Alfano AP, Conaway MR. Responsiveness of fibromyalgia clinical trial outcome measures. J Rheumatol 2000;27:2683–91.
10. Wolfe F, Hawley DJ, Goldenberg DL, Russell IJ, Buskila D, Neumann L. The assessment of functional impairment in fibromyalgia (FM): Rasch analyses of 5 functional scales and the development of the FM Health Assessment Questionnaire. J Rheumatol 2000;27:1989–99.
11. Schanberg LE, Keefe FJ, Lefebvre JC. Pain coping strategies in children with juvenile primary fibromyalgia syndrome: correlation with pain, physical function, and psychological disability. Arthritis Care Res 1996;9:89–96.

This measure can be found on the accompanying CD-ROM. Prior to using the measure, you are strongly advised to contact the developers for administration and scoring guidelines and revisions to the measure not available at time of publication.

FRENCHAY ARM TEST

Developers

The Frenchay Arm Test was first introduced by Heller and colleagues in 1986 as an adaptation of the Arm Function Test developed by Wade and colleagues in 1983. Affiliation: Frenchay Stroke Unit, Department of Neurology, Frenchay Hospital, Bristol, United Kingdom.

Purpose

To measure recovery in arm function after stroke. It was meant to be an evaluative measure; however, in many ways it is more like a screening tool.

Description

This viewed performance measure consists of five pass or fail tasks. The tasks consist of (1) stabilizing a ruler while drawing a line with a pencil held in the other hand, (2) grasping a cylinder, (3) picking up a glass half full of water and drinking from it, (4) removing and replacing a sprung clothes peg from a 10-mm diameter dowel, and (5) combing hair (or imitating combing). For each of the successfully completed tasks, the subject is given a score of 1.

Conceptual/Theoretical Basis of Construct Being Measured

None reported.

Groups Tested with This Measure

Chronic stroke patients[1] and acute and subacute stroke patients[1,2]

Language

English

Application/Administration

Subjects are asked to sit at a table with their hands in their lap; each task starts from this position.[1] Subjects use their affected upper extremity to complete each of the five tasks. The test takes less than 3 minutes to administer. No specific training is required. No sig-

nificant differences were noticed between the raters who had some experience with the test and those who did not. Furthermore, there were no significant differences in the score given by rehabilitation health care professional raters and other raters.[3]

Typical Reliability Estimates

Internal Consistency
Not available

Interrater
Spearman's rho: 0.68 to 0.90*

Test–Retest
Spearman's rho: 0.75 to 0.99*

Typical Validity Estimates

Content
No reference to content validity in the literature

Criterion
No gold standard exists for the construct being measured.

Construct—Cross-sectional

Convergent. The hypothesis was that sensation, as measured by the depth sense aesthesiometer, would be associated with arm function 3 months following the stroke. The analysis was done using a chi-square test for a 2×2 table. Sensation was classified as either normal/fair or abnormal and arm function was classified as 0 to 2 or better. The association was highly significant: chi-square test (1 df) = 40 ($p < 0.001$).[2] Correlation coefficients were 0.71 with the Barthel Index score and 0.90 with the Motricity Index score.[2]

Known Groups. Fourteen stroke survivors who had achieved a score of 5 out of 5 on the Frenchay Arm Test within 8 weeks following the event of the stroke as well as 2 to 3 years later were assessed on five selected tasks that normally would require the use of both upper extremities. Use of both arms for all five tasks was observed for 12 of 14 subjects and

---

*In their article, Heller et al describe the interrater reliability of four tests including the Frenchay Arm Test. However, no distinction is made when reporting the results. Although there is a range of reliability, it is impossible to establish the exact value for the Frenchay Arm Test. All were statistically significant.[1]

use for four of five tasks was observed for 1 of 14 subjects. These observations indicated that scoring 5 out of 5 on the Frenchay Arm test is a good indicator of spontaneous use of the affected upper extremity when necessary.[1]

Discriminant. Not available

Construct—Longitudinal/Sensitivity to Change

Convergent. In the study from Parker and colleagues (n = 187), the results showed that, 3 months following stroke, the majority of the subjects either failed or passed all of the tasks, with only 20% of the subjects falling in the middle range.[2] These data indicate poor sensitivity especially in the upper limit. Heller and colleagues had similar findings (n – 117).[1]

Known Groups and *Discriminant* are not available.

Interpretability

General Population Values
(Customary or Normative Values)

Sixty-three subjects recruited from senior citizens' social clubs (average age = 72 years; range = 47 to 92 years) were evaluated to provide normative values. All scored 5 out of 5 with both the dominant and the nondominant upper extremity.[1]

Typical Responsiveness Estimates

Not available

Comments

There seems to be some confusion in the literature about what would have been the first version of the Frenchay Arm Test. Wade and colleagues published an article referring to a simple test containing seven items that would measure upper extremity function.[4] In their article, the test was referred to as the Arm Function Test. However, Heller and colleagues referred to the seven-item test as being the long version of the Frenchay Arm Test and proposed a shorter version, containing five of the original items.[1] Okkema and Culler, in their review of the functional evaluation of upper extremity following a stroke, made the distinction between the two tests and clearly identified the Frenchay Arm Test as containing five items.[5]

The literature in regard to the Frenchay Arm Test is limited. The information provided in regard to the psychometric properties of the test is often buried with information about other tests, making it impossible to determine the specific attributes of the Frenchay Arm Test. Some of the conclusions of the authors in regard to validity and reliability are not supported by the results provided in the articles.

The limited sensitivity of the Frenchay Arm Test at both ends of the range represents a significant drawback. This might explain, in part, why the test has not often been referred to in the literature; only one published article using this test was found through a MEDLINE search.

References

1. Heller A, Wade DT, Wood VA, Sunderland A, Hewer RL, Ward E. Arm function after stroke: measurement and recovery over the first three months. J Neurol Neurosurg Psychiatry 1987;50:714–9.
2. Parker VM, Wade DT, Langton Hewer R. Loss of arm function after stroke: measurement, frequency, and recovery. Int Rehabil Med 1986;8:69–73.
3. De Souza LH, Langton-Hewer R, Miller S. Assessment of recovery of arm control in hemiplegic stroke patients. 1. Arm function tests. Int Rehabil Med 1980;2:3–9.
4. Wade DT, Langton-Hewer R, Wood VA, Skilbeck CE, Ismail HM. The hemiplegic arm after stroke: measurement and recovery. J Neurol Neurosurg Psychiatry 1983;46:521–4.
5. Okkema KA, Culler KH. Functional evaluation of upper extremity use following stroke: a literature review. Top Stroke Rehabil 1998;4:54–75.

This measure can be found in reference 1.

FUGL-MEYER ASSESSMENT OF SENSORIMOTOR RECOVERY AFTER STROKE (FM)

Developers

A. R. Fugl-Meyer and associates from The Institute of Rehabilitation Medicine, University of Göteberg, Göteberg, Sweden[1,2]

Purpose

An evaluative instrument that quantifies motor recovery, balance, sensation, joint motion, and pain. It is used clinically and in research to measure the severity of disease, describe motor recovery, and plan and evaluate treatment.[1,2]

Description

The FM is a disease-specific performance-based measure with three independent impairment sections: voluntary movement of the upper and lower extremities, balance, and sensation. Passive range of motion and pain are also evaluated. All are scored on a 3-point ordinal scale, from 0 = no function" to 2 = "full function." The motor section of the FM is arranged hierarchically and evaluates aspects of movement, reflexes, coordination, and speed. The upper and lower limb subscales of movement can be used separately or combined into a total motor score. The upper extremity measure is scored out of 66, with subscores for the upper arm of 34, the wrist for 10, the hand for 14, and 6 for coordination and speed of movement; the lower limb is scored out of 34. The total motor score is 100.[1] The balance section contains seven tests, three in sitting and four in standing, and is scored out of 14. The sensation section evaluates both light touch (on two surfaces of the arm and leg) and position sense (eight joints) for a total score of 24, light touch contributing 8 and position sense 16.[1] Joint motion (eight joints) evaluates the passive range of motion based on the standards of the American Academy of Orthopaedic Surgeons. The joint pain section assesses the presence of pain at the end of range of motion. The total score for each is 44. The total score for the FM assessment is 226.[1]

Conceptual/Theoretical Basis of Construct Being Measured

The FM is based on patterns of motor recovery observed by Twitchel.[3] The items in the motor section are derived from Brunnstrom's stages of post-stroke motor recovery, although the specific stages are not used.[4] That is, the restoration of motor function follows a predictable stepwise course, with the return of reflexes preceding volitional movement in stereotypical synergistic movements of flexion and extension, with a progression to detailed isolated movements without synergies and a normalization of reflexes. The wrist and hand are thought to recover separately. Additionally, as sensation, joint motion, and pain can frequently influence the return of motor behavior, sections on pain, sensation, and range of motion were included.

Groups Tested with This Measure

The FM has been applied to both acute and chronic clients post stroke in settings from an acute care hospital[5] to the community.[6]

Languages

English[1,7] and French (Canadian)[8]

Application/Administration

The FM is a viewed performance-based measure. Most items consist of standardized motor activities performed independently by the client.[1] Reflex activity is tested at the beginning and end of the motor assessment. Each of the five FM sections tested can be partitioned to test a specific construct (eg, to test lower extremity function, the subsections on lower extremity movement, sensation, and the joint motion and pain of the hip, knee, and ankle could be used). The score depends on the number of items included in the subsection selected for testing. Scoring is based on direct observation of performance. Guidelines by Fugl-Meyer et al[1] suggest that the client be instructed verbally and/or with a demonstration of the test and by performing the test with the nonaffected limb. Assistance of the evaluator is allowed in the testing of the wrist and hand to stabilize the arm.[1] Equipment needed is a scrap of paper, a ball, a pencil, and a cylinder (small can) for testing in the hand subsection. In bedridden patients, the joint range of shoulder abduction is performed only to 90 degrees and extension of the hip to "0." The experienced therapist takes 30 to 40 minutes to complete the entire 155 items; it may take longer and be more difficult to administer in aphasic or severely affected patients.[9,10]

Typical Reliability Estimates

Internal Consistency
Not available

Interrater
In 18 chronic stroke survivors with 5 therapists, pairwise Pearson product-moment correlations between therapists for each component of the upper extremity ranged from 0.96 to 0.97. Lower extremity subsections correlations varied from 0.83 to 0.95; the total score correlated at 0.99. No significant differences were found between the raters across the test times, except for the reflex and coordination subscores in the upper extremity, suggesting that they were unreliable.[7]

Reliability was also established in 12 patients, 6 days to 6 months post stroke, who were tested by three therapists (Table 1).

Test–Retest
In 49 chronic stroke patients tested twice, 3 weeks apart by one therapist, the ICC for the lower extremity was 0.86 and for balance 0.34. Although the test–retest reliability of balance is not very reliable, indicating that the patient performance was inconsistent, the inter-rater agreement was high. The standard error of the measure for the lower extremity was 1.76 points and for balance 1.17 points.[12]

Other
In 19 chronic patients tested by one therapist on three separate occasions, the Pearson correlation coefficients for the total FM score were high ($r > 0.99$) and ranged from $r = 0.86$ to $r = 0.99$ for the subscales.[7] There were no significant differences across times as assessed by a repeated measures analysis of variance.

Typical Validity Estimates

Content
The recovery patterns assessed in 28 clients followed from 6 weeks to 1 year were consistent with the concept of sequential recovery, confirming content validity.[1,12] The mean correlation, in 9 clients, between upper and lower extremity scores over a year was $r = 0.88$.[1] However, in 24 patients, 3 months post stroke, no relationship was seen between the present pain intensity and FM upper extremity motor score, as was theorized.[8] Preliminary findings in 10 chronic stroke clients indicate a negative correlation between the degree of spasticity (Ashworth) and voluntary movement ($r = -0.83$), as would be expected from the pattern of recovery.[13]

Criterion

Concurrent. A 1982 study found a relationship between sensory function and subsequent motor recovery demonstrated by high correlations between sensory evoked potentials (SEPs) 14 days post stroke. This relationship was strongest between SEP and the FM upper extremity and less strong for the FM lower extremity subsection. The strength of the relationship did not depend on whether the FM was assessed at 1 week, 3 months, or 6 months post stroke.[9] Recently, in a study of 64 patients followed from 2 weeks to 12 months post stroke, this relationship was weak.[14]

Predictive. The lower extremity FM admission score at 6 weeks post stroke in 48 patients predicted the rehabilitation discharge Functional Independence Measure (FIM) mobility ($r = 0.63$) and locomotion scores ($r = 0.74$).[14] Additionally, the admission FM motor score predicted length of stay in rehabilitation ($r = 0.42$) better than the FIM.

The FM has been considered the criterion measure against which a number of measures have

TABLE 1 Reliability of FM Assessment in Chronic Stroke Patients

Fugl-Meyer Section	ICC (95% Confidence Limits)[11]	Standard Error of the Measure [11]
Total instrument	0.96 (0.91–0.99)	9.4
Total motor		
Upper limb	0.97 (0.94–0.99)	3.6
Lower limb	0.92 (0.81–0.96)	3.2
Balance	0.93 (0.82–0.97)	1.0
Sensation	0.85 (0.67–0.94)	2.9
Joint motion	0.85 (0.67–0.94)	2.0
Pain	0.61 (0.29–0.85)	3.7

been validated: the Motor Assessment Scale,[15] the Action Research Arm test,[16] and the Bobath Assessment upper limb section.[8]

Acute populations: The FM correlated to activities of daily living (ADL) scores ($r = 0.64$) in 109 clients measured within 2 weeks of stroke.[17] In 161 acute stroke clients, the FM subscale scores and total scores were highly correlated at admission and follow-up (5 weeks), demonstrating a relationship between motor and functional recovery.[5] Additionally, the balance subscore was highly correlated with motor performance and ADL measures.[5] In 16 acute clients tested 3 to 8 weeks post stroke, the FM lower extremity scores correlated with cadence over 10 meters ($r = -0.50$), the FM total and balance subscores correlated with the Berg Balance Scale ($r = 0.62$ and $r = 0.77$, respectively), and gait speed correlated with the FM pain score ($r = -0.53$).[17]

Chronic population: Cross-validation between the FM upper extremity measure and the DeSouza arm test in 88 stroke clients showed that the two tests covaried and explained 90% of the variation in the total scores and 80% in the motor scores.[18]

The Bobath Assessment upper limb section correlated with the FM upper extremity arm subscore on admission ($r = 0.73$), during rehabilitation ($r = 0.62$), and at discharge ($r = 0.85$).[8] The lower extremity subscore correlated with measures of gait speed ($r = 0.66$) and cadence (fewer steps) ($r = 0.59$) in 15 males with chronic stroke. Significant correlations were also found between the upper limb and balance scores ($r = 0.68$). No correlations were found between gait measures and FM sensation scores.[10] This may be attributable to the characteristics of the particular sample or the fact that there is not a strong relationship between lower extremity motor and sensory recovery. Another study of 16 individuals with chronic stroke showed that FM sensation correlated poorly with both comfortable ($r = 0.14$) and maximal gait speeds ($r = 0.05$).[6] In ambulatory individuals with chronic stroke, an FM sensation score below 12 combined with the strength of the hip flexors, and ankle plantar flexors determined maximal gait speed but not the loss of sensation (FM) alone.[6] The FM total motor score in the same group of patients, however, correlated to comfortable (mean 0.76 m/sec; $r = 0.61$) and maximal speeds (mean 1.09 m/sec; $r = 0.61$).[6]

When tested concurrently in 32 persons, 2 months post stroke, the FM and the Motor Assessment Scale (MAS) total scores correlated highly at $r = 0.96$. Correlations with the MAS for selected subscales varied from 0.65 to 0.92, but there was no correlation with the sitting balance section ($r = -0.10$).[15] FM items were significantly intercorrelated with MAS items, except for sitting balance ($r = 0.28$).[19] FM sensation scores of light touch (0.64) and position sense (0.67) correlated with MAS balance score but not with the FM sitting balance items (0.12 and -0.10, respectively). The correlation difference could be because the MAS measures dynamic balance and the FM measures displacement.[15]

Construct—Cross-sectional

Convergent. The FM distinguishes between persons with minimal recovery better than the MAS. Significantly negative correlations between score differences and levels of recovery (upper extremity $r = -0.50$ and lower extremity $r = -0.69$) were found, indicating that the largest differences between the two measures were in earlier stages of recovery or among more disabled individuals.[15]

Known Groups. At gait speeds of < 0.34 m/sec, the FM lower extremity score distinguished the need for assistance in walking better than gait speed ($r = 0.62$).[19] The FM has been shown to distinguish three levels of self-care ability 2 weeks after stroke (N = 109).[20]

Discriminant. Not available

Construct—Longitudinal/Sensitivity to Change

Convergent. Over a 2-month period of rehabilitation, the FM was correlated to the Bobath Assessment of upper extremity pre- ($r = 0.73$) and post-rehabilitation ($r = 0.85$), with both measures showing a change across the time period.[8] Over a 5-week period of rehabilitation in an acute care hospital, the mean change in FM scores correlated to mean change scores in the BI (upper extremity: $r = 0.57$; lower extremity: $r = 0.57$; balance: $r = 0.68$; total score: $r = 0.68$). The effect sizes owing to 5 weeks of rehabilitation were small (0.2 upper, 0.19 lower, 0.33 balance, 0.24 total score).[5]

Known Groups and *Discriminant* are not available.

Interpretability

General Population Values (Customary or Normative Values)
Not available

Typical Responsiveness Estimates

Individual Patient. For the FM lower extremity, a change of greater than 5 points reflects a change greater than measurement error.[12] Similarly, for balance, the critical value of change is 4 points.

TABLE 2 Stroke Severity by Various FM Total Motor Scores

Fugl-Meyer[2]	Fugl-Meyer[1]	Duncan[21]
< 50 Severe		0–35 Very severe
50–84 Marked	≤ 84 Hemiplegia	36–55 Severe
85–94 Moderate	85–95 Hemiparesis	56–79 Moderate
95–99 Slight	96–99 Slight motor dyscoordination	> 79 Mild

Between Group. Table 2 shows indications of FM total motor scores that have been used to categorize the groups of stroke patients.

Comments

The FM is a frequently used measure of motor deficits. The most commonly used subscale of the FM is the total motor score; the sensory, balance, or joint motion subscales are used less often. Validity of the FM sections varies according to the populations and times tested. The above instrument measures only gross limb movement and not fine or complex movements or coordination. Consideration should be given to the construct being tested in selecting either the entire measure or its subsections.

References

1. Fugl-Meyer AR, Jääskö L, Leyman I, Olsson S, Steglind S. The post-stroke hemiplegic patient 1. A method for evaluation of physical performance. Scand J Rehabil Med 1975;7:13–31.
2. Fugl-Meyer AR. Post-stroke hemiplegia assessment of physical properties. Scand J Rehabil Med 1980;7(Suppl):85–93.
3. Twitchell TE. The restoration of motor function following hemiplegia in man. Brain 1951;74:443–80.
4. Brunnstrom S. Movement therapy in hemiplegia: a neurophysiological approach. New York: Harper and Row; 1970.
5. Wood-Dauphinee SW, Williams JI, Shapiro SH. Examining outcome measures in a clinical study of stroke. Stroke 1990;21:731–9.
6. Nadeau S, Arsenault AB, Gravel D, Bourbonnais D. Analysis of the clinical factors determining natural and maximal speeds in adults with stroke. Am J Phys Med Rehabil 1999;78:123–30.
7. Duncan PW, Propst M, Nelson SG. Reliability of the Fugl-Meyer assessment of sensorimotor recovery following cerebrovascular accident. Phys Ther 1983;63:1606–10.
8. Arsenault AB, Dutil E, Lambert J, Corriveau H, Guarna F, Drouin G. An evaluation of the hemiplegic subject based on the Bobath approach. Scand J Rehabil Med 1988;20:13–6.
9. Kusoffsky A, Wadell I, Nilsson BY. The relationship between sensory impairment and motor recovery in patients with hemiplegia. Scand J Rehabil Med 1982;14:27–32.
10. Dettman MA, Linder MT, Sepic SB. Relationships among walking performance, postural stability, and functional assessments of the hemiplegic patient. Am J Phys Med 1987;66:77–90.
11. Sanford J, Moreland J, Swanson LR, Stratford PW, Gowland C. Reliability of the Fugl-Meyer assessment for testing motor performance in patients following stroke. Phys Ther 1993;73:447–54.
12. Beckerman, Vogelaar TW, Lankhorst GJ, Verbeek AL. A criterion for stability of the function of the lower extremity in stroke patients using the Fugl-Meyer Assessment Scale. Scand J Rehabil Med 1996;28:3–7.
13. Lin FM, Sabbahi M. Correlation of spasticity with hyperactive stretch reflexes and motor dysfunction in hemiplegia. Arch Phys Med Rehabil 1999;80:526–30.
14. Feys H, Van Hees J, Bruyninck F, Mercelis R, De Weerdt W. Value of somatosensory and motor evoked potentials in predicting arm recovery after a stroke. J Neurol Neurosurg Psychiatry 2000;68:323–31.
15. Malouin F, Pichard L, Bonneau C, Durand A, Corriveau C. Evaluating motor recovery early after stroke: comparison of the Fugl Meyer and the Motor Assessment Scale. Arch Phys Med Rehabil 1994;75:1206–12.
16. deWeerdt WJG, Harrison MA. Measuring recovery of arm-hand function in stroke patients: a comparison of the Brunnstrom-Fugl-Meyer test and the Action Research Arm test. Physiother Can 1985;37:65–70.
17. Nilsson L, Carlsson JY, Grimby G, Nordholm LA. Assessment of walking, balance and sensorimotor performance of hemiplegic patients in the acute stage after stroke. Physiother Theory Pract 1998;14:149–57.
18. Berglund K. Fugl-Meyer upper extremity function in hemiplegia. Scand J Rehabil Med 1986;18:155–7.
19. Poole JL, Whitney SL. Motor assessment scale for stroke patients concurrent validity and interrater reliability. Arch Med Rehabil 1988;69:195–7.
20. Bernspang B, Asplund K, Eriksson S, Fugl-Meyer AR. Motor and perceptual impairments in acute stroke patients: effects on self-care ability. Stroke 1987;18:1081–6.
21. Duncan PW, Goldstein LB, Horner RD, Landsman PB, Samsa GP, Matchar DB. Similar motor recovery of upper and lower extremities after stroke. Stroke 1994;25:1181–8.

This measure can be found in reference 1 or by contacting the developers.

FUNCTIONAL ASSESSMENT SYSTEM OF LOWER-EXTREMITY DYSFUNCTION (FAS)

Developers

Ulrika Öberg,[1] ulrika.oberg@hoegland.ltjkpg.se

Purpose

The FAS is an instrument for evaluation of lower extremity dysfunction. It is developed for clinical use to measure present functional status, for goal setting, to design individual training programs, and for treatment evaluation.

Description

The FAS is a performance- and self-report-based measure developed for use by physiotherapists. It consists of 20 variables, representing major lower extremity dysfunction related to daily life activities. The variables are divided into five groups: hip impairment, knee impairment, physical disability, social variables, and pain. The variables are transformed to a uniform, dimensionless score on a 5-point scale according to a key for every variable. Zero means no disability; four means severe disability or total lack of function. The scores are plotted onto a diagram, giving a disability profile.[2]

Conceptual/Theoretical Basis of Construct Being Measured

A simplified model of the physiotherapy process has been used as a theoretical framework for assessment, diagnosis, goal setting, and outcome analysis. The grouping of the variables corresponds with the World Health Organization Classification of Impairment, Disabilities, and Handicaps.[1]

Groups Tested with This Measure

The FAS has been tested on patients with osteoarthritis (OA) in the hip or knee who are accepted for arthroplasty[2–6] or tibial osteotomy[7]; also used on persons with unspecific lower extremity problems and healthy people.[4]

Languages

Swedish, English, Finnish, Danish, Norwegian, Icelandic, Polish, and Spanish. No information is available about cultural adaptation or validation.

Application/Administration

The FAS is conducted close to a corridor. Active range of motion in the hip and knee is measured with a standard manual goniometer. Muscle strength is tested as isometric extension and flexion forces in the knee at 45 degrees flexion with the client in a fixed sitting position and a strain gauge dynamometer applied to the leg 16 cm distal to the knee joint space. Rising from a half-standing position is measured as the maximum number of times the patient can rise from a high chair with a hip angle of about 135 degrees. Rising/sitting down is recorded as the lowest possible sitting height from a chair with adjustable heights (corresponding to an ordinary chair, sofa, car seat) and without armrests. Step height is measured with the client ascending different step heights, corresponding to ordinary bus, and train stairs, with the affected leg and no support. The time standing on one leg is the number of seconds the client is able to stand on the affected leg wearing no shoes. Gait speed is tested on a 65-m indoor corridor in m/sec, in a self-selected speed. The social variables and pain are evaluated by a personal interview of the patient. The test results are converted to scores according to a key, which explains how to grade the measurements. The scores are plotted in a diagram, thus constituting an individual profile of lower extremity dysfunction. The total time needed to complete the profile is about 30 minutes. The FAS can be completed with or without a computer. Equipment needed includes a goniometer, a stopwatch, a strain gauge dynamometer, an adjustable chair, adjustable step heights, and a bench.[2] There is no need for special training.

Typical Reliability Estimates

Internal Consistency
Not available

Interrater
Goodman-Kruskal gamma coefficient values for the different variables are 0.99 to 1.00.[2]

Test–Retest
Not available

Typical Validity Estimates

Content

Content validity is tested with principal-components factor analysis with varimax rotation. The analysis indicated five subgroups consistent with the primary grouping: hip impairment, knee impairment, physical disability, social disability, and pain.[2]

Criterion

No gold standard for lower extremity dysfunction.

Construct—Cross-sectional

Convergent

- Goodman-Kruskal gamma coefficients between FAS (hip, pain, and disability) variables in OA clients and healthy controls and AIMS physical activity variables are 0.71 to 0.91 and with AIMS pain variable are 0.60 to 0.86[3]
- Rosser–Kind index between FAS (hip, pain, and disability) variables in OA clients and healthy controls and AIMS physical variables are 0.72 to 0.93 and with AIMS pain variable are 0.58 to 0.86

Known Groups. Not available

Discriminant

- Goodman-Kruskal gamma coefficients between FAS (hip, pain, and disability) variables and psychological and social variables of AIMS are 0.10 to 0.52 and with radiologic classification are 0.04 to 0.46[3]

Construct—Longitudinal/Sensitivity to Change

Not available

Other Validity Coefficients

Discriminatory power is evaluated with Kruskal-Wallis one-way analysis of variance (ANOVA) and the Ferguson delta on patients and a healthy group. For the whole group, there is a statistically significant difference ($p < 0.01$ to 0.001) between patients and controls in all variables. The ability of most variables to discriminate between different degrees of dysfunction had a high delta value. All physical and social disability variables and pain have high sensitivity. The specificity is high for all variables except for the muscle strength variables. When all variables are weighted together in Youden's index, most impairment variables have a low index, but most physical and social variables and pain have a high index. Exceptions are standing on one leg and use and type of walking aid.[4] Differences in functional status between younger and older people were explored with one-way ANOVA on 709 patients with OA. Older people showed higher dysfunction scores in almost all variables, except for pain, for which there was an inverse relationship.[5]

Interpretability

To evaluate improvements in functional variables after arthroplasty, 271 consecutive patients with hip or knee arthroplasty were examined with the FAS preoperatively and 6 months postoperatively using Wilcoxon's signed rank test. At group level, there was a significant reduction in disability scores for most variables ($p < 0.001$).

Individual patient goals set out preoperatively showed a high level of achievement in most variables postoperatively. Goal achievement in patients with high tibial osteotomy showed that the goals were not reached on group level for almost every variable. On the individual level, only 20 to 40% of the patients achieved the goals.[6]

General Population Values (Customary or Normative Values)

Not available

Typical Responsiveness Estimates

Not available

Comment

As there are few data to support this measure's ability to detect change in individuals or groups, the FAS needs to be used as an outcome measure with caution until sensitivity to change and responsiveness have been tested.

References

1. Öberg U. Functional Assessment System of Lower Extremity Dysfunction [thesis]. Linköping (Sweden): Linköping University; 1996.
2. **Öberg U, Öberg B, Öberg T. Validity and reliability of a new assessment of lower-extremity dysfunction. Phys Ther 1994; 74:861–71.**
3. Öberg U, Öberg B, Öberg T. Concurrent validity of a new assessment of lower extremity dysfunction. Eur J Phys Med Rehabil 1996;6:51–8.
4. Öberg U, Öberg T. Discriminatory power, sensitivity and specificity of a new assessment system (FAS). Physiother Can 1997;49:40–7
5. Öberg U, Öberg T. Worse functional status among old people when admitted for arthroplasty. Scand J Caring Sci 1996;10:96–102.
6. Öberg U, Öberg T, Hagstedt B. Functional improvement after hip and knee arthroplasty. Physiother Theory Pract 1996;12:3–13.
7. Öberg U, Öberg T. Functional outcome after high tibial osteotomy: a study using individual goal achievement as the primary outcome variable. J Rehabil Res Dev 2000;37:501–9.

This measure can be found on the accompanying CD-ROM. Prior to using the measure, you are strongly advised to contact the developers for administration and scoring guidelines and revisions to the measure not available at time of publication.

FUNCTIONAL AUTONOMY MEASUREMENT SYSTEM (SMAF)

Developers

R. Hébert, R. Carrier, and A. Bilodeau.[1] Copies of the SMAF are available upon request from Dr. R. Hébert, Sherbrooke Geriatric University Institute, 1036 Belvédère S, Sherbrooke, QC J1H 4C4; rhebert@courrier.usherb.ca.

Purpose

To measure functional performance in elderly people. The SMAF was originally designed to determine the need for and allocation of community services and to identify the level of supported residence required.[1]

Description

The SMAF is a 29-item interviewer-administered questionnaire examining five functional performance subscales: Activities of Daily Living (ADL) (7), Instrumental ADL (IADL) (8), Mobility (6), Communication (3), and Mental Function (5).[1,2] The scale rates an individual's limitation in functional performance (disability), the resources (type and stability) available in the environment to assist with the activity being evaluated, and the subsequent effect of the resources on the observed disability (handicap). Each item is rated from 0 (autonomy/complete independence) to –3 (total dependence), with a potential total of –87. A total disability SMAF score is calculated using the disability scores in the five subscales; a total SMAF score is calculated using the disability and handicap scores. A revised SMAF was developed to assist with the planning of rehabilitation intervention and the determination of adequate support service.[3] It includes a –0.5/–1.5 rating (independent but with difficulty) to some ADL, mobility, and IADL items. Both a total revised SMAF score (disability and handicap) and a total revised SMAF disability score can be calculated.

Conceptual/Theoretical Basis of Construct Being Measured

The SMAF is based on the International Classification of Impairment, Disability and Handicap model developed in 1980 and adopted by the World Health Organization (WHO).

Groups Tested with This Measure

Geriatric clients across supported residential sites,[1,4] health delivery sites,[3,5–7] and community-dwelling elderly people[7,8]

Languages

French,[1] English,[1] Dutch,[3] and Spanish[3]

Application/Administration

The SMAF is administered as a questionnaire to the older adult, a family member, or a caregiver.[1,8] The tasks may also be directly observed or tested at the discretion of the administrator.[8] The length of time to administer is estimated at 40 minutes.[1] Disability scores for each item are tracked on the left side of the scoring sheet. Handicap scores for each item are tracked on the right side of the scoring sheet once consideration has been given to the resources present in the older adult's home. There is no training manual.

Typical Reliability Estimates

Internal Consistency
Not available

Interrater
- Mean Cohen's weighted kappa of 0.75 for the total disability SMAF[1]
- ICC of 0.96 to 0.97 for the revised disability SMAF (ranging from 0.74 to 0.96 for each SMAF subscale)[3,6]

Test–Retest
- 0.95 for a total revised SMAF score (ranging from 0.78 to 0.95 for each subscale)[3]

Typical Validity Estimates

Content
The content was determined by reviewing existing functional performance scales published in the literature.[1] The individual SMAF items selected were then compared to the WHO's classification of disabilities pertaining to the elderly.

Criterion
No gold standard exists for the measurement of functional performance in the elderly.

Predictive

The mobility and the ADL subscale scores of the disability SMAF were independently associated with the length of stay in physical rehabilitation in clients with anxiety, depression, and cognitive disorders.[5]

Construct—Cross-sectional

Convergent

- Older Americans Resources and Services Scale (OARS) ADL questionnaire: $r = 0.80$ (disability SMAF) among older clients in emergency departments[6]
- New Handicap Scale: $r = 0.64$ to 0.77 (revised disability SMAF) among day hospital and inpatients[9]
- Timed Up and Go: $r = 0.42$ (revised disability SMAF) among home care clients[7]
- Modified Barthel Index: $r = 0.43$ (revised disability SMAF) among home care clients[7]
- Recorded amount of nursing care time: $r = 0.88$ (disability SMAF) across different care settings.[1] Note that the IADL subscale and outdoor mobility item were excluded.

Known Groups. The disability SMAF discriminated between older adults living in licensed and unlicensed homes for the aged ($p < 0.001$).[4]

Discriminant. Not available

Construct—Longitudinal/Sensitivity to Change

Convergent. Not available

Known Groups. The disability SMAF demonstrated change with rehabilitation in an inpatient acute/rehabilitation unit for the elderly ($t = 10.98$, $p < 0.0001$). The IADL subscale and outdoor mobility were excluded in the SMAF measurement.[2] The disability SMAF has been used to describe change over time in large epidemiologic studies of community-dwelling older adults.[8]

Divergent. Not available

Interpretability

General Population Values (Customary or Normative Values)
Not available

Typical Responsiveness Estimates

Individual Patient. The minimal metrically detectable change score for the total SMAF disability score is estimated to be ± 5.0 (method 1) for community-dwelling older adults over 75 years of age.[8,10]

Between Group. Not available

Comments

Although the SMAF was designed for evaluating service needs in older adults across health delivery sites, it has mainly been used as a disability scale.

References

1. Hébert R, Carrier R, Bilodeau A. The Functional Autonomy Measurement System (SMAF): description and validation of an instrument for the measurement of handicaps. Age Ageing 1988;17:293–302.

2. Rai GS, Gluck T, Weintjes HJFM, Rai SGS. The Functional Autonomy Measurement System (SMAF): a measure of functional change with rehabilitation. Arch Gerontol Geriatr 1996;22:81–5.

3. Desrosiers J, Brava G, Hébert R, Dubuc N. Reliability of the revised Functional Autonomy Measurement System (SMAF) for epidemiological research. Age Ageing 1995;24:402–6.

4. Bravo G, Charpentier M, Dubois M, DeWals P, Émond A. Profile of residents in unlicensed homes for the aged in the Eastern Townships of Quebec. Can Med Assoc J 1998;159:143–8.

5. Clerc Berod A, Klay M, Santos-Eggimann B, Paccaud F. Anxiety, depressive, or cognitive disorders in rehabilitation patients. Am J Phys Med Rehabil 2000;79:266–73.

6. McCusker J, Bellavance F, Cardin S, Belzile E. Validity of an activities of daily living questionnaire among older patients in an emergency department. J Clin Epidemiol 1999;52:1023–30.

7. Elliott K. The construct validity of the Functional Autonomy Measurement System (SMAF) for the older adult on home care [thesis]. Edmonton (AB): Univ. of Alberta; 1999.

8. Hébert R, Brayne C, Spiegelhalter D. Incidence of functional decline and improvement in a community-dwelling, very elderly population. Am J Epidemiol 1997;145:935–44.

9. Rai G, Kiniorns M, Burns W. New handicap scale for elderly in hospital. Arch Gerontol Geriatr 1998;28:99–104.

10. Hébert R, Spiegelhalter D, Brayne C. Setting the minimal metrically detectable change on disability rating scales. Arch Phys Med Rehabil 1997;78:1305–8.

This measure can be found on the accompanying CD-ROM. Prior to using the measure, you are strongly advised to contact the developers for administration and scoring guidelines and revisions to the measure not available at time of publication.

(FIM™) FUNCTIONAL INDEPENDENCE MEASURE

Developers

A national task force was struck in 1984 to develop a functional measure and to design a patient databank sponsored by the American Congress of Rehabilitation Medicine and the American Academy of Physical Medicine and Rehabilitation. The task force was co-chaired by Steven Forer (from the Congress) and Carl V. Granger (from the Academy).[1] The FIM™ is a proprietary measure. For further information on the scale, syllabus, and training materials, contact Uniform Data System for Medical Rehabilitation (UDS$_{MR}$), 232 Parker Hall, University at Buffalo, 3435 Main Street, Buffalo, NY 14214-3007; Tel: 716 829-2076; Fax: 716-829-2080; e-mail: fimnet@ubvms.cc. buffalo.edu or info@udsmr.org; Website: www. udsmr.org[2]

Purpose

Provides an estimate of the burden of care.[3] It can be used for the purpose of clinical, administrative management, external accountability, and clinical/epidemiologic research.[1]

Description

Eighteen items (13 motor, 5 cognition) are rated on a seven-level ordinal scale that describes stages of complete dependence to complete independence in performance of basic daily living activities.[3] Total scores range from 18 (lowest) to 126 (highest) level of independence.[2] A Rasch rating scale analysis has been applied to transform the FIM's ordinal ratings to an equal-interval rating scale that can then be used for linear regression models.[4]

Conceptual/Theoretical Basis of Construct Being Measured

The FIM assesses disability construct according to the International Classification of Impairments, Disabilities and Handicaps. It is not a measure of impairment.[5]

Groups Tested with This Measure

Individuals with stroke, traumatic brain injury (TBI), spinal cord injury (SCI), multiple sclerosis, and elderly individuals undergoing inpatient rehabilitation.

Languages

The guide for the Uniform Data Set for Medical Rehabilitation (UDS$_{MR}$) has been translated into 10 national versions.[6] The FIM instrument has been translated in the following languages (Smith M, personal communication, 2001): French, German, Italian, Spanish, Canadian French, Swedish, Finnish, Australian, Portuguese, and South African (Afrikaans).

Application/Administration

Time to administer is 45 minutes, with 7 minutes to gather demographic information. The site—clinic or community—where the FIM is performed must be licensed. Scores are based on clinical observation, although the FIM can also be used for telephone interviews (see reliability section). It is a discipline-free assessment, but the evaluator must be trained.[2] Different parts of the test can be administered by different disciplines.[1]

The UDS$_{MR}$ collects data from voluntary subscribers that include more than 1,300 facilities; over 3 million client records have been processed, and more than 70,000 clinicians have been credentialed to collect FIM data. These data are maintained in a national database for various purposes such as generating performance reports, research, and consulting work. The data can also be interfaced with a facility's information system and can generate facility-specific or patient-specific profiles.[7] To establish a threshold for acceptable interrater reliability for the purpose of reporting aggregate data, the UDS$_{MR}$ has established four statistical criteria, including a total FIM score ICC between raters of 90% or greater.[8]

Typical Reliability Estimates

Internal Consistency
- Cronbach's value of 0.93 for overall admissions and 0.95 for discharges[9]

Interrater
From meta-analysis,[10] see Table 1.

TABLE 1 Reliability Estimates of the FIM

Lead Author	Diagnosis	Type of Reliability	Statistic	Total FIM
Chau[11]	Mixed	Interrater	ICC	0.94
Ottenbucher[12]	Mixed	Interrater	κ	0.90
Hamilton[8]	Mixed	Interrater	ICC	0.92
				(motor = 0.96
				cognitive = 0.91)
Jaworski[13]	Mixed	Interrater	ICC	0.99
Kidd[14]	Mixed	Interrater	r	0.92
Segal[15]	Stroke	Interrater	ICC	0.96
Brosseau[16]	MS	Interrater	ICC	0.83

In a more recent study of 64 clients with multiple sclerosis (MS), ICC = 0.99.[17]

Test–Retest

See Table 2.

Other

See Table 3.

Intrarater reliability in 35 clients with multiple sclerosis was ICC = 0.94.[17]

Typical Validity Estimates

Content

Developed through a literature review of published and unpublished instruments and expert panels. It was then piloted in 11 centers for face and content validity (114 clinicians from eight different disciplines and 110 patients evaluated).[1] Face and content validity were both determined by the Delphi method polling rehabilitation expert opinion on the inclusiveness and appropriateness of the items.[21]

Criterion

Concurrent. Not available

Predictive. A bivariate regression analysis demonstrated the FIM's ability to predict the amount of help (assistance) in minutes among people with multiple sclerosis; a 1-point improvement in FIM raw score predicted a 3.4-minute reduction of care time.[22] The ability of the FIM to predict the amount of direct assistance and/or supervision and whether predictions could be improved with measures of neurobehavioral impairment was evaluated among individuals with TBI. Findings[24] are reported in Table 4.

TABLE 2 Reliability Estimates of the FIM

Lead Author	Diagnosis	Type of Reliability	Statistic	Total FIM
Chau[11]	Mixed	Test–retest	ICC	0.93
Segal[18]	SCI	Test–retest	r	0.84
Kidd[14]	Mixed	Test–retest	r	0.90

TABLE 3 Reliability Estimates of the FIM

Lead Author	Diagnosis	Type of Reliability	Statistic	Total FIM
Grey[19]	Spinal cord injury	Equivalence (nurse/self-report)	r	0.84
Jaworski[13]	Mixed	Equivalence (observe/telephone)	ICC	0.94
Smith[20]	Mixed	Equivalence (observe/telephone)	ICC	0.97
Segal[15]	Stroke	Equivalence (team/caregiver/proxy)	ICC	0.87

TABLE 4

Type of Assistance to Be Predicted	Accuracy of Prediction	Use of Neurobehavioral Impairment Measures
Assistance	Motor FIM → 83%	No improved accuracy
Supervision	Cognitive FIM → 77%	FIM motor and cognitive with somatic/anxiety factor → 82%
Both (ie, any assistance)	FIM motor and cognitive scores → 78%	No improved accuracy

Construct—Cross-sectional

Convergent. Among TBI clients, total (nursing) contact time was correlated –0.54 with the motor measure and –0.35 with the cognitive measure at admission and –0.51 and –0.47 at discharge ($p < .001$). Among SCI clients, total contact time was correlated –0.46 with the motor measure at admission and –0.52 at discharge ($p < 0.001$), whereas the cognitive measure was not related significantly to total contact time at admission or discharge.[25] Among clients with multiple sclerosis, there was high correlation between the FIM and the Barthel Index ($r = 0.88$) and with the physical functioning item of the 36-Item Short-Form Health Survey ($r = 0.88$). Correlations were also reported between the FIM and the clients' ability to work (–0.59*), do their housework (-0.64*), and look after themselves (–0.44**) and their perceived disability rank (–0.83*) (*$p < 0.001$; **$p = 0.001$ to 0.002).[17]

Known Groups. Dodds et al tested three hypotheses to demonstrate the construct validity of the FIM (Table 5).[9]

TABLE 5 Construct Validity of FIM

Hypothesis	Mean FIM Scores	Percent (N = 11,102)	*p* Value (test)
FIM scores should decrease with increasing age or comorbidity	Age < 45: FIM = 101	17	None reported
	Age > 74: FIM = 92	33	
	Scores decreased with age monotonically		
	Comorbidity: FIM = 95	*	< 0.005 (ANOVA)
	No comorbidity: FIM = 97		
SCI client FIM scores should decrease with ascending injury level	Incomplete paraplegic: FIM = 105	(n = 786)	< 0.005 (ANOVA)
	Complete paraplegic: FIM = 97	†	
	Incomplete quadriplegic: FIM = 95		
	Complete quadriplegic: FIM = 72		
Right body–involved stroke patients should have lower FIM communication subscale scores than left body-involved patients	Right = 66	‡	< 0.005 (*t*-test)
	Left = 68		
	(admission scores reported)		

*The authors note that although a statistically significant difference was found, they could not ensure clinical significance; they stated that "a two point difference in FIM score based on comorbidity status is difficult to interpret clinically."[9]

†The authors identify some limitations in the classification of impairment categories used (eg, a person with an incomplete quadriplegia is not always more impaired than a person with a complete paraplegia). This clinical similarity may explain the small difference in discharge FIM scores of these two groups of patients (95 and 97).[9]

‡A total of 5,717 patients with stroke were included. The authors state that most score differences between right and left stroke patients were in the communication domain.[9]

Discriminant. Not available

Construct—Longitudinal/Sensitivity to Change
Not available

Interpretability

**General Population Values
(Customary or Normative Values)**
Not available

Typical Responsiveness Estimates

Individual Patient. There were significant improvements between admission and discharge FIM scores ($p < 0.0005$). Temporal changes between admission and discharge FIM scores were assessed by paired *t*-tests (Table 6).[9]

Sensitivity to change: Among clients with multiple sclerosis, total FIM effect size reported was 0.30 ($p < 0.0001$), FIM motor was 0.34 ($p < 0.0001$), and FIM cognitive was 0 (p value 0.961 was not significant).[26] Among clients with stroke, the total FIM effect size was 0.82, FIM motor was 0.91, and FIM cognitive was 0.61 ($p < 0.0001$ for all estimates).[26] The FIM sum score was weakly sensitive to clinical change (effect size 0.46; $p < 0.001$).[17] Many "motor" items (eating, grooming, sphincter control, bed and toilet transfer, and locomotion) were also weakly to moderately responsive (effect size 0.25 to 0.67; $p = 0.44$ to 0.039), but none of the cognitive items were responsive.[17]

Between Group. Not available

Other
The distribution of FIM scores in a multiple sclerosis sample was found to be skewed toward "normal," with a cluster about the "severely disabled" end of the scale, suggesting a ceiling and floor effect of the instrument.[17]

Comments

A modified version of this instrument is available for acute patients: the AlphaFIM™ system.[7] This measure seems best suited for classifying individuals regarding how much care they currently require or will require in the future.

Websites of Interest

- UDS_MR Website: www.udsmr.org
- C. Granger Web page: www.smbs.buffalo.edu/frp/HTML/284.HTM
- Center on Outcome Measurement in Brain Injury (COMBI): www.tbims.org/combi/list.html
- Quality Enhancement Research Initiative (QUERI) - Spinal Cord Injury (SCI): www.sci-queri.research.med.va.gov/fim.htm

TABLE 6 Change in Admission and Discharge FIM Scores[9]

Patient Populations	Admit	Discharge	Change
All patients	72	96	24
Traumatic brain injury	65	100	35
Spinal cord injury	71	97	26
Stroke	68	93	25
Cardiac	79	103	24
Orthopedic conditions	82	104	22
Other neurologic conditions	76	98	22
Rheumatoid arthritis	81	101	20
Amputee subjects	85	105	20
Osteoarthritis	93	112	19
Pulmonary	90	108	18
Low back pain	110	119	9

References

1. **Keith RA, Granger CV, Hamilton BB, Sherwin FS. The Functional Independence Measure: a new tool for rehabilitation. In: Eisenberg MG, Grzesiak RC, editors. Advances in clinical rehabilitation. New York: Springer Publishing Company; 1987. p. 6–18.**

2. COMBI. Functional Independence Measure: description, background, properties and references. The Center for Outcome Measurement in Brain Injury; 2000. http://www.tbims.org/combi/list.html

3. Granger CV. The emerging science of functional assessment: our tool for outcomes analysis. Arch Phys Med Rehabil 1998; 79:235–40.

4. Heinemann AW, Linacre JM, Wright BD, Hamilton BB, Granger CV. Relationships between impairment and physical disability as measured by the Functional Independence Measure. Arch Phys Med Rehabil 1993;74:566–73.

5. Veterans Affairs. Functional Independence Measure. http://www.sci-queri.research.med.va.gov/fim.htm. 2000.

6. Uniform Data System for Medical Rehabilitation. Guide for the Uniform Data Set for Medical Rehabilitation (UDS$_{MR}$). Version 5. Buffalo (NY): State University of New York at Buffalo; 1996.

7. Uniform Data System for Medical Rehabilitation. http://www.udsmr.org/. 2001.

8. Hamilton BB, Laughlin JA, Fiedler RC, Granger CV. Interrater reliability of the 7-level functional independence measure (FIM). Scand J Rehabil 1994;26:115–9.

9. Dodds TA, Martin TP, Stolov WC, Deyo RA. A validation of the functional independence measurement and its performance among rehabilitation inpatients. Arch Phys Med Rehabil 1993; 74:531–6.

10. Ottenbacher KJ, Hsu Y, Granger CV, Fiedler RC. The reliability of the functional independence measure: a quantitative review. Arch Phys Med Rehabil 1996;77:1226–32.

11. Chau N, Daler S, Andre JM, Patris A. Inter-rater agreement of two functional independence scales: the Functional Independence Measure (FIM) and a subjective uniform continuous scale. Disabil Rehabil 1994;16:63–71.

12. Ottenbacher KJ, Mann WC, Granger CV, Tomita M, Hurren D, Charvat B. Inter-rater agreement and stability of functional assessment in the community-based elderly. Arch Phys Med Rehabil 1994;75:1297–301.

13. Jaworski DM, Kult T, Boynton PR. The Functional Independence Measure: a pilot study comparison of observed and reported ratings. Rehabil Nur Res 1994;3:141–7.

14. Kidd D, Stewart G, Baldry J, Johnson J, Rossiter D, Petruckevitch A, et al. The Functional Independence Measure: a comparative validity and reliability study. Disabil Rehabil 1995;17:10–4.

15. Segal ME, Schall RR. Determining functional/health status and its relation to disability in stroke survivors. Stroke 1994;25:2391–7.

16. Brosseau L, Wolfson C. The inter-rater reliability and construct validity of the Functional Independence Measure for multiple sclerosis subjects. Clin Rehabil 1994;8:107–15.

17. Sharrack B, Hughes RAC, Soudain S, Dunn G. The psychometric properties of clinical rating scales used in multiple sclerosis. Brain 1999;122(Pt 1):141–59.

18. Segal ME, Ditunno JF, Staas WE. Interinstitutional agreement of individual functional independence measure (FIM) items measured at two sites on one sample of SCI patients. Paraplegia 1993;31:622–31.

19. Grey N, Kennedy P. The Functional Independence Measure: a comparative study of clinician and self ratings. Paraplegia 1993;31:457–61.

20. Smith PM, Illig SB, Fiedler RC, Hamilton BB, Ottenbacher KJ. Intermodal agreement of follow-up telephone functional assessment using the functional independence measure in patients with stroke. Arch Phys Med Rehabil 1996;77:431–5.

21. Granger CV, Hamilton BB, Keith RA, Zielezny M, Sherwins FS. Advance in functional assessment for medical rehabilitation. Top Geriatr Rehabil 1986;1:59–74.

22. Granger CV, Cotter AC, Hamilton BB, Fiedler RC, Hens MM. Functional assessment scales: a study of persons with multiple sclerosis. Arch Phys Med Rehabil 1990;71:870–5.

23. Corrigan JD, Smith-Knapp K, Granger CV. Validity of Functional Independence Measure for persons with traumatic brain injury. Arch Phys Med Rehabil 1997;78:828–34.

24. Corrigan JD, Granger CV, Smith K. Functional Assessment Scales: a study of persons with traumatic brain injury. J Rehabil Outcomes Measurement 2000;4:8–9.

25. Heinemann AW, Kirk P, Hastie BA, Semik P, Hamilton BB, Linacre JM, et al. Relationships between disability measures and nursing effort during medical rehabilitation for patients with traumatic brain and spinal cord injury. Arch Phys Med Rehabil 1997;78:143–9.

26. van der Putten JJ, Hobart JC, Freeman JA, Thompson AJ. Measuring change in disability after inpatient rehabilitation: comparison of the responsiveness of the Barthel Index and the Functional Independence Measure. J Neurol Neurosurg Psychiatry 1999; 66:480–4.

This measure or ordering information can be found at the Website address included in this review, or by contacting the developers.

FUNCTIONAL REACH (FR) TEST

Developers

P. W. Duncan, D. K. Weiner, J. Chandler, S. Studenski, Graduate Program in Physical Therapy and Centre for the Study on Aging and Human Development, Duke University; Veterans Administration Medical Center, Durham, North Carolina[1]

Purpose

To assess dynamic postural control for clinical use, which corresponded with center of pressure excursion during forward lean, a dynamic balance test requiring the use of sophisticated laboratory equipment. It was originally developed and tested among well individuals across a wide age range (21 to 87 years)[1] to identify community-dwelling elderly individuals at risk for recurrent falls[2] and to evaluate clinical change over time.[3]

Description

The FR test is a performance-based test to assess postural responses to voluntary movement performed during a daily activity.[1] It is a measurement of the maximal distance one can reach forward beyond arm's length (in the horizontal plane) while maintaining a fixed base of support in the standing position.

Conceptual/Theoretical Basis of Construct Being Measured

"Dynamic balance" is defined as the ability to maintain equilibrium in response to either self-motivated or external perturbation.

Groups Tested with This Measure

Community-living elderly,[2,4,5] frail elderly,[6] clients with multiple sclerosis (MS),[7] cerebrovascular accident (CVA),[8] hemiparesis,[9] traumatic brain injury (TBI),[10] low back pain,[11] Parkinson's disease (PD),[12,13] diabetes, transmetatarsal amputations,[14] healthy children,[15] children with balance dysfunction,[16] and children with lower extremity (LE) spasticity.[17]

Language

English

Application/Administration

A level yardstick is secured to a wall at the height of the individual's acromion. Individuals stand in a relaxed stance, make a fist, and raise their dominant arm until it is parallel with the yardstick (approximately 90 degrees of shoulder flexion). The placement of the end of the third metacarpal along the yardstick is recorded (position 1). Individuals then reach as far forward as they can without taking a step or touching the wall. The position of the third metacarpal along the yardstick is again recorded (position 2). No attempt is made to control the individual's method of reach. Two practice trials and three test trials are completed, with FR defined as the mean difference between positions 1 and 2 over the last three trials. Neither shoes nor socks are worn. Equipment and space needed include a yardstick and mounting materials, enough wall space to hang the yardstick, and floor area for the subject.

Typical Reliability Estimates

Internal Consistency
Not applicable

Interrater
ICC = 0.98 in healthy adults,[1] ICC = 0.98 in healthy children[15]

Test–Retest
ICC = 0.92 in healthy adults,[1] 0.75 in healthy children,[15] 0.98 in subjects with low back pain,[11] 0.89 in subjects with MS,[7] 0.84 in early and middle stages of PD,[12] 0.93 in PD and a history of falls,[13] 0.42 in PD and no history of falls,[13] and 0.62 among controls without neurologic impairment[13]

Other
Intrarater ICC = 0.92 not affected by cognitive impairment in community-dwelling, elderly subjects[19]; ICC = 0.87 to 0.98 among children with LE spasticity[17]

Typical Validity Estimates

Content
Not available

Criterion

Concurrent. Center of pressure excursion (difference between relaxed stance and maximum forward reach): $r = 0.71$.[1] Conversely, Wallman found no correlation between FR and anterior limits of stability in older nonfallers ($r = -0.009$) and fallers ($r = 0.17$).[21]

Predictive. A FR score of less than 6 inches predicted recurrent falls in elderly male veterans.[2] However, Brauer et al did not find FR to be predictive of falling in a 6-month prospective study of community-dwelling older women.[22]

Construct—Cross-sectional

Convergent

- Walking speed: $r = 0.71$ ($p < 0.05$) in community-dwelling seniors,[4] $r = 0.08$ ($p > 0.05$) in healthy elderly,[23] $r = 0.39$ ($p > .05$) in elderly with vestibular hypofunction[23]
- Tandem walking: $r = 0.67$[4]
- One foot standing: $r = 0.66$[4]
- Frailty scale: $r = -0.51$[19]
- Cumulative illness rating scale: $r = -0.24$[19]
- Older Americans Resources and Services Instrumental Activities of Daily Living (OARS-IADL): $r = 0.60$,[19] OARS-ADL: $r = 0.58$[19]
- Lawton-Brody IADL index: $r = 0.48$[4]
- Modified Katz PADL Index: $r = 0.65$[4]
- Mobility skills: $r = 0.65$[4]

Known Groups

- Lower scores for elderly fallers compared with nonfallers,[6] lower scores among persons with PD with a history of falls compared with persons with PD and no history of falls ($p < 0.05$) and control group ($p < 0.05$),[13] lower scores among persons with MS than controls (analysis of variance, $p = 0.12$).[7]
- Children with LE spasticity scored lower than age-related norms (percent difference 25.9 to 47.8)[17]
- FR did not distinguish between a group with low back pain and controls ($F_{1,72} = 2.07$, $p = 0.155$).[11]

Discriminant. Not available

Construct—Longitudinal/Sensitivity to Change Estimates

Convergent

- The change score correlation between FR and other physical performance variables was modest for mobility skills (0.38; $p = 0.01$) and Functional Independence Measure (FIM) (0.37; $p = 0.02$) and poor for walking time (–0.20; $p > 0.05$).[3]
- Correlation between postural sway indices and FR was 0.03 to 0.21 among TBI patients following rehabilitation.[10]
- Correlation of baseline FR with change in FR among subjects with multiple rehabilitative diagnoses: $r = 0.38$.[3]

Known Groups

- Greater FR change score in veterans (multiple diagnoses) following rehabilitation compared to a control group.[3]
- Improvement found in FR scores following rehabilitation among subjects with a CVA.[8]
- No improvement in FR scores following rehabilitation among subjects with TBI.[10]

Discriminant

- Not available

Other Validity Estimates

- Lower scores on FR as age increases ($p < 0.05$) and height decreases ($p < 0.05$)[1,20]

Interpretability

General Population: Adult Means[1]

- 20 to 40 years: males 16.73 in ± 1.94 (n = 16); females 14.64 in ± 2.18 (n = 28)
- 41 to 69 years: males 14.98 in ± 2.21 (n = 22); females 13.81 in ± 2.2 (n = 28)
- 70 to 87 years: males 13.16 in ± 1.55 (n = 20); females 10.47 in ± 3.5 (n = 14)

General Population: Child Means[15]

- 5 to 6 years: 21.17 cm; 95% CI 16.79 to 24.91
- 7 to 8 years: 24.21 cm; 95% CI 20.56 to 27.96
- 9 to 10 years: 27.97 cm; 95% CI 25.56 to 31.64
- 11 to 12 years: 32.79 cm; 95% CI 29.68 to 36.18
- 13 to 15 years: 32.30 cm; 95% CI 29.58 to 36.08

Responsiveness Estimates

Individual Patient. Not available

Between Group

- Responsiveness Index = 0.97 (change due to treatment = 2 inches); 21 subjects per group needed to detect a meaningful difference in performance.[3]

Other

- FR has a floor effect (35.9% of community-dwelling population of seniors over 65 years were unable or unwilling to complete the test or could not safely perform the test).[19]

Comments

The FR test is not a feasible measure for use in representative studies of elderly people, particularly those with cognitive impairment.[19] People with spinal cord injuries have been tested in a seated position using a modified FR.[3]

References

1. **Duncan PW, Weiner DK, Chandler J, Studenski S. Functional reach: a new clinical measure of balance. J Gerontol 1990;45:M192–7.**

2. Duncan PW, Studenski S, Chandler J, Prescott B. Functional reach: predictive validity in a sample of elderly male veterans. J Gerontol 1992;47:M93–8.

3. Weiner DK, Bongiorni DR, Studenski SA, Duncan PW, Kochersberger GG. Does functional reach improve with rehabilitation? Arch Phys Med Rehabil 1993;74:796–800.

4. Daubney ME, Culham EG. Lower-extremity muscle force and balance performance in adults aged 65 years and older. Phys Ther 1999;79:1177–85.

5. O'Brien K, Culham E, Pickles B. Balance and skeletal alignment in a group of elderly female fallers and nonfallers. J Gerontol A Biol Sci Med Sci 1997;52:B221–6.

6. **Weiner DK, Duncan PW, Chandler J, Studenski SA. Functional reach: a marker of physical frailty. J Am Geriatr Soc 1992; 40:203–7.**

7. Frzovic D, Morris ME, Vowels L. Clinical tests of standing balance: performance of persons with multiple sclerosis. Arch Phys Med Rehabil 2000;81:215–21.

8. Hill K, Ellis P, Bermjardt J, Maggs P, Hull S. Balance and mobility outcomes for stroke patients: a comprehensive audit. Aust J Phys Ther 1997;43:173–80.

9. Fishman MN, Colby LA, Sachs LA, Nichols DS. Comparison of upper-extremity balance tasks and force platform testing in persons with hemiparesis. Phys Ther 1997;77:1052–62.

10. Wade LD, Canning CG, Fowler V, Felmingham KL, Baguley IJ. Changes in postural sway and performance of functional tasks during rehabilitation after traumatic brain injury. Arch Phys Med Rehabil 1997;78:1107–11.

11. Simmonds MJ, Olson SL, Jones S, Hussein T, Lee CE, Novy D, et al. Psychometric characteristics and clinical usefulness of physical performance tests in patients with low back pain. Spine 1998;23:2412–21.

12. Schenkman M, Cutson TM, Kuchibhatla M, Chandler J, Pieper C. Reliability of impairment and physical performance measures for persons with Parkinson's disease. Phys Ther 1997;77:19–27.

13. Smithson F, Morris ME, Iansek R. Performance on clinical tests of balance in Parkinson's disease. Phys Ther 1998;78:577–92.

14. Mueller MJ, Salsich GB, Strube MJ. Functional limitations in patients with diabetes and transmetatarsal amputations. Phys Ther 1997;77:937–43.

15. Donahoe B, Turner D, Worrell T. The use of Functional Reach as a measurement of balance in boys and girls without disabilities: ages 5-15 years. Pediatr Phys Ther 1994;6:189–93.

16. Wheeler A, Shall M, Lewis A, Sheperd J. The reliability of measurements obtained using Functional Reach in children with cerebral palsy aged 3-16 years. Pediatr Phys Ther 1996;8:182–3.

17. Niznik TM, Turner D, Worrell TW. Functional Reach as a measurement of balance for children with lower extremity spasticity. Phys Occup Ther Pediatr 1995;15:1–15.

18. Lynch SM, Leahy P, Barker SP. Reliability of measurements obtained with a modified Functional Reach test in subjects with spinal cord injury. Phys Ther 1998;78:128–33.

19. Rockwood K, Awalt E, Carver D, MacKnight C. Feasibility and measurement properties of the Functional Reach and the Timed Up and Go tests in the Canadian Study of Health and Aging. J Gerontol A Biol Sci Med Sci 2000;55:M70–3.

20. Franzen H, Hunter H, Landreth C, Reling G, Greenberg M, Canfield J. Comparison of functional reach in fallers and nonfallers in an independent retirement community. Phys Occupat Ther Geriatr 1998;15:33–41.

21. Wallmann HW. Comparison of elderly nonfallers and fallers on performance measures of functional reach, sensory organization, and limits of stability. J Gerontol A Biol Sci Med Sci 2001; 56:M580–3.

22. Brauer SG, Burns YR, Galley P. A prospective study of laboratory and clinical measures of postural stability to predict community-dwelling fallers. J Gerontol A Biol Sci Med Sci 2000; 55:M469–76

23. Wernick-Robinson M, Krebs DE, Giorgetti MM. Functional Reach: does it really measure dynamic balance? Arch Phys Med Rehabil 1999;80:262–9.

To obtain this measure, contact the developers, or it can be found in references 1 and 6.

151

GAIT SPEED

Developers

Unknown

Purpose

Gait speed is a temporal distance parameter that has been traditionally measured in the laboratory setting to quantify one aspect of normal and pathologic gait.[1]

Description

Gait speed is based on the performance of individuals on a timed walk test. It is computed by dividing the distance a person walks by the time it takes him/her to cover that distance. Thus, gait speed is commonly reported in units of meters/second (m/s), feet/second, centimeters/second, or meters/minute.

Conceptual/Theoretical Basis of Construct Being Measured

Gait speed is not a construct but a physical characteristic derived from directly measuring the parameters of distance and time. Different authors refer to gait speed as an indicator of "walking ability,"[2] "activity of daily living (ADL) function,"[3] and "mobility."[4] Gait speed is distinguished from tests that record the distance walked in a set period of time, such as the 2-, 6-, and 12-Minute Walk Tests,[5] which were originally developed to evaluate exercise tolerance.

Groups Tested with This Measure

Gait speed has been used extensively in many populations that include individuals with acute[6–8] and chronic stroke,[9] multiple sclerosis,[10] lower limb amputation,[11] rheumatoid arthritis,[12] osteoarthritis,[13] Alzheimer's disease,[14] spinal cord injury,[15,16] renal transplantation,[17] Parkinson's disease,[18] and cerebral palsy.[19] It has also been used in healthy adult[20] and elderly individuals.[3,21,22]

Languages

Canadian English and Canadian French instructions for the 5-m and 10-m walk tests performed at a comfortable and maximum pace have recently been published.[8]

Application/Administration

In the clinical setting, testing usually takes less than 1 minute and is conducted in a quiet location. The middle test distance of a longer walkway typically ranges from 2 to 20 m[3,4,8,13,14] and may be marked on the floor. Acceleration and deceleration distances commonly range from 1 to 3 m,[8,23–27] and these are also marked. A pylon placed at the finish line may provide an easily visualized goal.[8] The subject wears supportive footwear and comfortable clothing and may walk with his/her usual orthosis and/or ambulatory aid. Standardized instructions to walk at a "comfortable," "preferred," "normal," or "maximum" speed are given. Timing procedures vary, but in one report,[8] the evaluator walked alongside the subject and began timing with a digital stopwatch when the subject's first foot crossed the start line. Timing was stopped when the first foot crossed the stop line, although the subject continued to walk the final deceleration distance. Gait speed can then be computed manually by dividing the test distance by the time in seconds that the subject has taken to walk that distance. In the laboratory setting, electronic timing methods are used.[6,20]

Typical Reliability Estimates

Unless otherwise specified, values are for "comfortable" or "normal" gait speed.

Internal Consistency
Not applicable

Interrater and Test-Retest
See Table 1.

TABLE 1 Interrater and Test–Retest Reliability

Population	Test Distance	Interrater Reliability	Test Distance	Test–Retest Reliability (time interval between assessments)
Stroke			6 m	$r = 0.93$, ICC = 0.92 (1-day interval)[28]
			10 m	ICC = 0.96 (1-wk intervals)[29]
			5 m, 5 m, and return	$r = 0.95$ to 0.99 (interval varied from 1 to 3 wk)[30]
			8 m	ICC = 0.99 (1-day interval)[31]
	10 m	$r = 0.99$[2]	10 m	$r = 0.89$ to 0.90 (interval not reported)[2]
	6.1 m	$r = 1.00$[24]	6.1 m	$r = 0.97$ (15-min interval)[24]
Osteoarthritis of the knee	8 m			NGS: ICC = 0.88 to 0.94
				FGS: ICC = 0.91 to 0.95 (1-wk intervals)[13]
Alzheimer's disease	25 ft (7.6 m)	ICC = 0.83 to 0.94[14]		
Rheumatoid arthritis			2 m	Best 95% CI - ICC reported NGS: 0.94 to 0.99
				FGS:0.90 to 0.98 (1-wk intervals)[12]
Healthy individuals			25 feet (7.6 m)	CGS: ICC = 0.90
				MGS: ICC = 0.91 (2 consecutive tests)[32]

NGS = normal gait speed; FGS = fast gait speed; CGS = comfortable gait speed; MGS = maximum gait speed.

Typical Validity Estimates

Unless otherwise specified, values are for "comfortable" or "normal" gait speed.

Content

Not applicable

Criterion

Gait speed has been used as the gold standard to validate numerous outcome measures in different patient populations. A comprehensive appraisal of this literature, however, is beyond the scope of this review.

Construct—Cross-sectional

Convergent. Among Healthy Individuals Aged 20 to 79 Years[32]
- Age: CGS $r = -0.1$, MGS $r = -0.56$
- Gender: CGS $r = 0.08$, MGS $r = 0.16$
- Weight: CGS $r = 0.07$, MGS $r = 0.09$
- Height: CGS $r = 0.22$, MGS $r = 0.32$
- Strength of four lower extremity muscles: CGS $r = 0.19$ to 0.25, MGS $r = 0.29$ to 0.50

Among Elderly Individuals
- Exercise tolerance (6-Minute Walk Test): $r = 0.73$ (retirement home residents and community center participants)[21]
- Strength of five lower extremity muscles: CGS $r = 0.07$ to 0.31, MGS $r = 0.08$ to 0.37[22]

Among Individuals with Renal Transplantation[17]
- Repetitions of sit-to-stand-to-sit: CGS $r = 0.41$, MGS $r = 0.74$

- Nondominant knee extension force: CGS $r = 0.33$, MGS $r = 0.54$
- Dominant knee extension force: CGS $r = 0.31$, MGS $r = 0.54$

Among Individuals with Stroke
- Strength of the affected lower extremity: CGS $r = 0.25$ to 0.67,[26,31,33] MGS $r = 0.76$, 0.85[26,27]
- Cadence and stride length: MGS $r = 0.75$ to 0.94[25]
- Balance (Balance Scale): $r = 0.60$[34]
- Degree of lower extremity motor recovery (Fugl-Meyer Assessment of Sensorimotor Recovery): $r = 0.62$[34]
- Functional mobility (Timed Up and Go): $r = -0.61$[35]

Correlations have been reported between gait speed and numerous temporal, kinematic, power, and work variables measured for each lower extremity.[36] These include proportion of time spent in stance ($r = -0.52$ to -0.77), maximum flexion of the knee during swing phase ($r = 0.32$ to 0.49), and maximum ankle power bilaterally ($r = 0.75$), among others.[36]

Known Groups. Among Elderly Individuals
- Degree of habitual activity at home, $p < 0.05$[38]
- Use of ambulatory aids, $p < 0.01$[38]
- Discharge destination, $p < 0.01$[39]

Among Individuals with Stroke
- Degree of independence in walking ability, $p < 0.001$[23]

TABLE 2 One to Five Weeks Post Stroke[8]

Walk Test	SRM (95% CI)	ES
5 m, Comfortable speed	1.22 (0.93, 1.50)	0.83
5 m, Maximum speed	1.00 (0.68, 1.30)	0.66
10 m, Comfortable speed	0.92 (0.64, 1.18)	0.74
10 m, Maximum speed	0.83 (0.52, 1.12)	0.55

SRM = standardized response mean; ES = effect size.

Discriminant. Not available

Construct—Longitudinal/Sensitivity to Change
Not available

Other Validity Coefficients
Among Individuals with Stroke
- Sensitivity to change of gait speed in acute stroke patients participating in a randomized controlled pilot trial of early, intensive, task-specific gait therapy: effect size = 0.58[6]
- See Table 2

Among Inpatients of Rehabilitation Facilities[41]
- 6m, comfortable speed: SRM 1.17; Guyatt's Change Index 3.41; Norman's S Coefficients ICC = 0.57

Interpretability

Age- and gender-specific norms for healthy individuals walking at slow, comfortable, and maximum speeds are available.[20,22,32] It has also been report-ed that in large American cities, walking speeds ranging from 0.71 and 1.38 m/s are required to cross street intersections. Ranges for smaller cities have also been provided.[41]

Typical Responsiveness Estimates

Individual Patient. Table 3 presents the limits of repeat-ed measurement error when measuring gait speed in different populations. In repeated testing, patients must demonstrate a change greater than the lower limit provided for this to be considered an important deterioration. Conversely, patients must demonstrate a change greater than the upper limit provided for this to be considered an important improvement.

Standard deviations of change in normal and fast gait speed in stable subjects with rheumatoid arthri-tis have been reported to indicate the responsive-ness of gait speed in this patient population.[12]

Between Group. Not available

TABLE 3 Limits of Repeated Measurement Error When Measuring Gait Speed in Different Populations

Population	Speed	Confidence Interval (%)	Limits of Repeated Measurement Error
Stroke	Comfortable	95	−0.11 m/s to 0.17 m/s[42]
Oteoarthritis of the knee	Normal	90	−0.12 to 0.12 m/s[13]
	Fast	90	−0.12 to 0.12 m/s[13]

References

1. Murray MP. Gait as a total pattern of movement. Am J Phys Med 1967;46:290–333.
2. Wade DT, Wood VA, Heller A, Maggs J, Langton, Hewer R. Walking after stroke. Measurement and recovery over the first 3 months. Scand J Rehabil Med 1987;19:25–30.
3. Potter JM, Evans AL, Duncan G. Gait speed and activities of daily living function in geriatric patients. Arch Phys Med Rehabil 1995;76:997–9.
4. Wade DT. Measurement in neurological rehabilitation. New York: Oxford University Press; 1996.
5. Butland RJ, Pang J, Gross ER, Woodcock AA, Geddes DM. Two-, six-, and 12-minute walking tests in respiratory disease. BMJ 1982;284:1607–8.
6. Richards CL, Malouin F, Wood-Dauphinee S, Williams JI, Bouchard JP, Brunet D. Task-specific physical therapy for opti-mization of gait recovery in acute stroke patients. Arch Phys Med Rehabil 1993;74:612–20.

7. Duncan P, Richards L, Wallace D, Stoker-Yates J, Pohl P, Luchies C, et al. A randomized, controlled pilot study of a home-based exercise program for individuals with mild and moderate stroke. Stroke 1998;29:2055–60.

8. Salbach NM, Mayo NE, Higgins J, Ahmed S, Finch LE, Richards CL. Responsiveness and predictability of gait speed and other disability measures in acute stroke. Arch Phys Med Rehabil 2001;82:1204–12.

9. Dean CM, Richards CL, Malouin F. Task-related circuit training improves performance of locomotor tasks in chronic stroke: a randomized, controlled pilot trial. Arch Phys Med Rehabil 2000;81:409–17.

10. Taylor PN, Burridge JH, Dunkerley AL, Wood DE, Norton JA, Singleton C, et al. Clinical use of the Odstock dropped foot stimulator: its effect on the speed and effort of walking. Arch Phys Med Rehabil 1999;80:1577–83.

11. Boonstra AM, Fidler V, Eisma WH. Walking speed of normal subjects and amputees: aspects of validity of gait analysis. Prosthet Orthot Int 1993;17:78–82.

12. Fransen M, Edmonds J. Gait variables: appropriate objective outcome measures in rheumatoid arthritis. Rheumatology 1999; 38:663–7.

13. Fransen M, Crosbie J, Edmonds J. Reliability of gait measurements in people with osteoarthritis of the knee. Phys Ther 1997;77:944–53.

14. Tappen RM, Roach KE, Buchner D, Barry C, Edelstein J. Reliability of physical performance measures in nursing home residents with Alzheimer's disease. J Gerontol A Biol Sci Med Sci 1997;52:M52–5.

15. Ladouceur M, Barbeau H. Functional electrical stimulation-assisted walking for persons with incomplete spinal injuries: longitudinal changes in maximal overground walking speed. Scand J Rehabil Med 2000;32:28–36.

16. Melis EH, Torres-Moreno R, Barbeau H, Lemaire ED. Analysis of assisted-gait characteristics in persons with incomplete spinal cord injury. Spinal Cord 1999;37:430–9.

17. Bohannon RW, Smith J, Hull D, Palmeri D, Barnhard R. Deficits in lower extremity muscle and gait performance among renal transplant candidates. Arch Phys Med Rehabil 1995; 76:547–51.

18. Stolze H, Kuhtz-Buschbeck JP, Drucke H, Johnk K, Illert M, Deuschl G. Comparative analysis of the gait disorder of normal pressure hydrocephalus and Parkinson's disease. J Neurol Neurosurg Psychiatry 2001;70:289–97.

19. White R, Agouris I, Selbie RD, Kirkpatrick M. The variability of force platform data in normal and cerebral palsy gait. Clin Biomechanics 1999;14:185–92.

20. Oberg T, Karsznia A, Oberg K. Basic gait parameters: reference data for normal subjects, 10-79 years of age. J Rehabil Res Dev 1993;30:210–23.

21. Harada ND, Chiu V, Stewart AL. Mobility-related function in older adults: assessment with a 6-minute walk test. Arch Phys Med Rehabil 1999;80:837–41.

22. Bohannon RW, Andrews AW, Thomas MW. Walking speed: reference values and correlates for older adults. J Orthopaed Sports Phys Ther 1996;24:86–90.

23. Holden MK, Gill KM, Magliozzi MR. Gait assessment for neurologically impaired patients. Standards for outcome assessment. Phys Ther 1986;66:1530–9.

24. Holden MK, Gill KM, Magliozzi MR, Nathan J, Piehl-Baker L. Clinical gait assessment in the neurologically impaired. Reliability and meaningfulness. Phys Ther 1984;64:35–40.

25. Nakamura R, Handa T, Watanabe S, Morohashi I. Walking cycle after stroke. Tohoku J Exp Med 1988;154:241–4.

26. Bohannon RW, Walsh S. Nature, reliability, and predictive value of muscle performance measures in patients with hemiparesis following stroke. Arch Phys Med Rehabil 1992;73:721–5.

27. Suzuki K, Nakamura R, Yamada Y, Handa T. Determinants of maximum walking speed in hemiparetic stroke patients. Tohoku J Exp Med 1990;162:337–44.

28. Evans MD, Goldie PA, Hill KD. Systematic and random error in repeated measurements of temporal and distance parameters of gait after stroke. Arch Phys Med Rehabil 1997;78:725–9.

29. Liston RA, Brouwer BJ. Reliability and validity of measures obtained from stroke patients using the Balance Master. Arch Phys Med Rehabil 1996;77:425–30.

30. Collen FM, Wade DT, Bradshaw CM. Mobility after stroke: reliability of measures of impairment and disability. Int Disabil Stud 1990;12:6–9.

31. Bohannon RW, Andrews AW. Correlation of knee extensor muscle torque and spasticity with gait speed in patients with stroke [published erratum appears in Arch Phys Med Rehabil 1990;71:464]. Arch Phys Med Rehabil 1990;71:330–3.

32. Bohannon RW. Comfortable and maximum walking speed of adults aged 20-79 years: reference values and determinants. Age Ageing 1997,26:15–9.

33. Bohannon RW. Strength of lower limb related to gait velocity and cadence in stroke patients. Physiother Can 1986;38:204–6.

34. Richards CL, Malouin F, Dumas F, Tardif D. Gait velocity as an outcome measure of locomotor recovery after stroke. In: Craik RL, Oatis C, editors. Gait analysis: theory and application. St. Louis: Mosby; 1995. p. 355–64.

35. Podsiadlo D, Richardson S. The Timed "Up & Go": a test of basic functional mobility for frail elderly persons. J Am Geriatr Soc 1991;39:142–8.

36. Olney SJ, Griffin MP, Monga TN, McBride ID. Work and power in gait of stroke patients. Arch Phys Med Rehabil 1991;72:309–14.

37. Olney SJ, Griffin MP, McBride ID. Temporal, kinematic, and kinetic variables related to gait speed in subjects with hemiplegia: a regression approach. Phys Ther 1994;74:872–85.

38. Imms FJ, Edholm OG. Studies of gait and mobility in the elderly. Age Ageing 1981;10:147–56.

39. Friedman PJ. Gait recovery after hemiplegic stroke. Int Disabil Stud 1990;12:119–22.

40. Goldie PA, Matyas TA, Evans OM. Deficit and change in gait velocity during rehabilitation after stroke. Arch Phys Med Rehabil 1996;77:1074–82.

41. Robinett CS, Vondran MA. Functional ambulation velocity and distance requirements in rural and urban communities. A clinical report. Phys Ther 1988;68:1371–3.

This measure can be found in reference 8.

GROSS MOTOR FUNCTION MEASURE (GMFM)

Developers

For GMFM-88: D. Russell, P. Rosenbaum, C. Gowland, S. Hardy, M. Lane, N. Plews, H. McGavin, D. Cadman, and S. Jarvis. For GMFM-66: D. Russell, P. Rosenbaum, L. Avery, and M. Lane, canchild@mcmaster.ca

Purpose

To assess change in gross motor function for children with cerebral palsy (CP). It is used for both research and clinical purposes.

Description

There is the original 88-item GMFM (GMFM-88)[1,2] and the newer 66-item measure (GMFM-66).[3,4] The original GMFM is a performance-based measure arranged into five dimensions: (1) lying and rolling; (2) crawling and kneeling; (3) sitting; (4) standing; and (5) walking, running, and jumping. Each item is scored on a 4-point scale (0 to 3) with specific descriptors for scoring items contained in a manual. Percent scores are calculated within each dimension and averaged to obtain a total score that ranges from 0 to 100. For children with Down syndrome, the authors advocate an alternate scoring method incorporating parent report of activities that the child can do but are not demonstrated during the assessment.[5] The GMFM-66 was developed using Rasch analysis and identifies 66 of the original 88 items that form a unidimensional construct. The item scoring is the same as for the GMFM-88; however, the scores must be entered into a computer program (called the Gross Motor Ability Estimator) for analysis and conversion to an interval-level total score. The user-friendly program allows tracking of clients over time and plots scores on an item map; it provides estimates of the standard error and 95% confidence interval around the total score and calculates change scores between assessments.

Conceptual/Theoretical Basis of Construct Being Measured

The GMFM is a criterion-referenced measure designed to evaluate gross motor function skills that are observable and important and have the potential to change over time.

Groups Tested with This Measure

Children with CP, Down syndrome,[5] and osteogenesis imperfecta.[6] The GMFM-88 has been used (but not validated) for children with developmental delay, acquired brain injury, and acute lymphoblastic leukemia. The GMFM-66 is designed for use only with children with CP because the item weights are derived from a large sample of children with CP and may be different for children with other diagnoses.

Languages

English. The GMFM-88 has been translated (and back-translated for verification) into French, Dutch, German, and Japanese.

Application/Administration

The GMFM is designed for use by pediatric therapists familiar with assessing the motor skills of children. Children perform gross motor tasks identified in the administration and scoring guidelines. The original validation sample included children 5 months to 16 years old, but the GMFM is appropriate for children whose motor skills are at or below those of a 5 year old without any motor difficulties. Administration of the measure takes approximately 45 to 60 minutes. A mat, bench, toys, and access to stairs (with at least five steps) are required. The GMFM-66 should take less time to administer than the GMFM-88. The GMFM-66 requires a computer scoring program that provides an estimate of the child's gross motor ability even when all of the items have not been administered. The more items tested, the more accurate is the estimate. Training is not required; however, evidence from evaluating training workshops has shown improved reliability of workshop participants following training.[7] A CD-ROM self-teaching program is available with the GMFM-88 and GMFM-66 user's manual.[3]

Typical Reliability Estimates

Internal Consistency

Established with the GMFM-66 using Rasch analysis by demonstrating the unidimensionality of the measure (removing items with a standardized infit statistic > 3.0 until less than 5% of the items misfit) and satisfying the assumptions of sample-free and test-free measurement.[3]

Interrater

- ICCs = 0.87 to 0.99[1]
- When comparing therapist versus expert scoring of a videotaped GMFM assessment κw = 0.58 to 0.86 pretraining and 0.82 to 0.93 following training were obtained.[7] Spearman rank order correlations ranged from 0.75 to 0.99.[8]

Test–Retest

ICCs = 0.92 to 0.99[1] and 0.76 to 1.00.[9] Physical therapists with no previous experience with the GMFM rating videotaped assessments of items from the first three dimensions over two time points had a rank order correlation of 0.68.[10]

Typical Validity Estimates

Content

Items were selected based on a review of the literature and clinical judgment. Face validity was established by pediatric therapists at two children's treatment centers who provided feedback on early versions of the measure.

Criterion

No gold standard exists for the attribute being measured.

Construct—Cross-sectional

Convergent

- GMFM-88 scores and the Gross Motor Function Classification System (GMFCS) $r = -0.91$.[11]
- GMFM-88 scores and gait parameters showed cadence (0.79) and normalized velocity (0.72)[12]
- Gait velocity and GMFM scores in dimension D (standing) ($r = 0.91$) and dimension E (walking, running and jumping) ($r = 0.93$).[13]

Known Groups and *Discriminant* are not available.

Construct—Longitudinal/Sensitivity to Change

Convergent. Correlation of change on the GMFM-88 with change as judged by parents (0.54), by the child's treating therapist (0.65), and by a "masked" videotape-based evaluation (0.82).[1] For a sample of children with spastic diplegia, correlations of change in GMFM-88 score with a "masked" videotape-based evaluation were 0.66 at 12 months and 0.79 at 24 months follow-up.[14]

Known Groups. There was a gradient of change as hypothesized between a "large change" group (children recovering from acute brain injury), a

"moderate change" group (young children < 5 years old without motor disabilities), and a "small change" group of children with CP. There was a significant difference between the GMFM-88 change scores of older (3 to 5 years old) and younger (< 3 years) children without motor disabilities as hypothesized ($t (29) = 4.5$, $p < 0.05$).[1]

Discriminant. A two-way analysis of variance of age (< 3 years, 3 to 5 years, ≥ 6 years) and severity groups (mild/moderate/severe) for children with CP showed an age by severity interaction ($F_{4,101} = 2.49$, $p < 0.05$), indicating that the change in each age group was dependent on the severity of motor disability.[1]

Interpretability

General Population Values
(Customary or Normative Values)

The GMFM manual provides tables of GMFM-88 and GMFM-66 scores and change scores for a sample of children with CP (N = 652) broken down by age and severity.[3]

Typical Responsiveness Estimates

Individual Patient. The GMFM-66 has a computer scoring program that calculates the child's score and the 95% confidence intervals around the score. Error is specific to a child's score and is larger at the extremes of the scale (eg, for GMFM-66 scores of 0 and 100, the standard error of measurement is 8.36 and 8.24, respectively) and lower for total GMFM-66 scores in the middle of the scale (eg, for a GMFM-66 score of 50, the standard error of measurement is 1.18).

Between Group. Initial validation of the GMFM-88[1] examined responsiveness over 6 months by contrasting change scores between stable (mean change = 1.3) and responsive groups (mean change = 6.2) ($p < 0.01$). The GMFM-88 has been used to evaluate a variety of interventions including physiotherapy (PT)[15] [significant change of 4.3 in favor of goal-directed PT versus generalized PT over 2 weeks ($p < 0.05$, 95% CI = −0.134 to 8.542)], therapeutic electrical stimulation[16] [mean change of 5.5 over 1 year in the treatment group versus 1.9 in the control ($p < 0.001$)], and surgical intervention (rhizotomy). A summary of five studies (total 99 cases) showed mean improvement in GMFM-88 scores ranging from 3.2 to 12.1.[17]

Comments

The recent application of Rasch analysis to convert the ordinal scaling to an interval measure with fewer items (GMFM-66) should improve the interpretability of scores, allow for the use of more robust parametric statistics, and improve the overall clinical utility.

References

1. Russell D, Rosenbaum P, Cadman D, Gowland C, Hardy S, Jarvis S. The Gross Motor Function Measure: a means to evaluate the effects of physical therapy. Dev Med Child Neurol 1989;31:341–52.

2. Russell D, Rosenbaum P, Gowland C, Hardy S, Lane M, Plews N, et al. The Gross Motor Function Measure Manual. 2nd ed. Hamilton (ON): CanChild Centre for Childhood Disability Research, IAHS, McMaster University; 1993.

3. Russell D, Rosenbaum P, Avery L, Lane M. "Gross Motor Function Measure (GMFM-66 and GMFM-88) User's Manual." Clinics in Developmental Medicine No. 159. London: Mac Keith Press. In press. 2002.

4. Russell DJ, Avery LM, Rosenbaum PL, Raina PS, Walter SD, Palisano RJ. Improved scaling of the Gross Motor Function Measure for children with cerebral palsy: evidence of reliability and validity. Phys Ther 2000;80:873–85.

5. Russell D, Palisano R, Walter S, Rosenbaum P, Gemus M, Gowland C, et al. Evaluating motor function in children with Down syndrome: validity of the GMFM. Dev Med Child Neurol 1998;40:693–701.

6. Ruck-Gibis J, Plotkin H, Hanley J, Wood-Dauphinee S. Reliability of the Gross Motor Function Measure for children with osteogenesis imperfecta. Physiother Can 2001;53:S16.

7. Russell DJ, Rosenbaum PL, Lane M, Gowland C, Goldsmith CH, Boyce WF, et al. Training users in the Gross Motor Function Measure: methodological and practical issues. Phys Ther 1994;74:630–6.

8. Bjornson KF, Graubert CS, McLaughlin JF, Astley SJ. Inter-rater reliability of the Gross Motor Function Measure. Dev Med Child Neurol 1994;36 Suppl 70:27–8.

9. Bjornson KF, Graubert CS, McLaughlin JF, Kerfeld CI, Clark EM. Test-retest reliability of the Gross Motor Function Measure in children with cerebral palsy. Phys Occup Ther Pediatr 1998;18:51–61.

10. Nordmark E, Hagglund G, Jarnlo GB. Reliability of the Gross Motor Function Measure in cerebral palsy. Scand J Rehabil Med 1997;29:25–8.

11. Palisano RJ, Hanna SE, Rosenbaum PL, Russell DJ, Walter SD, Wood EP, et al. Validation of a model of gross motor function for children with cerebral palsy. Phys Ther 2000;80:974–85.

12. Damiano DL, Abel MF. Relation of gait analysis to gross motor function in cerebral palsy. Dev Med Child Neurol 1996; 38:389–96.

13. Drouin LM, Malouin F, Richards C, Marcoux S. Correlation between the Gross Motor Function Measure scores and gait spatiotemporal measures in children with neurological impairments. Dev Med Child Neurol 1996;38:1007–19.

14. Bjornson KF, Graubert CS, Burford VL, McLaughlin JF. Validity of the Gross Motor Function Measure. Pediatr Phys Ther 1998;10:43–7.

15. Bower E, McLellan DL, Arney J, Campbell MJ. A randomised controlled trial of different intensities of physiotherapy and goal-setting procedures in 44 children with cerebral palsy. Dev Med Child Neurol 1996;38:226–37.

16. Steinbok P, Reiner A, Kestle J. Therapeutic electrical stimulation following selective dorsal rhizotomy in children with spastic diplegic cerebral palsy: a randomised clinical trial. Dev Med Child Neurol 1997;39:515–20.

17. Steinbok P. Outcomes after selective dorsal rhizotomy for spastic cerebral palsy. Childs Nerv Syst 2001;17:1–18.

For a copy of the measure and guidelines, contact www. cambridge.org/medicine/mackeith and quote ISBN 1 898 683 298.

GROSS MOTOR PERFORMANCE MEASURE (GMPM)

Developers

The Gross Motor Measures Group: W. Boyce,* C. Gowland,[†] S. Hardy,[‡] M. Lane,[†] N. Plews,[†] C. Goldsmith,[†] and D. Russell.[†] Affiliated with *Queen's University, Kingston, Ontario; [†]McMaster University, Hamilton, Ontario; and [‡]Bloorview MacMillan Children's Centre, Toronto, Ontario

Purpose

To evaluate quality of movement of children (infancy through adolescence) with cerebral palsy (CP) and to assess change over time. The GMPM was designed as an evaluative measure to be used in both clinical practice and research.[1]

Description

A performance-based measure that was developed as a companion measure to the Gross Motor Function Measure (GMFM)[2] to evaluate how well a child is able to perform a subgroup of 20 items from the GMFM. There are four items each from the GMFM's lie, sit, kneel, stand, and walk dimensions. Performance is assessed for five quality attributes: alignment, coordination, dissociated movement, weight shift, and stability. Each attribute is scored using an attribute-specific 5-point degree of difficulty response scale that varies from severely abnormal to consistently normal performance. Average attribute and total scores are calculated as percentages and can vary from a minimum score of 20%, indicating that a child had a severely abnormal quality of movement on all items performed, to 100%, indicating that the child has consistently normal performance for each attribute on all 20 items.

Conceptual/Theoretical Basis of Construct Being Measured

It is based on inductive grounded theory, combining theory, clinical observation, and research and expert opinion (described by its authors as a clinical epidemiology approach to measurement).[3]

Groups Tested with This Measure

Children with CP (mild to severe disability),[4–6] acquired brain injury,[4,6] or no disability.[4,6]

Language

English

Application/Administration

The physical therapist (PT) or occupational therapist (OT) conducts a practice trial and three test trials for each of the GMPM's items, observing all three quality attributes each time and then scoring average performance. The child's GMFM must have been recently completed prior to the GMPM administration. The child is assessed on only the GMPM items that he/she was at least able to initiate. The time to administer varies from 45 to 60 minutes.[1] If necessary, the assessment can be done over two sessions within the same week. Equipment needed is the GMPM test manual,[1]* a mat, a small bench, a table, small toys, and a stopwatch. Physical or occupational therapists, experienced in working with children with neuromotor conditions, should have passed criterion testing on the GMFM. GMPM training is recommended but not essential.[1] GMPM training and criterion testing have been done in the past by the Gross Motor Measures Group at McMaster University in a 1- or 2-day workshop format (a fee is charged for training and testing). Missing scores (owing to an inability to initiate the item or behavioral issues) are scored as a 5 and subtracted from the denominator of the raw score calculation.

Typical Reliability Estimates

Internal Consistency

Not available

---

*The GMPM test manual can be obtained from Dr. William Boyce, School of Rehabilitation Therapy, Faculty of Health Sciences, Queen's University, Kingston, ON K7L 3N6; 613-533-6000, ext. 77405; boycew@post.queensu.ca for $30 US plus $10 US handling charges. It is permissible to photocopy score sheets.

Test–Retest

Children with CP (n = 25), acquired brain injury (n = 1), or no disability (n = 2), aged 1 to 10 years, assessed by one PT assessor twice over a 2-week retest interval[4]: attribute scales ICC = 0.89 to 0.96 and total score ICC = 0.96 (95% CI: 0.93 to 0.98).

Interrater

Children with CP (same sample as the test–retest evaluation) were assessed simultaneously by two PTs (one handling and one observing) at the time of the repeat GMPM[4]: attribute scales ICC = 0.84 to 0.94 and total score ICC = 0.92 (95% CI: 0.85 to 0.97). Ambulatory children with CP (n = 36) were assessed by a PT and kinesiologist in the sit, crawl/kneel, stand, and walk dimensions of the GMPM: ICCs for GMPM dimensions = 0.67 for the crawl/kneel dimension to 0.88 for the stand dimension; kappa estimates = 0.53 for the crawl/kneel dimension to 0.68 for the walk dimension. For the quality attributes, ICCs = 0.79 for alignment to 0.86 for stability; kappa estimates = 0.64 for alignment to 0.66 for dissociation. For the 20 individual items, ICCs = 0.20 to 1.00, and kappa estimates = 0.11 to 0.77. The two assessors' reliability scores for individual items tended to improve over the 3 years of the study (ie, from fair/good to excellent).[5]

Other

Live performance and a videotape of the same assessment performance were scored by the same PT, separated by an 8-week period (same sample as the test–retest evaluation)[4]: attribute scales ICC = 0.90 to 0.97 and total score ICC = 0.96 (95% CI: 0.92 to 0.98).

Typical Validity Estimates

Content

Evaluated through Delphi consensus methodology with a panel of 13 experts in developmental therapy and research.[7] Clarity, completeness, and potential for evaluation of change were confirmed. Face validity: confirmed by nominal group process meetings with therapists and Q-sort tasks.[7]

Criterion

No gold standard exists for the attribute being assessed.

Construct—Cross-sectional

Convergent. Not available

Known Groups. The GMPM was able to differentiate between children with mild (n = 23), moderate (n = 53), and severe impairment (n = 23) (F = 62.8; $p = 0.0001$).[6]

Discriminant. There was moderate to strong correlation between GMFM and GMPM total scores for children without disability and those with CP ($r = 0.64$ and 0.72, respectively).[6] There was no correlation between GMFM and GMPM scores in the acquired brain injury group ($r = 0.18$).[6]

Construct—Longitudinal/Sensitivity to Change

Convergent. The group of children (n = 60) rated by therapists as having changed showed change on total GMPM score (F = 12.3; $p < 0.001$) from first to second assessment, whereas the stable group's (n = 36) scores were unchanged (F = 2.13; $p = 0.15$).[6] There was no comparable relationship between parents' ratings of change and GMPM score changes, with the groups designated by parents as stable (n = 17) and changed (n = 66) on the GMPM both showing change (minimum F = 8.97; maximum $p < 0.01$).[6]

Known Groups. The GMPM was able to differentiate between different magnitudes of change for a variety of severity and age group comparisons (eg, younger children changed less than older children).[6] In a diagnostic group comparison, GMPM scores changed for children with CP over a 1-month retest interval (t[98] = 3.79; $p = 0.003$) and for children with acquired brain injury (t[16] = 3.22; $p = 0.005$) and did not change for children without a disability (t[26] = 2.02; $p = 0.05$).[6]

Discriminant. There was a lack of relationship change between GMFM total change scores and GMPM total change scores in the three diagnostic groups (maximum $r < 0.25$), supporting the authors' hypothesis that function and quality are different constructs.[6]

Interpretability

General Population Values (Customary or Normative Values)
Not available

Typical Responsiveness Estimates
Not available

Comments

The GMPM has started to appear in publications about the effectiveness of rehabilitation interventions in CP,[8,9] but, for the most part, studies that evaluate motor function following spasticity-reducing procedures such as rhizotomy or botulinum toxin injections rely on the GMFM to assess changes in motor function and do not tackle the quality of movement issue. Potential limitations of the GMPM in terms of responsiveness, interpretation of changes in scores over time, and difficulties with the scoring algorithm have been noted.[10] An expanded version of the GMPM (contact Virginia Wright, vwright@bloorviewmacmillan.on.ca) focusing on evaluating all of the stand and walk/run/jump dimension items from the GMFM is in the process of development and testing. This version will be targeted for use with children with CP who are ambulatory and are undergoing interventions (rehabilitation or spasticity-reducing procedures) that may have considerable impact on quality of movement as well as on gross motor abilities. Some of the issues in scoring protocols that were noted by Sienko Thomas et al[5] in their reliability work will be addressed in the expanded GMPM.

References

1. Boyce W, Gowland C, Rosenbaum P, Hardy S, Lane M, Plews N, et al. Gross Motor Performance Measure manual. Kingston (ON): Queen's University, School of Rehabilitation Therapy; 1998.

2. Russell DJ, Rosenbaum PL, Cadman DT, Gowland C, Hardy S, Jarvis S. The Gross Motor Function Measure: a means to evaluate the effects of therapy. Dev Med Child Neurol 1989;31:341–52.

3. Boyce W, Gowland C, Hardy S, Rosenbaum P, Lane M, Plews N, et al. Development of a quality of movement measure for children with cerebral palsy. Phys Ther 1991;71:802–32.

4. Gowland C, Boyce WF, Wright V, Russell DJ, Goldsmith CH, Rosenbaum PL. Reliability of the Gross Motor Performance Measure. Phys Ther 1995;75:597–602.

5. Sienko Thomas S, Buckon C, Aiona MD, Sussman MD, Phillips DS. Interobserver reliability of the Gross Motor Performance Measures: preliminary results. Dev Med Child Neurol 2001;43:97–102.

6. Boyce WF, Gowland C, Rosenbaum PL, Lane M, Plews N, Goldsmith CH, et al. The Gross Motor Performance Measure: validity and responsiveness of a measure of quality of movement. Phys Ther 1995;75:603–13.

7. Boyce W, Gowland C, Russell D, Goldsmith C, Rosenbaum P, Plews N, et al. Consensus methodology in the development and content validation of a Gross Motor Performance Measure. Physiother Can 1993;45:94–100.

8. Bower E, Michell D, Burnett M, Campbell MJ, McLellan DL. Randomized controlled trial of physiotherapy in 56 children with cerebral palsy followed for 18 months. Dev Med Child Neurol 2001;43:4–15.

9. Buckon CE, Sienko Thomas S, Jakobson-Huston S, Moor M, Sussman M, Aiona M. Comparison of three ankle-foot orthosis configurations for children with spastic hemiplegia. Dev Med Child Neurol 2001:43:371–8.

10. Boyce W, King C, Olney S. Evaluating instruments of motor assessment in international practice. La Riabilitazione del Bambino con Paralisi Cerebrale 1998;2 Suppl:17–34.

To obtain the measure and the test manual, see ordering information at the bottom of page 159.

HEALTH UTILITIES INDEX (HUI)

Developers

G. W. Torrance, M. Boyle, D. Feeny, W. Furlong, www.healthutilities.com

Purpose

The HUI Mark1 system was developed for use in evaluating outcomes for very low birthweight infants.[1,2] It was then modified to assess the health status of survivors of childhood cancer, becoming the HUI Mark2 and one of the first systems with a set of preferences for the seven-attribute system.[3] This second version was subsequently adapted for use in population health surveys and became the HUI Mark3.[4] This final version can be used to describe and monitor the health of the general population. The HUI is designed to provide a single summary score of health-related quality of life that can then be transposed into quality weights for calculating quality-adjusted life-years.[2,4] For this reason, it can be used as an outcome in cost effectiveness and cost utility analyses.

Description

The HUI is a generic multiattribute system for the assessment of health status. In its latest combined version, the HUI Mark2/3 covers nine attributes: emotion, cognition, self-care, pain, vision, hearing, speech, ambulation, and dexterity.

Each attribute contains between four and six levels of ability. Each possible combination of response choice describes a health state. Using a scoring algorithm, each health state is then assigned a utility value that ranges from 0 (worst possible health state) to 1.0 (best possible health state). The scoring algorithm integrates general population preference weights obtained from using the standard gamble technique.

Conceptual/Theoretical Basis of Construct Being Measured

The developers agree that health status is multidimensional, yet they narrowed their definition of health status to physical and emotional dimensions, excluding social interactions, which they felt were "outside the skin" of the construct being measured.[2] Assessment of the different attributes is based on capacity rather than performance.[4] The HUI is based on multiattribute utility theory, which allows the estimation of preference scores for all of the possible health states generated by the multiattribute index.

Groups Tested with This Measure

First developed for neonatal intensive care infants, it has been extensively used in childhood cancers. The latest versions of the HUI have been used in arthritis, asthma, Alzheimer's disease, multiple sclerosis, human immunodeficiency virus (HIV), and stroke. The HUI systems (HUI Mark2, HUI Mark3, HUI Mark2/3) can be used in any population aged 5 years and over.[5] The Website provides an exhaustive list of clinical areas or health problems that have used the HUI.

Languages

The HUI was originally developed in Canadian English. The English version has been successfully used in the United Kingdom, the United States, and Australia. The HUI has been translated in French (Canadian and European), Spanish, German, Italian, Dutch, and Japanese (refer to Website for other languages presently in the process of translation).

Application/Administration

The HUI has three modes of administration: self-report, face-to-face interview, and telephone interview. The HUI Mark2/3 version comprises 10 domains, covered on 41 questions. The HUI uses a "skip pattern," thus reducing the number of questions for a person with few health problems. When used with the general population, it is estimated to take 8 to 10 minutes if the questionnaire is self-completed and 3 to 5 minutes if it is interviewer based. With face-to-face interviews, stroke subjects take approximately 20 minutes to complete the HUI Mark2/3.[6] A choice of four recall periods (usual, 1 week, 2 weeks, 4 weeks) is available for each questionnaire. Values from any HUI versions typically range from 0 to 1, where 0 represents the worst possible health state and 1 the best possible state.

Typical Reliability Estimates

Internal Consistency

Not available

Interrater

- General population[7] (HUI Mark2): kappa = 0.29 on emotion and 0.31 on pain domains (respondent-proxy)
- Intensive care unit childhood[8] (HUI Mark2): ICC = 0.82 to 0.96 on the different domains (parents-investigator), 0.34 (emotional domain) to 0.89 (parents-clinician), 0.39 (emotional domain) to 0.93 (clinician-investigator)
- Stroke[6] (HUI Mark2/3): ICC = 0.39 (pain domain) to 0.81 (patient-caregiver) (HUI Mark2) and 0.63 (pain and cognition domains) to 0.78 (patient-caregiver) (HUI Mark3)

Test–Retest

- General population[2,9] (HUI Mark2): kappa = 0.53 on emotion and 0.47 on pain domains; ICC = 0.77 at 1 month[4]
- Lupus[10] (HUI Mark2): kappa = 0.32 (pain domain) to 0.88 on the different domains at 2- to 4-week intervals
- Musculoskeletal disorders[11] (HUI Mark2): ICC = 0.78 at 1 to 6 weeks

Typical Validity Estimates

Content

All levels on every attribute appearing at least once in a general population health survey support the content validity.[2]

Criterion

No gold standard measure exists.

Construct—Cross-sectional

Convergent. In lupus patients,[10] domains of HUI Mark2 correlated moderately with related domains of the 36-Item Short-Form Health Survey (SF-36), for example, Mobility with Physical Function (0.61) and Emotion with Role Emotional (0.66).

Known Groups. The HUI Mark3 was found to distinguish between stroke and arthritic subjects (mean utility score was 0.538 for stroke compared with 0.765 for arthritis). The main differences were for ambulation and cognition that were more severely affected in stroke. No differences were seen for pain.[12]

Discriminant. In lupus clients,[10] SF-36 sensation and general health domains: $r = 0.08$, SF-36 mental health: $r = 0.05$

Construct—Longitudinal/Sensitivity to Change

Not available

Interpretability

General Population Values (Customary or Normative Values)

The HUI Mark2/3 has population-based utility weights. These weights provide a standard set of utility values for HUI-generated health states. For example, mean HUI Mark3 scores for persons with stroke were estimated from a general population survey as 0.68 compared with 0.58 for someone with Alzheimer's disease.[13] A move of 0.03 to 0.06 on the overall utility score has been identified as a clinically important change in health-related quality of life.[9]

Typical Responsiveness Estimates

Standardized response mean = 0.57, and standardized effect size = 0.40 among injured workers with musculoskeletal disorders who improved over 3 to 6 weeks following return to work or a physiotherapy program (HUI2).[11]

Comments

The HUI is a comprehensive, generic measure of health-related quality of life. Although evidence of validity is gathering in various population groups, further knowledge is required regarding its validity for use as an outcome measure in rehabilitation. In addition, a computerized program is essential to calculate the utility value of a health state. The HUI may therefore not be readily accessible for day-to-day clinical practice.

References

1. Feeny D, Torrance G, Furlong W. Health Utilities Index. In: Spilker B, editor. Quality of life and pharmacoeconomics in clinical trials. 2nd ed. Philadelphia: Lippincott-Raven Press; 1996. p. 239–52.

2. Feeny D, Furlong W, Boyle M, Torrance GW. Multi-attribute health status classification systems: Health Utilities Index. Pharmacoeconomics 1995;7:490–502.

3. Cadman D, Goldsmith C. Construction of social values or utility-based health indices: the usefulness of factorial experimental design plans. J Chron Dis 1986;39:643–51.

4. Torrance GW, Furlong W, Feeny D, Boyle M. Multi-attribute preference functions: Health Utilities Index. Pharmacoeconomics 1995;7:503–20.

5. Furlong W, Feeny D, Torrance GW, Barr D. The Health Utilities Index (HUI) system for assessing health-related quality of life in clinical studies. Ann Med 2001;33:375–84.

6. Mathias S, Bates M, Pasta D, Cisternas M, Feeny D, Patrick D. Use of the Health Utilities Index with stroke patients and their caregivers. Stroke 1997;28:1888–94.

7. Grootendorst P, Feeny D, Furlong W. Does it matter whom and how you ask? Inter- and intra-rater agreement in the Ontario Health Survey. J Clin Epidemiol 1997;50:127–35.

8. Gemke R, Bonsel G. Reliability and validity of a comprehensive health status measure in a heterogeneous population of children admitted to intensive care. J Clin Epidemiol 1996;49:327–33.
9. Samsa G, Edelman D, Rothman M, Williams G, Lipscomb J, Matchar D. Determining clinically important differences in health status measures: a general approach with illustration using the Health Utilities Index Mark II. Pharmacoeconomics 1999;15:141–55.
10. Moore A, Clarke A, Danoff D, Joseph L, Bélisle P, Neville C, et al. Can health utility measures be used in lupus research? A comparative validation and reliability study of 4 utility indices. J Rheumatol 1999;26:1285–90.

11. Beaton D, Hogg-Johnson S, Bombardier C. Evaluating changes in health status: reliability and responsiveness of five generic health status measures in workers with musculoskeletal disorder. J Clin Epidemiol 1997;50:79–93.
12. Grootendorst P, Feeny D, Furlong W. Health Utilities Index Mark 3: evidence of construct validity for stroke and arthritis in a population health survey. Med Care 2000;38:290–9.
13. Mittman N, Trakas K, Risebrough N, Liu B. Utility scores for chronic conditions in a community-dwelling population. Pharmacoeconomics 1999;15:369–76.

This measure or ordering information can be found at the Website address included in this review.

LOWER EXTREMITY ACTIVITY PROFILE (LEAP)

Developers

Elspeth Finch and Deborah Kennedy.[1,2] Contact: Deborah Kennedy, Research Associate/Clinical Coordinator of Inpatient Rehabilitation, Centre for Studies of Physical Function, Orthopaedic and Arthritic Institute, 43 Wellesley Street East, Toronto, Ontario M4Y 1H1, e- mail: d.kennedy@utoronto.ca

Purpose

To measure health status related to lower extremity function[1,2]; originally developed for clients with lower extremity osteoarthritis (OA).

Description

The LEAP is a 23-item self-administered condition-specific questionnaire designed to assess perceived difficulty and satisfaction within the activity categories of self-care and mobility and the participation categories of household, work, leisure, and social activities. Questions concerning pain severity and frequency, the effect and subsequent satisfaction of knee disability on emotional health, sleep and rest patterns, and appearance are also included. Two items are descriptive questions regarding work and leisure activities. There is a visual analogue scale (VAS) response version (using a 10-cm horizontal VAS with terminal descriptors) and a numeric rating scale version (using a 0 to 10 scale with terminal descriptors). A score of 10 represents maximal difficulty, complete dissatisfaction, and maximal pain; 0 represents no pain or difficulty and full satisfaction. A total LEAP score and aggregate difficulty, satisfaction, and pain scores are calculated by summing the related scores in each category and dividing the total by the number of items used.

Conceptual/Theoretical Basis of Construct Being Measured

The LEAP was developed to reflect the physical, emotional, and social components of lower extremity function and to address both the individual's difficulty and satisfaction with their ability in these domains. It recognizes the importance of both the disability and handicap domains of the original International Classification of Impairment, Disability, and Handicap model.

Groups Tested with This Measure

Individuals with end-stage hip or knee OA and total knee arthroplasty (TKA). Also used but not validated in those individuals with patellofemoral disorders, rheumatoid arthritis, and traumatic injuries of the lower extremity.

Language

English

Application/Administration

The questionnaire requires individuals to think about their function over the previous week. In a more chronic population, this time frame can be changed to 1 month. A full explanation of format and examples should be reviewed with the respondent. Responses reflecting only lower extremity disability should be emphasized. Respondents must be able to read and comprehend English and be mentally competent to complete the questionnaire. The questionnaire takes approximately 20 minutes to complete and 5 minutes to score.

Typical Reliability Estimates

Internal Consistency
Cronbach's alpha = 0.73

Interrater
Not applicable

Test–Retest
Not available

Typical Validity Estimates

Content
Original categories and items were based on the MACTAR Patient Preference Disability Questionnaire, originally developed from patient interviews.

Criterion
No gold standard exists for the attribute being assessed.

Construct—Cross-sectional

Convergent. LEAP scores preoperatively ($\leq$ 1 month before surgery) showed low to moderate correlations ($r = 0.21$ to 0.37) with physical performance measures (Fast Self-Paced Walk [SPW], Timed Up and Go, and Stair Performance Measure) in TKA and total hip arthroplasty (THA) candidates.[3] LEAP scores 1 year post-TKA showed moderate correlations with normal and fast SPW velocity (0.41 to 0.71)[2] and with stair performance time (0.62 to 0.71).[2]

Known Groups and *Discriminant* are not available.

Construct—Longitudinal/Sensitivity to Change

Convergent. Sensitivity to change was demonstrated in TKA and THA clients preoperatively to 3 months postoperatively in all categories and subscales of the LEAP ($0.001 < p < 0.01$).[1]

Known Groups and *Discriminant* are not available.

Interpretability

General Population Values (Customary or Normative Values)
The scores of healthy males aged 63.6 ± 6.3 and healthy females aged 61.9 ± 4.5 years for difficulty, pain, and satisfaction are available.[2]

Typical Responsiveness Estimates
Not available

Comments
The LEAP has been mainly used with the THA and TKA populations. In a recent study,[3] preoperative LEAP quartile values on more than 1,800 TKA and THA subjects were provided according to gender and group for comparative purposes.

References
1. Finch E, Kennedy D. The Lower Extremity Activity Profile: a health status instrument for measuring lower extremity disability. Physiother Can 1995;47:239–46.
2. Finch E, Walsh M, Thomas SG, Woodhouse LJ. Functional ability perceived by individuals following total knee arthroplasty compared to age-matched individuals without knee disability. J Orthopaed Sports Phys Ther 1998;27:255–63.
3. Kennedy D, Stratford PW, Pagura SMC, Walsh M, Woodhouse LJ. Comparison of gender and group differences in self-report and physical performance measures in total hip and knee arthroplasty candidates. J Arthroplasty 2002;17:70–7.

This measure (NRS version) can be found on the accompanying CD-ROM. Prior to using the measure, you are strongly advised to contact the developers for administration and scoring guidelines and revisions to the measure not available at time of publication. To obtain the VAS version, contact the developers.

LOWER EXTREMITY FUNCTIONAL SCALE (LEFS)

Developers

J. Binkley and P. Stratford[1]

Purpose

To assess functional status in clients with musculoskeletal conditions of the lower extremity for both clinical decision making on individual clients and as an outcome measure for clinical research.

Description

The LEFS is a 20-item self-report condition-specific functional status measure intended for clients with musculoskeletal conditions of the lower extremity. Each item is scored on a 5-point scale (0 to 4). Total LEFS scores can vary from 0, the lowest functional level, to 80, the highest functional level.

Conceptual/Theoretical Basis of Construct Being Measured

The conceptual basis for functional status is not addressed. The conceptual basis for initial development of the LEFS is defined as the need for a measure of functional status that is easy to administer and score, applicable to a wide range of clients with lower extremity orthopedic conditions, and appropriate for clinical decision making and research.[1]

Groups Tested with This Measure

Outpatients with acute and chronic musculoskeletal conditions of the lower extremity (sample included only two clients with hip problems)[1] and clients following total hip and knee joint arthroplasty attending an outpatient physical therapy rehabilitation program.[2]

Language

English

Application/Administration

The LEFS is a self-report measure in which clients respond by circling relevant responses for each of 20 items. Responses range from 0 (extreme difficulty or inability to perform activity) to 4 (no difficulty). Most clients can complete the LEFS in 3 to 5 minutes. The score is the sum of the numbered responses and can be determined by the clinician in approximately 30 seconds without computational aids.

Typical Reliability Estimates

Internal Consistency
- 0.93 to 0.96[1,2]

Interrater
Not applicable

Test–Retest
R = 0.85[1,2] (lower 95% CI 0.80[1] and 0.69[2]) and R = 0.94 in a subset of clients with more chronic conditions.[1]

Typical Validity Estimates

Content
No reference in the literature.

Criterion
No gold standard exists for the construct being measured.

Construct—Cross-sectional

Convergent. Correlation with the 36-Item Short Form Health Survey (SF-36) Physical Function subscale was 0.80[1] and with Functional Independence Measure (FIM) ambulation was 0.45.[2] Correlations with functional performance measures such as Timed Up and Go of 0.51 and a Pooled Index of Function (FIM, Timed Up and Go, Pain, 6-Minute Walk Test) of 0.68.[2]

Known Groups. Capable of discriminating between acute and chronic ($F_{2,28} = 3.8$),[1] surgery/no surgery patient subgroups ($F_{1,41} = 7.8$),[1] and clients receiving/not receiving home care ($t_{56} = 2.19$)

Discriminant. Correlations with SF-36 Mental Health subscale and Mental Component summary score: 0.23 to 0.30.

Construct—Longitudinal/Sensitivity to Change

Convergent. Change score correlation with SF-36 Physical Function subscale of 0.57[1] and Pooled Index of Function of 0.64.[2] Correlation with prognostic rating of change: $r = 0.36$.[1]

Known Groups and *Discriminant* are not available.

Interpretability

General Population Values
(Customary or Normative Values)
Not available

Typical Responsiveness Estimates

Individual Patient

- Confidence in a measured score: ± 6 scale points (90% CI)
- True change estimates: MDC_{90} = 9 points (90% of stable clients display a difference of less than 9 LEFS points on retest)
- Minimal clinically important difference: 9 LEFS points

Between Group. Not available

Other

No ceiling or floor effect reported; appears to be applicable to all levels of function.[1,2]

References

1. Binkley JM, Stratford PW, Lott SA, Riddle DL, and the North American Orthopaedic Rehabilitation Research Network. The Lower Extremity Functional Scale (LEFS): scale development, measurement properties and clinical application. Phys Ther 1999;79:371–83.

2. Stratford PW, Binkley JM, Watson J, Heath-Jones T. Validation of the LEFS on patients with total joint arthroplasty. Physiother Can 2000;52:97–105.

This measure can be found on the accompanying CD-ROM. Prior to using the measure, you are strongly advised to contact the developers for administration and scoring guidelines and revisions to the measure not available at time of publication.

MOTOR ASSESSMENT SCALE (MAS)

Developers

Janet H. Carr and Roberta B. Shepherd

Purpose

The MAS was developed to assess individuals with stroke using relevant and functional motor activities. It was designed for clinical practice and research.[1]

Description

The MAS is a performance-based measure and consists of eight items intended to measure motor function and one item related to muscle tone on the affected side. Each item is scored on a 7-point scale from 0 to 6. The motor functions tested are (1) supine to side lying, (2) supine to sitting over the side of the bed, (3) balanced sitting, (4) sitting to standing, (5) walking, (6) upper arm function, (7) hand movements, and (8) advanced hand activities. The category of general tonus was included to gain an impression about the presence of excessive or depressed motor activity. For all items except general tonus, a score of 6 indicates the optimal motor behavior. For general tonus, a score of 4 indicates a consistently normal response; more than 4 points indicates persistent hypertonus and less than 4 points indicates various degrees of hypotonus.[1]

A modified version of the MAS has also been developed (MMAS). The modifications of item descriptions were made by S. C. Loewen and reviewed by three physical therapists experienced in the care of stroke clients. The item for general tonus was removed from the MMAS owing to the subjective nature of muscle tone testing. This modified version is still scored on a 7-point scale from 0 to 6.[2]

Conceptual/Theoretical Basis of Construct Being Measured

The developers' aim was to address the concern that existing assessments were too time consuming for clinical practice and lacked numeric scoring and that some assessments were based on an assumption that recovery is initially characterized by stereotyped movements performed within flexor and extensor synergies, which may not always be the case. The measure is based on the principles guiding the Motor Relearning Program for treating stroke clients.[3,4]

Groups Tested with This Measure

Individuals with stroke with various degrees of disability at different periods of recovery,[1] in rehabilitation[5] and hospital settings.

Languages

Australian English.[1] They have also been translated into French and were tested in preliminary trials.[3]

Application/Administration

Criteria for each point on the MAS are provided to assist the examiners in reliably grading the performance of each item together with general rules for administering the MAS. This measure takes approximately 15 minutes to administer.[1]

Typical Reliability Estimates

Internal Consistency

Not available

Interrater

Interrater reliability of the MAS and MMAS was assessed in three separate studies:

1. *MAS*: Five subjects at various stages of recovery were selected for interrater reliability testing. The assessments were videotaped, and a time was visible on the tape. Twenty physical therapists and physical therapy undergraduate students were raters (general tonus excluded), r = 0.89 to 0.99.[1]

2. *MAS*: Twenty-four individuals with stroke; the post-stroke average time was 12 months. Two examiners observed and scored each subject independently. Correlation for the total MAS was 0.99 and ranged from 0.92 to 1.0 for the individual items, excluding general tonus, which was 0.29.[5]

3. *MMAS*: Seven hospitalized subjects with stroke were assessed by a trained physical therapist, and the assessments were videotaped. Another 14 trained physical therapists rated the seven videotaped assessments. Mean kappa coefficients for the total MMAS ranged from 0.79 to 0.96, and Spearman's rank-order correlation coefficients ranged from 0.88 to 1.0. For the individual items, the mean kappas ranged from 0.56 (balanced sitting) to 1.0 (hand movements and advanced hand activities).[2]

Test–Retest

1. *MAS*: Fourteen individuals, an average of 55 months post stroke, were evaluated by the same rater on two occasions separated by 4 weeks. Test–retest correlations ranged from 0.87 to 1.0, with an average correlation of 0.98.[1]

2. *MMAS*: The procedure was the same as for the MAS above, but, in addition, the videotaped assessments were rated 1 month later by the 14 therapists. Mean kappa coefficients for the total MMAS ranged from 0.72 to 0.97, and Spearman's rank-order correlation coefficients ranged from 0.81 to 1.0. For the individual items, the Kendell's tau rank-order correlation coefficients were all significant except for 4% of the 112 values.[2]

Typical Validity Estimates

Content
Carr and Shepherd based items and scoring options on observations of the progress of a large number of patients. No formal content validation is available.[1]

Criterion

Concurrent
Not available

Predictive
Individual items from MMAS have been shown to be good predictors of stroke outcome; for example, arm function scores at 1 week and 1 month were a good predictor of functional arm recovery at discharge from the medical or rehabilitation ward.[6] See Table 1.

Construct—Cross-sectional

Convergent
Study 1 assessed the validity of the MAS compared to the Fugl-Meyer Assessment (FM) early after stroke (mean time post stroke = 64.5 days) and reported high and significant Spearman's correlations for total scores as well as for individual items, except for balanced sitting.[3] Study 2 assessed the validity of the MAS compared to the FM in a more chronic group and found similar results.[5]

TABLE 1 Spearman Correlations of MMAS Scores of Stroke Patients at Discharge from Rehabilitation with Other Measures

	MMAS	Barthel Index	Walking Component MMAS	Walking Component Barthel Index	Upper Arm Function	Combined Arm Score
Balanced sitting						
1 wk	0.81	0.72	0.71	NS	—	—
1 mo	0.74	0.72	NS	NS	—	—
Sitting to standing						
1 wk	0.75	NS	NS	NS	—	—
1 mo	NS	0.77	NS	0.71	—	—
Combined arm score						
1 wk	0.80	NS	NS	NS	NS	0.86
1 mo	0.90	NS	NS	NS	NS	0.94
Upper arm function						
1 wk	—	—	—	—	0.84	0.81
1 mo	—	—	—	—	0.91	0.87

NS = not significant.

TABLE 2 Validity Estimates of MAS Compared to FM

MAS	FM	Spearman's Correlation Study 1 (n = 32)	Study 2 (n = 30)
Total MAS (excluding general tonus)	Total FM: upper and lower motor + balance + sensation	0.96*	0.88‡
Total MAS (excluding general tonus)	Upper and lower motor + balance	0.91*	Not assessed
Walking (item 5)	Lower motor + standing balance	0.79*	0.64‡
Walking (item 5)	Lower motor	0.65*	Not assessed
Walking (item 5)	Standing balance	Not assessed	0.64‡
Upper extremity total (items 6, 7, 8)	Upper motor	0.93*	0.91‡
Upper extremity proximal (item 6)	Upper motor proximal (shoulder, elbow, and forearm)	0.92*	0.89‡
Upper extremity distal (items 7 and 8)	Upper motor distal (wrist and hand)	0.89*	0.92‡
Balanced sitting (item 3)	Sitting balance	−0.10	0.28
Sitting to standing (item 4)	Standing balance	0.69†	0.77‡

*$p < 0.001$; †$p < 0.002$; ‡$p < 0.01$.

FM = Fugl-Meyer Assessment of Sensorimotor Recovery After Stroke.

In addition to the data in Table 2, results from study 1 indicated that FM sensation scores of light touch (0.64) and position sense (0.67) correlated with MAS balance score but not with FM balance items (0.12 and −0.10, respectively).

Known Groups and *Discriminant* are not available.

Construct—Longitudinal/Sensitivity to Change
Not available

Other Validity Coefficients
1. A study that assessed change in scores on each item of the MAS between admission and discharge from rehabilitation found that there were statistically significant differences between mean scores after an average of 71 days of rehabilitation, as shown in Table 3.[7]

TABLE 3

Item	Admission Mean ± SD	Discharge Mean ± SD
1	4.0 ± 2.6	5.3 ± 1.7
2	4.5 ± 2.1	5.5 ± 1.4
3	4.3 ± 1.6	5.3 ± 1.1
4	2.6 ± 2.1	4.5 ± 1.9
5	2.3 ± 2.4	4.1 ± 1.9
6	3.0 ± 2.5	4.3 ± 2.2
7	2.8 ± 2.6	3.9 ± 2.6
8	2.3 ± 2.7	3.4 ± 2.8

2. A moderate and statistically significant correlation ($r = 0.45$, $p < 0.01$) was found between the number of repetitions of a weight-bearing exercise (designed to strengthen the leg extensor muscles) and the change in the MAS score for the walking item among 25 subjects in inpatient rehabilitation. To be included in the study, subjects had to have a score greater than 0 but less than 6 on the walking item.[8]

Interpretability

General Population Values (Customary or Normative Values)
Not available

Typical Responsiveness Estimates
Not available

Comments
Other studies have used the MAS to quantify motor function when evaluating issues related to stroke rehabilitation[9] and the use of health services after discharge from the hospital.[10]

References
1. Carr JH, Shepherd RB, Nordholm L, Lynne D. Investigation of a new motor assessment scale for stroke patients. Phys Ther 1985;65:175–80.
2. Loewen SC, Anderson BA. Reliability of the Modified Motor Assessment Scale and the Barthel Index. Phys Ther 1988;68:1077–81.

3. Malouin F, Pichard L, Bonneau C, Durand A, Corriveau D. Evaluating motor recovery early after stroke: comparison of the Fugl-Meyer Assessment and the Motor Assessment Scale. Arch Phys Med Rehabil 1994;75:1206–12.

4. Carr J, Shepherd R. Neurologic rehabilitation: optimizing motor performance. Boston: Butterworth Heinemann; 1998.

5. Poole JL, Whitney SL. Motor Assessment Scale for stroke patients: concurrent validity and interrater reliability. Arch Phys Med Rehabil 1988;69:195–7.

6. Loewen SC, Anderson BA. Predictors of stroke outcome using objective measurement scales. Stroke 1990;21:78–81.

7. Dean C, Mackey F. Motor Assessment Scale scores as a measure of rehabilitation outcome following stroke. Aust Physiother 1992;38:31–5.

8. Nugent JA, Schurr KA, Adams RD. A dose-response relationship between amount of weight-bearing exercise and walking outcome following cerebrovascular accident. Arch Phys Med Rehabil 1994;75:399–402.

9. Esmonde T, McGinley J, Wittwer J, Goldie P, Martin C. Stroke rehabilitation: patient activity during non-therapy time. Aust J Physiother 1997;43:43–51.

10. Geerts MJP, De Witte LP, Visser-Meily JMA, Tilli DJP, Lindeman E, Bakx WGM. Daily functioning during the first year after stroke: living arrangements and use of rehabilitation and other care facilities after discharge from hospital. J Rehabil Sci 1995; 8:39–45.

This measure can be found in reference 1.

NECK DISABILITY INDEX (NDI)

Developers

H. Vernon and S. Mior[1]; Dr. H. Vernon, Division of Research, Canadian Memorial Chiropractic College, Toronto, Ontario M4G 3E6

Purpose

To assess pain-related disability associated with activities of daily living in persons with neck pain.

Description

The NDI consists of 10 items. Each item is scored on a 6-point scale (0 to 5). Higher scores represent more disability. Total scores can vary from 0 to 50, and some authors have elected to present the score as a percentage.

Conceptual/Theoretical Basis of Construct Being Measured

None reported

Groups Tested with This Measure

Acute, subacute, and chronic neck pain client groups; various conservative, surgical, and behavioral intervention groups.

Language

English

Application/Administration

Most clients can complete this measure in less than 3 minutes. Clinicians can score the measure without the use of computational aids in less than 20 seconds.

Typical Reliability Estimates

Internal Consistency

Coefficient alpha values: 0.80 to 0.87.[1,2]

Interrater

Not applicable

Test–Retest

ICC: 0.89 to 0.94[1–3]

Typical Validity Estimates

Content

No reference to content validity in the literature

Criterion

No gold standard exists for the construct being measured.

Construct—Cross-sectional

Convergent

- Correlation with pain intensity: 0.44 to 0.60[1,3]
- Correlation with pain limitation: 0.74 to 0.79[3]
- Correlation with Patient Specific Functional Scale (PSFS) activities: 0.73 to 0.81[3]
- Correlation with 36-Item Short-Form Health Survey (SF-36) Mental Component Scale: 0.47[4]
- Correlation with SF-36 Physical Component Scale: 0.53[4]
- Correlation with cervical range of motion: 0.27 to 0.40[4]

Known Groups

- Discriminates between work status levels: $t_{143} = 4.05$[4]
- Discriminates between litigation levels: $t_{142} = 4.65$

Discriminant. Not available

Construct—Longitudinal/Sensitivity to Change

Convergent

- Correlates with prognostic rating of change: 0.54 to 0.70[2,3]
- Correlates with PSFS rating of change: 0.79 to 0.81[3]
- Correlates with pain intensity change: 0.66[3]
- Correlates with pain limitation change: 0.68[3]

Known Groups

- Discriminates between litigation levels: $F_{1,69} = 4.21$[4]
- Discriminates between work status levels: $F_{1,70} = 11.91$[4]
- Discriminates between goals met levels: $F_{1,67} = 16.92$[4]
- Discriminates between dichotomized prognostic rating of change: receiver operating characteristic curve area: 0.90[2]

Discriminant. Not available

Interpretability

Values below are presented for a 0 to 50 scale.

General Population Values (Customary or Normative Values)

Typical admission scores are less than 35 NDI points.[1,2]

Typical Responsiveness Estimates

Individual Patient

Standard error of the mean $(SEM)_{internalconsistency} = 2.7$ NDI points, $SEM_{test-retest} = 2.0$ NDI points.[2] Rule in a change if the change score is ≥ 7 NDI points; rule out a change if the change score is < 3 NDI points.[2]

Between Group. Not available

Comments

Because some authors present scores on a 0 to 50 scale and other investigators present scores on a 0 to 100 scale, care must be taken when interpreting the meaning of score values.

References

1. Vernon H, Mior S. The Neck Disability Index: a study of reliability and validity. J Manipulative Physiol Ther 1991; 14:409–15.
2. Stratford PW, Riddle DL, Binkley JM, Spadoni G, Westaway MD, Padfield B. Using the Neck Disability Index to make decisions concerning individual patients. Physiother Can 1999; 51:107–12, 119.
3. Westaway MD, Stratford PW, Binkley JM. The Patient Specific Functional Scale: validation of its use in persons with neck dysfunction. J Orthop Sport Phys Ther 1998;27:331–8.
4. Riddle DL, Stratford PW. Use of generic versus region-specific functional status measures on patients with cervical spine disorders: a comparison study. Phys Ther 1998;78: 951–63.

To obtain this measure, contact the developers, or it can be found in reference 1.

NOTTINGHAM HEALTH PROFILE (NHP)

Developers

Carlos J. Martini and Ian McDowell, from the Department of Community Health, University Hospital and Medical School, University of Nottingham, England, led the initial research team in 1975 (earlier versions were referred to as the Nottingham Health Index [NHI]). Since October 1978, the development of the NHP has been under the direction of Sonja M. Hunt and James McEwen.[1]

Purpose

The most prevalent use of the NHP is to measure perceived health status in population surveys.[1,2] The NHP can also be used as a tool for evaluating outcomes of interventions by clinicians and researchers (eg, in clinical trials on individuals).[3-5]

Description

The NHP is a self-report, yes/no answer, two-part, generic quality of life measure. Part one includes a 38-item questionnaire with six subscales: emotional reactions (9 items), physical mobility (8 items), pain (8 items), sleep (5 items), social isolation (5 items), and energy level (3 items). Statements refer to problems with "normal" functioning a person may be experiencing at the moment owing to ill health. Each affirmative answer is scored and weighted. Scores range from 0 (no perceived distress) to 100 for each subscale. Part two contains seven questions regarding the effect of health problems on occupation, jobs around the house, personal relationships, social life, sex life, hobbies, and holidays.[3,4,6,7]

Conceptual/Theoretical Basis of Construct Being Measured

According to Hunt et al, subjective assessment of health status may be a better indicator of satisfaction with outcomes and use of medical services than mortality and morbidity statistics.[8] The design and content of the NHP was influenced by the Sickness Impact Profile (SIP), a generic quality of life measure developed in the United States. Whereas the SIP asks about changes in behavior owing to ill health, the NHP asks directly about feelings and emotional states.[7] The questions reflect the World Health Organization definition of disability. The profile is an indicator of perceived distress.[7] The

developers contend that it is easier to identify departures from normal functioning than it is to define normal functioning.[2]

Groups Tested with This Measure

The NHI was tested on individuals with arthritis with a variety of acute and chronic ailments,[1] clients before and after hip replacement operations,[9] and rehabilitation center clients.[5] Reliability was reported for clients with osteoarthritis,[10] peripheral vascular disease,[11] and musculoskeletal disorders.[12] Validation studies were performed on individuals with eczema, low back pain, depression, peptic ulcer, and hypertension[1]; groups of elderly people differing in health status[2]; rehabilitation center clients[5]; women throughout pregnancy[3]; persons undergoing minor surgery[13]; clients with fractures[14]; clients with rheumatoid arthritis.[15] In addition, this measure has been used with people after a stroke,[16,17] coronary bypass surgery,[17] and heart transplant[18]; community dwellers[19]; those with myocardial infarction,[20,21] chronic obstructive pulmonary disease (COPD),[22] multiple sclerosis, and Parkinson's disease[23]; chronic care populations[24]; and those with coronary artery disease,[25] severe physical disabilities,[26] diabetes,[27] zoster,[28] and angina pectoris.[29] This list is not exhaustive.

Languages

English, French, Swedish, Spanish, Italian, German, Finnish, Danish, Turkish, Arabic, and Urdu.[4,7] The developers have guided the international adaptation procedures using an independent item translation by a panel of experts in health, translation by bilingual individuals, and a back translation to review conceptual equivalence.[4,30] The Swedish NHP is the most widely used and psychometrically evaluated.[4,31] The Spanish, Dutch, and Turkish versions have been translated and culturally adapted, with information on their reliability and validity available.[4,7,26,32-34] The French version is translated and culturally adapted, but data on its reliability and validity are not reported.[4,35]

Application/Administration

The NHP takes 10 to 15 minutes to complete, is self-administered, can be used as a mailed questionnaire, and is sometimes administered by interview.[18,36] Scoring requires no special equipment. For part one, each affirmative answer is assigned a determined weight, and the weights for each subscale are summated. The developers recommend presenting part one as a profile (ie, the subscale scores are not summated), although some users present an overall score.[7] For part two, the number of positive responses is summed, and no weights are used. If part two of the questionnaire is not completed, the reliability and validity of part one are not affected.[4]

Typical Reliability Estimates

Internal Consistency
According to Hunt et al, the NHP does not meet the requirement for internal consistency that items in the instrument be homogeneous with respect to the attribute being measured.[10]

Interrater
Not applicable

Test–Retest
Four-week test–retest reliability of the NHP is reported for mailed questionnaires to 58 patients with osteoarthritis awaiting hip arthroplasty. Spearman's r reliability coefficients for part one of the NHP ranged from 0.77 for the energy subscale to 0.85 for the sleep and physical mobility subscales.[3,10] For part two of the NHP, Cramer's o reliability coefficients ranged from 0.44 to 0.86 for the area of hobbies and paid employment, respectively. In a similar postal survey, 4-week test–retest reliability was estimated on 93 patients with peripheral vascular disease; the Spearman's r reliability coefficients ranged from 0.75 for the emotional reactions subscale to 0.88 for the pain subscale.[3] For part two, Cramer's o reliability coefficients ranged from 0.55 to 0.89 for the areas of paid employment and family relationships, respectively. In 1-week test–retest reliability of the overall NHP score, an ICC was 0.95 (95% CI 0.91, 0.97) in a group of 49 people with work-related musculoskeletal disorders. The ICC for each subscale varied from 0.76 for physical mobility to 0.87 for pain.[7,12]

Typical Validity Estimates

Content
During the development of the NHI, the developers scrutinized interviews from clients with a variety of acute and chronic ailments for redundancy, ambiguity, reading age required, and esoteric expressions. Studies were then used to further refine the items between 1976 and 1978 and again after 1979.[1] Items were retained if they demonstrated some degree of correlation with pain and a physical rat-

ing; for the 33 retained items, Kendall's correlations with a pain score derived from the McGill Pain Questionnaire ranged from 0.21 to 0.66, and correlations with a physical score based on a physiotherapy assessment and Harris's recommendations ranged from 0.16 to 0.47. The statements were supplemented with items from the SIP. Factor analysis was also used to identify statements that did not cluster into interpretable groups.[9] When the NHI became the NHP, weighting and scoring of each domain were determined. Weighting the seriousness of perceived health problems was done through interviews of both outpatients and nonpatients.[36]

Criterion

Concurrent. Not available

Predictive. A study of 73 persons post heart transplant[18] suggested that a better score on the NHP pretransplant was indicative of a higher survival rate post-transplant. For every group of persons who differed by 20% in the number of questions affirmed, the risk of dying in the post-transplant period doubled. If 20% of the questions in the NHP were affirmed, the rate of death compared to persons with 0% affirmed was 2.07; if all questions were confirmed, the death rate was 38 times that of persons with none affirmed.

Construct—Cross-sectional

Convergent. Correlation between the NHI and the McGill Pain Questionnaire was 0.74, with a range from 0.50 for social activities to 0.78 for pain.[7,9] For cardiac patients, the NHP indicated a consistent relationship with the New York Heart Association (NYHA) classification and was statistically significant at $p < 0.0001$; higher NHP scores in each domain were associated with higher NYHA class.[20] The NYHA classification describes how heart disease affects the patient's physical activity and symptoms such as pain and fatigue.[20] The NHP subscales of physical mobility, energy, and pain correlated the highest with the NYHA classification, and Spearman's rank correlation coefficients were 0.45, 0.52, and 0.43, respectively, with $p < 0.0001$.[20] The NHP subscale scores were compared to the Karnofsky Performance Status Scale, and NHP scores decreased as the Karnofsky grade increased (ie, grade 7, unable to carry out normal activity, to grade 10, normal, no complaints), $p < 0.0004$.[20]

In stroke clients, the NHP emotional reactions subscale correlated highly (Spearman's $p = 0.71$) with scores on the General Health Questionnaire, used to detect important mood disturbance.[16] The NHP subscales of pain (r = 0.42 to 0.50), energy (r = 0.34 to 0.38), and sleep (r = 0.32 to 0.38) most highly correlated with pain measures in a group of zoster patients.[28]

Known Groups. The decision to consult a doctor for medical reasons differed significantly based on the mean rank of NHP scores: consulters' ranks were significantly greater than that of nonconsulters' ranks ($p < 0.01$).[8] Statistically significant differences for pain and physical scores were found between preoperative and postoperative hip arthroplasty patients.[9] The NHP was able to distinguish between persons with diagnosed chronic illness; persons with varying degrees of physical, social, and emotional disability; the physiologically fit; and persons not seeking medical intervention (Kruskal-Wallis tests were significant at $p < 0.001$).[2] The NHP was able to distinguish between "provisionally" accepted and "definitely" accepted patients awaiting heart transplant; the Mann-Whitney U statistic was significant at $p < 0.01$ for each subscale of the NHP.[18]

Discriminant. Not available

Construct—Longitudinal/Sensitivity to Change

Convergent. In long-term survivors of myocardial infarction, the 36-Item Short-Form Health Survey (SF-36) was better able to detect the impact of breathlessness than the NHP.[21] In COPD clients, the receiver operating characteristic curve and the area under the curve did not show a significant difference ($p > 0.10$) between the NHP and the SF-36 in discriminating among different levels of respiratory impairment.[22] When the NHP was compared with the Arthritis Impact Measurement Scales (AIMS), the Health Assessment Questionnaire (HAQ), and the Functional Limitations Profile, no single instrument was consistently the "best" at demonstrating change over all dimensions.[15] An overall NHP effect size of 0.52 was obtained in a group of 45 persons with work-related musculoskeletal injuries. The effect sizes varied from 0.18 for the emotional subscale to 0.57 for the pain subscale.[12] For the same group, the overall NHP standardized response mean (SRM) was 0.66 (95% CI 0.34, 0.98), whereas the subscale SRMs varied from 0.25 for emotional reactions to 0.70 for pain.[12]

Known Groups. Although no effect size estimates were calculated, the NHP showed significant improvement in all subscales ($p < 0.01$) in 62 patients before and after heart transplant.[18]

Alternatively, Hunt et al showed no contrast in the status of a group of patients before and after minor surgery.[13]

Discriminant. Not available

Interpretability

General Population Values
(Customary or Normative Values)

General population values on a random sample of 2,173 men and women[19] showed that the level of distress increased with increasing age and was higher among women than men. For the energy subscale, there was little variation across age up to the age of 54 years (men 4.0 to 11.6 across age groups, women 11.8 to 20.0, with the age group 25 to 29 years reporting the highest distress in energy). After the age of 55, there was a steep increase in energy distress level, with men 75 years of age and over reporting 29.3 and women 44.0. This pattern was similar for pain, sleep, social isolation, and physical mobility. The physical mobility values for men before 55 years ranged from 1.2 to 4.0 and for women from 1.0 to 4.8; for men and women aged 75 years of age and older, the corresponding values were 21.3 and 36.1. The state of emotional reactions in men ranged from 5.3 to 12.8, with both the lowest and highest values over the age of 65 years; the corresponding range for women was 9.3 to 17.9, with both the lowest and highest values in women under the age of 65 years. Typical values for various groups of individuals are given in Table 1.[3,16]

Typical Responsiveness Estimates
Not available

Other
A floor effect has been documented in several studies. Healthy people will score many zeroes, thus making the NHP unable to detect a change in this group.[6]

Comments

The NHP is best used to survey populations on perceived health status to determine the needs or levels of distress among different groups. The NHP may be more useful as an evaluative tool in populations with some level of disability.[4] The NHP was developed by asking persons with disabilities about the ill effects of health; however, it is being widely used on healthy populations. A European NHP group exists to follow the continued development and applicability of the NHP.[16] No data are available comparing telephone interview and self-administration of the NHP.[4]

TABLE 1 Mean Scores of Subscales of the NHP for Selected Groups

Group	Energy	Pain	Emotional Reactions	Sleep	Social Isolation	Physical Mobility
Mine rescue workers	1.0	1.4	1.3	4.2	0.4	0.5
Fit elderly	4.1	1.1	3.3	0.7	1.3	1.9
Pregnant women						
18 wk	31.4	2.1	15.7	11.3	6.4	7.3
37 wk	39.6	11.2	15.7	28.3	6.2	26.0
Minor or nonacute conditions	24.2	15.9	14.7	18.7	5.1	7.3
Fracture victims	25.8	26.5	13.7	28.0	8.0	27.6
Peripheral vascular disease	30.3	22.6	13.9	24.7	9.2	22.0
Chronically ill elderly	38.0	29.2	15.1	32.1	12.8	29.2
Osteoarthritis	63.2	70.8	11.0	48.7	12.5	54.8
Stroke						
1 mo	35.0	11.0	21.0	22.0	20.0	21.0
6 mo	40.0	13.0	25.0	26.0	23.0	Missing

A copy of the NHP with weights for scoring is available.[7,18]

References

1. Hunt SM, McEwen J. The development of a subjective health indicator. Sociol Health Illness 1980;2:231–46.
2. Hunt SM, McKenna SP, McEwen J, Beckett EM, Williams J, Papp E. A quantitative approach to perceived health status: a validation study. J Epidemiol Community Health 1980;34:281–6.
3. Hunt SM, McEwen J, McKenna SP. Measuring health status: a new tool for clinicians and epidemiologists. J R Coll Gen Pract 1985;35:185–8.
4. Anderson RT, Aaronson NK, Wilkin D. Critical review of the international assessments of health-related quality of life. Qual Life Res 1993;2:369–95.
5. Martini CJ, McDowell I. Health status: patient and physician judgments. Health Serv Res 1976;11:508–15.
6. Kind P, Carr-Hill R. The Nottingham Health Profile: a useful tool for epidemiologists? Soc Sci Med 1987;25:905–10.
7. McDowell I, Newell C. Measuring health: a guide to rating scales and questionnaires. 2nd ed. New York: Oxford University Press; 1996. p. 438–46.
8. Hunt SM, McKenna SP, McEwen J, Williams J, Papp E. The Nottingham Health Profile: subjective health status and medical consultations. Soc Sci Med 1981;15A:221–9.
9. McDowell IW, Martini CJM, Waugh W. A method for self-assessment of disability before and after hip replacement operations. BMJ 1978;2:857–9.
10. Hunt SM, McKenna SP, Williams J. Reliability of a population survey tool for measuring perceived health problems: a study of patients with osteoarthrosis. J Epidemiol Community Health 1981;35:297–300.
11. Hunt SM, McEwen J, McKenna SP, Beckett EM, Pope C. Subjective health of patients with peripheral vascular disease. Practitioner 1982;226:133–6.
12. Beaton DE, Hogg-Johnson S, Bombardier C. Evaluating changes in health status: reliability and responsiveness of five generic health status measures in workers with musculoskeletal disorders. J Clin Epidemiol 1997;50:79–93.
13. Hunt SM, McEwen J, McKenna SP, Beckett EM, Pope C. Subjective health assessments and the perceived outcome of minor surgery. J Psychosom Res 1984;28:105–14.
14. McKenna SP, McEwen J, Hunt SM, Papp E. Changes in the perceived health of patients recovering from fractures. Public Health 1984;98:97–102.
15. Fitzpatrick R, Ziebland S, Jenkinson C, Mowat A, Mowat A. Importance of sensitivity to change as a criterion for selecting health status measures. Qual Health Care 1992;1:89–93.
16. Ebrahim S, Barer D, Nouri F. Use of the Nottingham Health Profile with patients after a stroke. J Epidemiol Community Health 1986;40:166–9.
17. Wiklund I. The Nottingham Health Profile—a measure of health-related quality of life. Scand J Prim Health Care 1990; 8 Suppl 1:15–8.
18. O'Brien BJ, Buxton MJ, Ferguson BA. Measuring the effectiveness of heart transplant programmes: quality of life data and their relationship to survival analysis. J Chron Dis 1987;40 Suppl 1:137S–53S.
19. Hunt SM, McEwen J, McKenna SP. Perceived health: age and sex comparisons in a community. J Epidemiol Community Health 1984;38:156–60.
20. O'Brien BJ, Buxton MJ, Patterson DL. Relationship between functional status and health-related quality of life after myocardial infarction. Med Care 1993;31:950–5.
21. Brown N, Melville M, Gray D, Young T, Skene AM, Hampton JR. Comparison of the SF-36 health survey questionnaire with the Nottingham Health Profile in long-term survivors of a myocardial infarction. J Public Health Med 2000;22:167–75.
22. Prieto L, Alonso J, Ferrer M, Anto JM. Are results of the SF-36 Health Survey and the Nottingham Profile similar? A comparison in COPD patients. Quality of Life Study Group. J Clin Epidemiol 1997;50:463–73.
23. Sitzia J, Haddrell V, Rice-Oxley M. Evaluation of a nurse-led multidisciplinary neurological rehabilitation programme using the Nottingham Health Profile. Clin Rehabil 1998;12:389–94.

24. Albert SM. Assessing health-related quality of life in chronic care populations. J Mental Health Ageing 1997;3:101–18.

25. Lukkarinen H, Hentinen M. Assessment of quality of life with the Nottingham Health Profile among patients with coronary heart disease. J Adv Nurs 1997;26:73–84.

26. Post MW, Gerritsen J, Van Leusen ND, Paping MA, Prevo AJ. Adapting the Nottingham Health Profile for use in people with severe physical disabilities. Clin Rehabil 2001;15:103–10.

27. Bardsley MJ, Astell S, McCallum A, Home PD. The performance of three measures of health status in an outpatient diabetes population. Diabetic Med 1993;10:619–26.

28. Mauskopf J, Austin R, Dix L, Berzon R. The Nottingham Health Profile as a measure of quality of life in zoster patients: convergent and discriminant validity. Qual Life Res 1994;3:431–5.

29. Visser MC, Fletcher AE, Parr G, Simpson A, Bulpitt CJ. A comparison of three quality of life instruments in subjects with angina pectoris: the Sickness Impact Profile, the Nottingham Health Profile and the Quality of Well Being Scale. J Clin Epidemiol 1994;47:157–63.

30. Hunt SM. Cross-cultural issues in the use of socio-medical indicators. Health Policy 1986;6:149–58

31. Wiklund I, Romanus B, Hunt SM. Self-assessed disability in patients with arthrosis of the hip joint. Int Disabil Stud 1988;10:159–63.

32. Van Schayck CP, Rutten-van Molken MP, van Dooslaer EK, Folgering H, van Weel C. Two-year bronchodilator treatment in patients with mild airflow obstruction. Chest 1992;102:1384–91.

33. Deveci AA, McKenna SP, Kutlay S, Whalley D, Arasil T. The development and psychometric assessment of the Turkish version of the Nottingham Health Profile. Int J Rehabil Res 2000;23:31–8.

34. Erdman RA, Passchier J, Kooijman M, Stronks DL. The Dutch version of the Nottingham Health Profile: investigations of psychometric aspects. Psychol Rep 1993;72(3 Pt 1):1027–35.

35. Bucquet D, Condor S, Ritchie K. The French version of the Nottingham Health Profile: a comparison of item weights with those of the source version. Soc Sci Med 1990;30:809–35.

36. McKenna SP, Hunt SM, McEwen J. Weighting the seriousness of perceived health problems using Thurstone's method of paired comparisons. Int J Epidemiol 1981;10:93–7.

To obtain this measure, contact the developers, or it can be found in reference 7.

NUMERIC PAIN RATING SCALE (NPRS)

Description

The NPRS is a self-report or interviewer-administered measure. It consists of an 11-point scale (0 to 10) with the extreme anchors of "no pain" (0) and "pain as bad as it can be" (10). Clients are asked to rate their pain intensity over the previous 24 hours.

Conceptual/Theoretical Basis of Construct Being Measured

None reported.

Groups Tested with This Measure

Individuals with orthopedic[1,2] (neck, back, upper extremity, lower extremity) dysfunction, acute[3,4] (emergency department, postsurgical) and chronic[5,6] problems, and rheumatoid arthritis.[7]

Languages

English and Portuguese[7]

Application/Administration

Self-report: Clients are presented with a copy of the NPRS and are asked to circle the number corresponding to their perceived level of pain intensity (0 to 10). Scoring is simply the response circled out of 10 (eg, 7/10). Interviewer administered: The clinician verbally describes the NPRS and then asks the patient for a verbal rating of his/her perceived pain intensity score. The patient's verbal response is then his/her pain intensity rating out of 10.

Typical Reliability Estimates

Internal Consistency

Not applicable

Interrater

Not applicable for the self-administered version and not reported for the verbal format.

Test–Retest

- 0.67 to 0.96[1,5–7]

Typical Validity Estimates

Content

No reference in the literature.

Criterion

No gold standard exists for the attribute being assessed.

Construct—Cross-sectional

Convergent

- Correlated with the visual analogue scale: 0.79 to 0.95[3,4]

Known Groups and *Discriminant* are not available.

Construct—Longitudinal/Sensitivity to Change

Not available

Other Validity Coefficients

Effect size: 1.34 ("usual" pain: NPRS compared to the visual analogue scale and a verbal rating scale of pain)[2]

Interpretability

General Population Values (Customary or Normative Values)

Not available

Typical Responsiveness Estimates

Individual Patient

- Confidence in measured score: 90% CI = ± 2 points on scale[1]
- True change estimates: ± 3 points on scale (MDC$_{90}$)[1]

Between Group. Not available

Comments

Older and less literate persons have less difficulty responding to the NPRS compared with the visual analogue scale. More importantly, in a busy clinical setting, the NPRS is easier to administer and quicker to score. A change of 3 points is necessary to be confident of a true change in pain intensity; this value may present limitations given that it is 27% of the scale range.

References

1. Stratford PW, Spadoni G. The reliability, consistency, and clinical application of a numeric pain rating scale. Physiother Can 2001;53:88–91, 114.

2. Bolton JE, Wilkinson RC. Responsiveness of pain scales: a comparison of three intensity measures in chiropractic patients. J Manipulative Physiol Ther 1998;21:1–7.

3. Berthier F, Potel G, Leconte P, Touze M, Baron D. Comparative study of methods measuring acute pain intensity in an ED. Am J Emerg Med 1998;16:132–6.

4. DeLoach LJ, Higgins MS, Caplin AB, Stiff JL. The visual analogue scale in the immediate postoperative period: intrasubject variability and correlation with a numeric scale. Anesth Analg 1998;86:102–6.

5. Jenson MP, Turner JA, Romano JM, Fisher LD. Comparative reliability and validity of chronic pain intensity measures. Pain 1999;83:157–62.

6. Jensen MP, Karoly P, Braver S. The measurement of clinical pain intensity: a comparison of six methods. Pain 1986;27: 117–26.

7. Ferraz MB, Quaresma MR, Aquina LR, Atra E, Tugwell P, Goldsmith CH. Reliability of pain scales in the assessment of literate and illiterate patients with rheumatoid arthritis. J Rheumatol 1990;17:1022–4.

This measure can be found in reference 6.

OARS-IADL (OLDER AMERICANS RESOURCES AND SERVICES SCALE-INSTRUMENTAL ACTIVITIES OF DAILY LIVING)

Developers

Duke University Center for the Study of Aging and Human Development, Durham, North Carolina (1975); www.geri.duke.edu/service/oars.htm

Purpose

The Multidimensional Functional Assessment Questionnaire (MFAQ), of which the IADL scale is one component, was developed to provide a comprehensive profile of functioning and the need for services for older persons who live at home but who have some degree of impairment. It can be used as a screening instrument to evaluate outcomes and in modeling the cost effectiveness of alternative approaches to providing care.[1,2] The MFAQ is a multisection questionnaire consisting of scales to measure mental health, physical health, and basic and instrumental ADL as well as questionnaires to ascertain demographic, resource use, and economic information. Although the OARS team counsels against using the sections separately, they have commonly been used in this manner, particularly the IADL section.

Description

The OARS-IADL scale comprises seven items (using the telephone, getting to place out of walking distance, shopping, meal preparation, housework, medication, paying bills), each scored on a 3-point scale: 0 = unable, 1 = with help, 2 = without help. It has been used for clinical assessment, population surveys, program evaluation, personnel training and service planning, and in research. For the purposes of evaluation, a scoring system from 0 to 14 has evolved, but the original scoring was on a 6-point continuum from excellent function to total impairment. For other purposes, IADL profiles can be created and used to match services.[3]

Conceptual/Theoretical Basis of Construct Being Measured

The MFAQ is an information system to help ensure that services are tailored to needs. The conceptual basis permits the examination of function, service use, and the link between the two. The IADL section focuses on the capacity to perform tasks necessary to maintain an independent household.[1,3]

Groups Tested with This Measure

The OARS-IADL was tested with community residents aged 65 and over, persons with hip fracture, and persons with rheumatoid arthritis. However, many groups have been studied through the use of this instrument (eg, elderly people and those with stroke, hip fracture, and Alzheimer's disease).

Languages

English. The instrument has been translated into Canadian French but not formally tested for equivalence.[4,5]

Application/Administration

The OARS-IADL was originally developed as part of a comprehensive test battery administered through a face-to-face interview with the client or with a respondent who knows the client well. The measure has evolved to be used over the telephone or self-completed.

Typical Reliability Estimates

Internal Consistency
See content validity.

Interrater
The 6-point scoring system was tested on 11 raters reviewing a copy of 30 interviews; the ICC for self-care including ADL and IADL was 0.86.[2]

Test–Retest
The OARS-IADL was administered twice, 5 weeks apart, to a community sample of 30 elderly sub-

jects. The correlation (form not stated) between the two IADL assessments was 0.72. Persons tended to rate their performance higher on the first testing than on the second.[2]

Typical Validity Estimates

Content

Content validity was established using published measures with established validity and with items designed to ensure content validity.[2] Items were chosen for their relevance and because they met one of the following criteria: reliability and validity were known or could be tested or local or national (US) comparison standards were available or required because of accepted professional standards (manual). Two studies, an early one (results not accessible) and a more recent one, assessed the factor structure of the OARS items for ADL and IADL.[6] The factor structure of the 14 ADL/IADL items of the OARS was assessed on 668 persons participating in a clinical trial of case management to reduce hospital use for elderly medical patients recently discharged from acute care.[6] This study confirmed earlier work, and 3 + 1 dimensions emerged. The first and strongest dimension was labeled advanced ADL and included the IADL items of telephoning, finances, and medications, as well as the basic ADL item of eating. This dimension explained 37.4% of total variance, and Cronbach's alpha was 0.72. The second dimension was basic ADL (variance explained = 10%; Cronbach's alpha = 0.69). The third dimension was formed by the household IADL tasks (preparing meals, shopping, housework, and community travel) that explained 9% of the variance, and Cronbach's alpha was 0.78. A weak fourth dimension was incontinence. The dimensionality of the OARS ADL and IADL scales was examined on a convenient sample of 372 elderly persons.[7] Rasch analysis difficulty orderings and item separation indices indicated that the IADL items were more difficult than the ADL items, with the housework item being the most difficult followed by shopping, meal preparation and money management (tied), transportation and medication management (tied), and finally telephone use. This analysis confirmed the theoretical hierarchical relationship between basic ADL and IADL.

Criterion

No gold standard exists for the construct being measured.

Construct—Cross-sectional

Convergent. In a group of 83 seniors (mean age 76 years), a recent study[8] compared measures of function that have different formats for administration (viewed performance, interview administered, and self-completed). The OARS-IADL correlated 0.56 with a measure that scored seven performance-based mobility and dexterity tasks on a 5-point scale. Correlations were 0.36 with the 36-Item Short-Form Health Survey (SF-36) Physical Function (PF) subscale, 0.33 with the Katz, and 0.70 with the ADL section of the Functional Status Questionnaire (FSQ). The correlation with the self-administered rating of the FSQ IADL component was 0.59. All correlations were significantly different from 0 and were higher for more closely related constructs and lower for those more distantly related (PF). A community-based survey of elderly persons (N= 872) found an expected relationship between OARS-IADL score and depression and vision.[9] The probability of an IADL limitation was 10 times higher for a person with low vision (unable to read newsprint even with glasses) and 9 times higher among persons with significant depressive symptomatology measured using the Center for Epidemiologic Studies-Depression Scale (CES-D).

Among 20 persons with rheumatoid arthritis, the OARS-IADL correlated with the 11 performance-based items of the Arthritis Hand Function Test.[10] The lowest correlation of 0.46 was observed for the task manipulating coins and the highest correlation of 0.75 was observed for pouring water and manipulating pegs. In another study, the hypothesis that the advanced IADL factor (telephoning, finances, and medications) would relate to measures of cognitive status better than the other two factors (basic ADL and household ADL) was confirmed; a correlation of 0.33 was reported, larger than any other correlations with any other ADL scale.[6]

Known Groups. Among 312 older persons with hip fracture, the OARS-IADL distinguished, both pre and 6 months post-fracture, between groups defined by age, steadiness of gait, degree of disorientation, comorbidity, and nursing home admission.[11] For example, for persons with pre-fracture unsteady walking, the IADL score was 4.67 (SD 4.01) compared with 1.86 (SD 2.79) for persons with steady walking; 6 months post-fracture, these values were 6.99 (SD 4.45) for unsteady walkers and 3.88 (SD 3.73) for steady walkers; differences between groups ranged from 2 to 3 points.

Discriminant. See information for convergent validity.

Construct—Longitudinal/Sensitivity to Change

Convergent. A total of 619 community-dwelling elderly women (mean age 74 years) were assessed over 2 years for change in function.[12] The majority remained stable for IADL (67%), 20% declined, and 13% improved. Half of those who declined in IADL did so in one of the seven IADL items and the other half in two or more (n = 69). For more than 90% of the sample, the range of improvement or decline was −4 units to +4 units.

Known Groups. Community-dwelling elderly women who were older, in poorer health, and with lower cognitive scores were more likely to decline in IADL than other groups of women.[13]

Discriminant. Not available

Other Validity Coefficients

The OARS-IADL was sensitive to change occurring as a result of a hip fracture. Pre-fracture IADL score for persons between the ages of 75 and 84 years was 3.22 (SD 3.58) and 6 months post-fracture, the score was 5.59 (SD 4.25).[11] After a 1-year intervention of geriatric management (n = 194), 71% of persons in the intervention group had none or only one IADL dependency compared with 90% of controls.[14] In a study of the effectiveness of a 4-week comprehensive home-based rehabilitation program post–acute stroke (n = 114), persons in the home intervention group scored 11.0 (SD 3.5) on the OARS-IADL measure compared with 9.5 (SD 3.9) for persons having usual care.[4] This difference was statistically significant.

Interpretability

General Population Values
(Customary or Normative Values)

A community survey of 997 persons (> 65 years) from Durham County, North Carolina, indicated that the most difficult items were (1) housework (72% able, 12% unable) followed by (2) shopping (76% able, 9% unable), (3) community travel (76% able, 5% unable), (4) meal preparation (83% able, 7% unable), (5) handling finances (89% able, 5% unable), (6) using the telephone (90% able, 4% unable), and (7) taking medications (93% able, 3% unable).[1] In a comparative study of 434 community-dwelling individuals 6 months post-stroke and 486 age-matched controls, the difference in IADL score was 11.6 of 14; SD 3.2 in the mean stroke group and 13.8 of 14; SD 0.8 in the mean control group. Fifty-four percent of persons with stroke reported a limitation with one or more IADL items compared with only 7% for controls. The most challenging task for persons with stroke was housework (48% with limitation), followed by shopping, community travel, and meal preparation (36%, 32%, 29%, respectively). The values for the nonstroke group ranged from 5 to 2%.

Typical Responsiveness Estimates
Not available

Comments

Although developed primarily for screening and to discriminate among people with unmet needs for services, this measure has evolved as an evaluative measure because of its performance in longitudinal studies of populations that are changing over time; its short, easy-to-administer format; and its performance when used in evaluative studies. It also captures activities that are required for successful community living and reflect the impact of a wide range of impairments.

References

1. **Multidimensional Functional Assessment: the OARS methodology: a manual. Durham (NC): Center for the Study of Aging and Human Development; 1975.**
2. **Fillenbaum GG, Smyer MA. The development, validity, and reliability of the OARS multidimensional assessment questionnaire. J Gerontol 1981;36:428–34.**
3. **George LK, Fillenbaum GG. OARS methodology: a decade of experience in geriatric assessment. J Am Geriatr Soc 1985; 33:607–15.**
4. Mayo NE, Wood-Dauphinee S, Cote R, Gayton D, Carlton J, Buttery J, et al. There's no place like home: an evaluation of early supported discharge for stroke. Stroke 2000;31:1016–23.
5. Mayo NE, Wood-Dauphinee S, Cote R, Duncan L, Carlton J. Activity, participation, and quality of life six months post-stroke. Arch Phys Med. In press.
6. Fitzgerald JF, Smith DM, Martin DK, Freedman JA, Wolinsky FD. Replication of the multidimensionality of activities of daily living. J Gerontol 1993;48(1):S28–31.
7. Doble SE, Fisher AG. The dimensionality and validity of the Older American Resources and Services (OARS) Activities of Daily Living (ADL) scale. J Outcome Measurement 1998;2:4–24.
8. Reuben DB, Valle LA, Hays RD, Siu AL. Measuring physical function in community-dwelling older persons: a comparison of self-administered, interviewer-administered, and performance-based measures. J Am Geriatr Soc 1995;43:17–23.
9. Rovner BW, Ganguli M. Depression and disability associated with impaired vision: The MoVies project. J Am Geriatr Soc 1998;46:617–9.
10. Backman C, Mackie H. Reliability and validity of the arthritis hand function test in adults with osteoarthritis. Occup Ther J Res 1997;17:55–66.

11. Young Y, Brant L, German P, Kenzora J, Magaziner J. A longitudinal examination of functional recovery among older people with subcapital hip fractures. J Am Geriatr Soc 1997;45:288–94.

12. Freedman JD, Beck A, Robertson B, Calonge BN, Gade G. Using a mailed survey to predict hospital admission among patients older than 60. J Am Geriatr Soc 1996;44:689–92.

13. Sarwari AR, Freedman L, Langenberg P, Magaziner J. Prospective study on the relation between living arrangement and change in functional health status of elderly women. Am J Epidemiol 1998;147:370–8.

14. Rubin CD, Sizemore MT, Loftis PA, Loret de Mola N. A randomized, controlled trial of outpatient geriatric evaluation and management in a large public hospital. J Am Geriatr Soc 1993; 41:1023–8.

This measure or ordering information can be found at the Website address included in this review.

OSWESTRY LOW BACK PAIN DISABILITY QUESTIONNAIRE

Description
The Oswestry is a 10-item questionnaire. Each item is scored on a 6-point scale (0 to 5). Raw scores can vary between 0 and 50. The final score is expressed as a percentage. Higher scores represent more disability.

Conceptual/Theoretical Basis of Construct Being Measured
None reported.

Groups Tested with This Measure
Acute, subacute, and chronic back pain client groups; various conservative, surgical, and behavioral intervention groups.

Languages
English, Danish, Dutch, Finnish, French and French Canadian, German, Greek, Norwegian, Spanish, and Swedish.

Application/Administration
The Oswestry is self-administered, and most clients can complete the measure in less than 5 minutes. The measure can be scored without the use of computational aids in less than 1 minute.

Typical Reliability Estimates

Internal Consistency
Coefficient alpha values: 0.82 to 0.90[5]

Interrater
Not applicable

Test–Retest
ICC: 0.88 to 0.94[5]

Typical Validity Estimates

Content
No reference to content validity in the literature

Criterion
No gold standard exists for the construct being measured.

Construct—Cross-sectional

Convergent
- Correlations: Quebec Back Pain Scale 0.80,[5] Roland-Morris Questionnaire (RMQ) 0.82,[6] and Jan van Breeman (JVB) pain and function 0.62

Known Groups
- Medication use (yes/no) effect size = 1.00, work absence (yes/no) effect size = 0.89, compensation (yes/no) = 0.85[5]
- Radiculopathy (yes/no) 49.6 versus 33.0 ($p < 0.0001$)[7]

Discriminant. Not available

Construct—Longitudinal/Sensitivity to Change

Convergent
- Correlation with global rating of change: 0.31 to 0.57[5,6,8]
- Correlation with RMQ change scores: 0.79 and JVB change scores: 0.61 (pain) to 0.64 (function)[8]

Known Groups. Important change (yes/no) receiver operating characteristic curve area: 0.76[9] and 0.78[8]

Discriminant. Not available

Other Validity Coefficients
Effect size: 0.65[10]

Interpretability

General Population Values (Customary or Normative Values)
Zero to 20% minimal disability, 20 to 40% moderate disability, 40 to 60% severe disability, 61 to 80% crippled, and 80 to 100% either bed-bound or exaggerating their symptoms[1]

Typical Responsiveness Estimates

Individual Patient

- 4 to 6 percentage points[9]

Between Group

- 4 to 15 percentage points[4]

Comments

Many modified versions of the Oswestry exist. However, none of the modified versions have been shown—in a formal hypothesis testing study—to have better measurement properties than the original version. It is for this reason that the original version of the Oswestry is reviewed. A noted shortcoming of the Oswestry is that patients tend to leave more questions blank than competing measures.[5,8] The original version and more recent versions of the Oswestry contain double-barreled questions, and this may be one source of confusion for respondents.

References

1. Fairbank JC, Couper J, Davies JB, O'Brien JP. The Oswestry Low Back Pain Disability Questionnaire. Physiotherapy 1980; 66:271–3.

2. Baker DJ, Pynsent PB, Fairbank JCT. The Oswestry Disability Index revisited: its reliability, repeatability and validity, and a comparison with the St Thomas's Disability Index. In: Roland MO, Jenner JR, editors. Back pain: new approaches to rehabilitation and education. New York: Manchester University Press; 1989. p. 175–204.

3. Fairbank JCT, Pynsent PB. The Oswestry Disability Index. Spine 2000;25:2940–53.

4. Roland M, Fairbank J. The Roland-Morris Disability Questionnaire and the Oswestry Disability Questionnaire. Spine 2000;24:3115–24.

5. Kopec JA, Esdaile JM, Abrahamowicz M, Abenhaim L, Wood-Dauphinee S, Lamping DL, et al. The Quebec Back Pain Disability Scale: measurement properties. Spine 1995;20:341–52.

6. Stratford PW, Binkley JM. Measurement properties of the RM-18 a modified version of the Roland-Morris disability scale. Spine 1997;22:2416–21.

7. Leclaire R, Blier F, Fortin L, Proulx R. A cross-sectional study comparing the Oswestry and Roland-Morris functional disability scales in two populations of patients with low back pain of different levels of severity. Spine 1997;22:68–71.

8. Stratford PW, Binkley J, Solomon P, Gill C, Finch E. Assessing change over time in patients with low back pain. Phys Ther 1994;74:528–33.

9. Beurskens AJHM, de Vet HCW, Koke AJA. Responsiveness of functional status in low back pain: a comparison of different instruments. Pain 1996;65:71–6

10. Jette DU, Jette AM. Physical therapy and health outcomes in patients with spinal impairments. Phys Ther 1996;76:930–45.

This measure can be found on the accompanying CD-ROM. Prior to using the measure, you are strongly advised to contact the developers for administration and scoring guidelines and revisions to the measure not available at time of publication. This measure can also be found in references 3 and 4.

OXYGEN COST DIAGRAM (OCD)

Developers

C. R. McGavin, M. Artvinli, H. Naoe, and G. J. R. McHardy[1]

Purpose

The OCD is a self-assessment tool designed to allow clients with respiratory impairment to report their functional exercise limitation.

Description

The OCD is a linear analogue scale consisting of a 100-mm vertical line with descriptions of daily activities on either side. The descriptions are arranged from least oxygen cost at the bottom (sleeping) to highest at the top (brisk walking uphill). Subjects are asked by an interviewer to draw a line at the point above which their breathlessness will not let them go on, yielding a continuous variable with possible values ranging from 0 to 100 mm.

Conceptual/Theoretical Basis of Construct Being Measured

The scale was designed to assess the value of self-reported exercise limitation as an estimate of exercise performance.[1]

Groups Tested with This Measure

Validity has been tested in clients with mild to severe airflow limitation and acute pulmonary infiltrates[1] and restrictive lung diseases.[2] The OCD has been used but not validated in individuals with cancer,[3] eosinophilia myalgia syndrome,[4] heart disease,[5] and obesity.[5]

Languages

The OCD has been validated only in English,[1] although translations into German,[6] French,[7] and Japanese[8] have been reported.

Application/Administration

This measure requires a brief explanation by an interviewer, followed by a self-assessment by the client. The measure requires 1 to 2 minutes to complete. Clinicians use a ruler to obtain the score to the nearest millimeter.

Typical Reliability Estimates

Internal Consistency
Not applicable

Interrater
ICC = 0.68[5]

Test–Retest
ICC = 0.66[9]

Typical Validity Estimates

Content
No reference to content validity in the literature

Criterion

Concurrent
- VO_{2max}: $r = 0.56$ to 0.66[8,10] in individuals with chronic obstructive pulmonary disease (COPD)
- 6-minute walk distance: $r = 0.65$[11] in individuals with COPD
- 12-minute walk distance: $r = 0.68$[1] in individuals with COPD

Predictive. Not available

Construct—Cross-sectional

Convergent
- 36-Item Short-Form Health Survey (SF-36) physical domain: $r = 0.78$ in COPD[9]
- Forced expiratory volume in 1 second (FEV_1): $r = 0.48$[8]

Known Groups. In individuals with chronic lung disease, the OCD was able to distinguish clear differences between mild (69 mm), moderate (57 mm), and severe (46 mm) respiratory disease severity.[9]

Discriminant. Nonphysical domains of SF-36: $r = 0.27$ to 0.30[9]

Construct—Longitudinal/Sensitivity to Change

Convergent
- Change in 6-minute walk: $r = 0.37$ in COPD[12]
- OCD showed no difference (50 ± 12 mm versus 51 ± 15 mm) after 1-year follow-up despite a significant decline in 6-minute Walk Test (327 ± 96 m versus 319 ± 101 m) among patients noninvasively ventilated at home.[2] Following respiratory rehabilitation, 6-minute walk distance improved significantly from mean 328 m

to 356 m (effect size 0.6), whereas a small change in the OCD from 48 mm to 51 mm (effect size 0.1) was not significant.[13]

Known Groups and *Discriminant* are not available.

Interpretability

General Population Values (Customary or Normative Values)

Healthy people who are able to walk briskly uphill score 100 mm.

Typical Responsiveness Estimates

Not available

References

1. McGavin CR, Artvinli M, Naoe H, McHardy GJR. Dyspnoea, disability, and distance walked: comparison of estimates of exercise performance in respiratory disease. BMJ 1978;2:241–3.

2. Janssens JP, Bretenstein E, Rochat T, Fitting JW. Does the "Oxygen Cost Diagram" reflect changes in six minute walking distance in follow up studies? Respir Med 1999;93:810–5.

3. Farncombe M. Dyspnea: assessment and treatment. Support Care Cancer 1997;5:94–9.

4. Read CA, Clauw D, Weir C, Da Silva AT, Katz P. Dyspnea and pulmonary function in the L-tryptophan-associated eosinophilia-myalgia syndrome. Chest 1992;101:1202–6.

5. Mahler DA, Wells CK. Evaluation of clinical methods for rating dyspnea. Chest 1988;93:580–6.

6. Bergmann KC. Controlled clinical comparative evaluation of fluticasone powder inhalation versus flunisolide dose aerosol in patients with mild to moderate asthma. Pneumologie 1997; 51:27–32.

7. Noseda A, Yernault JC. Quantifying dyspnea. Presse Med 1994;23:1527–32.

8. Hajiro T, Nishimura K, Tsukino M, Ikeda A, Koyama H, Izumi T. Analysis of clinical methods used to evaluate dyspnea in patients with chronic obstructive pulmonary disease. Am J Respir Crit Care Med 1998;158:1185–9.

9. O'Brien B, Viramontes JL. Willingness to pay: a valid and reliable measure of health state preference? Med Decis Making 1994;14:289–97.

10. Robinson RW, White DP, Zwillich CW. Relationship of respiratory drives to dyspnea and exercise performance in chronic obstructive pulmonary disease. Am Rev Respir Dis 1987;136: 1084–90.

11. Chuang ML, Lin IF, Wasserman K. The body weight-walking distance product as related to lung function, anaerobic threshold and peak VO2 in COPD patients. Respir Med 2001;95:618–26.

12. Guyatt GH, Townsend M, Keller J, Singer J, Nograd S. Measuring functional status in chronic lung disease: conclusions from a randomized control trial. Respir Med 1989;83:293–7.

13. Guyatt GH, King DR, Feeny DH, Stubbing D, Goldstein RS. Generic and specific measurement of health-related quality of life in a clinical trial of respiratory rehabilitation. J Clin Epidemiol 1999;52:187–92.

This measure can be found in reference 1.

PATIENT SPECIFIC FUNCTIONAL SCALE (PSFS)

Developers

P. Stratford, C. Gill, M. Westaway, and J. Binkley,[1]
stratfor@mcmaster.ca

Purpose

Provides a standardized method for eliciting and recording functional status limitations that are most relevant to an individual client.

Description

The PSFS consists of an introductory statement, which is read by the clinician. Clients are asked to identify up to five important activities with which they are having difficulty or are unable to perform because of their problem. In addition to specifying the activities, clients are asked to rate, on an 11-point scale (0 = unable to perform to 10 = able to perform with no problem), the current level of difficulty associated with each activity.

Conceptual/Theoretical Basis of Construct Being Measured

The PSFS was conceived to be (1) applicable to a large number of clinical presentations (eg, conditions, problems, age groups); (2) efficient to administer, score, and record in the medical record; (3) reliable, valid, and sensitive to change; and (4) able to provide a comparison of a client's specific important activity level at a given point in time with respect to the preinjury or disability state.

Groups Tested with this Measure

Clients with back,[1] lower extremity,[2] and neck[3] problems of suspected musculoskeletal origin; acute, subacute, and chronic client groups; and various conservative and surgical intervention groups.

Language

English

Application/Administration

The PSFS is administered at a client's initial assessment, during the history taking and prior to the assessment of any impairment measures. The clinician's role is to read the script (instructions) to the client and record the activities and corresponding numeric difficulty ratings. At subsequent reassessments, the clinician reads the follow-up script, which reminds the client of the activities he/she identified previously. Once again, the clinician records the numeric difficulty ratings.

Typical Reliability Estimates

Internal Consistency
Coefficient alpha: 0.97[2]

Interrater
Not applicable

Test–Retest
ICC: individual item 0.84 to 0.91,[1,2] average score 0.87 to 0.97[1–3]

Typical Validity Estimates

Content
Important items most relevant to the client.

Criterion
No gold standard exists for the construct being measured.

Construct—Cross-sectional

Convergent
- Physical Function domain of the 36-Item Short-Form Health Survey (SF-36): $r = 0.39$ to 0.49
- Roland-Morris Questionnaire: $r = 0.59$ to 0.74[1]
- Neck Disability Index (NDI): $r = 0.74$ to 0.80

Known Groups. Easy items (walking) are given higher scores than more difficult activities (eg, running)[2]

Discriminant. Correlates higher with the SF-36 Physical Function domain ($r = 0.49$) compared with the Mental Health domain ($r = 0.09$)

Construct—Longitudinal/Sensitivity to Change

Convergent
- Correlates 0.77 with a retrospective global rating of change[2]
- Correlates 0.52 to 0.56 with a prognostic rating of change[3]
- Correlates 0.59 with the Physical Function domain of the SF-36[2]
- Correlates 0.66 with NDI change scores[3]

Known Groups. Easy activities (walking) change more rapidly than more difficult activities (eg, running)[2]

Discriminant. Not available

Interpretability

General Population Values (Customary or Normative Values)
Not applicable

Typical Responsiveness Estimates

Individual Patient. The SEM$_{test–retest}$ is 1.0 PSFS point.[2] Ninety percent of stable patients vary by less than 3.0 PSFS points (ie, MDC$_{90}$ = 2.5 PSFS change points)[2]

Between Group. Not available

Comment

Because clients are likely to identify different activities, patient-specific measures are not advocated for between-client comparisons.

References

1. **Stratford P, Gill C, Westaway M, Binkley J. Assessing disability and change on individual patients: a report of a patient specific measure. Physiother Can 1995;47:258–63.**
2. Chatman AB, Hyams SP, Neel JM, Binkley J, Stratford P, Schomberg A, et al. The Patient Specific Functional Scale: measurement properties in patients with knee dysfunction. Phys Ther 1997;77:820–9.
3. Westaway MD, Stratford PW, Binkley JM. The Patient Specific Functional Scale: validation of its use in persons with neck dysfunction. J Orthop Sport Phys Ther 1998;27:331–8.

This measure can be found on the accompanying CD-ROM. Prior to using the measure, you are strongly advised to contact the developers for administration and scoring guidelines and revisions to the measure not available at time of publication.

PEABODY DEVELOPMENTAL MOTOR SCALES (PDMS)

Developers

M. Rhonda Folio and Rebecca R. Fewell.
M. Rhonda Folio: rfolio@tntech.edu
Rebecca R. Fewell: EEU WJ-10, University of Washington, Seattle, Washington, 98195

Purpose

To measure gross and fine motor development in children 0 to 83 months.[1] Intended for use as both a discriminative and an evaluative tool.[1,2]

Description

The Peabody[1–3] is intended as an individually administered, observer-scored, performance-based measure of motor development for children 0 to 83 months. The test can be administered in groups but requires adherence to specific instructions outlined in the manual. The tool is divided into a gross motor scale (GMS) and a fine motor scale (FMS). Gross motor scale: 170 items split into 17 age levels with 10 items at each level. There are 5 skill categories: reflexes, balance, nonlocomotion, locomotion, and receipt and propulsion of objects. Each skill is not necessarily represented at every age level. Fine motor scale: 122 items split into 16 age levels with 6 to 8 items at each level. There are 4 skill categories: grasping, hand use, eye-hand coordination, and manual dexterity. Each skill is not necessarily represented at every age level. Scores on each item range from 0 (cannot do) to 2 (full performance). Raw summary scores can be converted into an age-equivalent score, a developmental motor quotient, and a percentile ranking or a standardized score, with a higher score reflecting greater skill acquisition.

Conceptual/Theoretical Basis of Construct Being Measured

The PDMS is based on the models of developmental theory, behavioral and learning theory, neurophysiology, and perceptual-motor theory.[1] Gross motor skills are defined as tasks involving the large muscles of the body. Fine motor skills require the smaller muscles of the body.

Groups Tested with This Measure

Children ages 0 to 83 months

Language

English

Application/Administration

The PDMS[1,3] is a performance-based measure with the GMS and FMS administered and scored separately. If both are done, it is recommended that they be completed within 5 days of each other. The PDMS is intended to be administered in a clinical or school setting using standardized tasks that are rated by the administrator. The manual contains administration instructions including start positions and task requirements, scales, and the response/scoring booklet. The administrator is instructed to begin each scale at one level below the expected motor age of the child. Basal and ceiling rules are given to eliminate unnecessary items. In a child with normal function, if all items are completed, each scale requires 20 to 30 minutes to complete. Scoring time varies depending on the type of score desired. Scaled scores are useful in making comparisons over time (not age dependent). Standardized scores allow for comparison of motor performance to age-expected norms. There is a large amount of equipment required for each scale; some of the FMS materials are included with the test kit. No specific training is required; however, the authors recommend familiarity with normal development and the test procedures as outlined in the manual. Incomplete items are used to determine the child's level of motor development.

Typical Reliability Estimates

Internal Consistency
Not assessed. The scales are not intended to measure one dimension.[1]

Interrater

FMS: ICC = 0.97 for delayed children and 0.76 for normal children[4]

ICC = 0.90 to 0.97 for subskills and 0.99 for total score in those with developmental delay[5]

Test–Retest

Total score ICC > 0.99 for both scales[1]; excluding basal items: GMS 0.95, FMS 0.80[1]

Typical Validity Estimates

Content

The PDMS is based on previously validated measures and research into the motor development of children.[1,3,6] It is also based on the taxonomy of the psychomotor domain by Harrow,[7] which lends reported strength to its content validity.[1,6]

Criterion

Concurrent. Not available

Predictive. Predictive validity at 18 months: $r = 0.25$ to 0.75[8]

Construct—Cross-sectional

Convergent

- Bayley Motor Scales: $r = 0.78$ to 0.96 (GMS), $r = 0.2$ to 0.57 (FMS)[8]
- FMS and Bayley Mental Subscale: $r = 0.26$ to 0.80[1,3,6]
- FMS and Bayley Psychomotor Subscale: $r = 0.31$ to 0.46[1,3,6]
- GMS and Bayley Psychomotor Subscale: $r = 0.37$ to 0.64[1,3,6]
- FMS and West Haverstrow FM: $r = 0.36$ to 0.62[1,3,6]
- GMS and West Haverstrow GM: $r = 0.27$ to 0.63[1,3,6]
- Posture and Fine Motor Assessment of Infants (PFMAI)[9]: $r = 0.84$ (GMS), 0.67 (FMS)
- Alberta Infant Motor Scale (AIMS): $r = 0.97$[10]
- Pediatric Evaluation of Disability Inventory (PEDI): $r = 0.24$ to 0.95[11]

Known Groups. The PDMS demonstrates a clear overall trend of improvement with increased chronologic age in normal children.[1] The mean standardized scores were significantly lower in children with developmental delay compared to normal except at the 0 to 5 months level.[1,6]

Discriminant

Not available

Construct—Longitudinal/Sensitivity to Change

Convergent. Gross Motor Function Measure and PDMS-GMS were comparable in measuring change in infants with motor delays and cerebral palsy.[12] The PDMS is more suitable for children younger than 18 months.

Known Groups and *Discriminant* are not available.

Interpretability

General Population Values (Customary or Normative Values)

Normative data are available.[1,3,6] Caution should be exercised when interpreting standardized scores from populations not well represented by the normative sample.[13]

Typical Responsiveness Estimates

Individual Patient. Not fully determined

Between Group. Not available

References

1. **Folio MR, Fewell RR. Peabody Developmental Motor Scales and Activity Cards manual. Allen (TX): DLM Teaching Resources; 1983.**
2. Palisano RJ, Kolobe TH, Haley SM, Lowes LP, Jones SL. Validity of the Peabody Developmental Gross Motor Scale as an evaluative measure of infants receiving physical therapy. Phys Ther 1995;75:939–51.
3. Palisano RJ, Lydic JS. The Peabody Developmental Motor Scales: an analysis. Phys Occup Ther Pediatr 1984;4:69–75.
4. Stokes NA, Deitz JL, Crowe TK. The Peabody Developmental Fine Motor Scale: an interrater reliability study. Am J Occup Ther 1990;44:334–40.
5. Gebhard AR, Ottenbacher KJ, Lane SJ. Interrater reliability of the Peabody Developmental Motor Scales: Fine Motor Scale. Am J Occup Ther 1994;48:976–81.
6. Hinderer KA, Richardson PK, Atwater SW. Clinical implications of the Peabody Developmental Motor Scales: a constructive review. Phys Occup Ther Pediatr 1989;9:81–106.
7. Harrow AJ. A taxonomy of the psychomotor domain. New York: D. McKay Co; 1972.
8. Palisano R. Concurrent and predictive validities of the Bayley Motor Scale and the Peabody Developmental Motor Scales. Phys Ther 1986;66:1714–9.
9. Case-Smith J. A validity study of the posture and fine motor assessment of infants. Am J Occup Ther 1992;47:597–605.
10. Darrah J, Piper M, Watt MJ. Assessment of gross motor skills of at-risk infants: predictive validity of the Alberta Infant Motor Scale. Dev Med Child Neurol 1998;40:485–91.

11. Nichols DS, Case-Smith J. Reliability and validity of the Pediatric Evaluation of Disability Inventory. Pediatr Phys Ther 1996;8:15–24.

12. Kolobe THA, Palisano RJ, Stratford PW. Comparison of two outcome measures for infants with cerebral palsy and infants with motor delays. Phys Ther 1998;78:1062–72.

13. Crowe TK, McClain C, Provost B. Motor development of Native American children on the Peabody Developmental Motor Scales. Am J Occup Ther 1999;53:514–8.

14. Green K, Deitz J, Kartin Brady D. Comparison of two scoring methods of the Peabody Gross Motor Scale. Phys Occup Ther Pediatr 1995;14:121–32.

15. Harris SR, Heriza CB. Measuring infant movement: clinical and technological techniques. Phys Ther 1987;67:1877–80.

16. Schmidt LS, Westcott SL, Crowe TK. Interrater reliability of the gross motor scale of the Peabody Developmental Motor Scales with 4 and 5 year old children. Pediatr Phys Ther 1993;5:169–75.

To obtain this measure, contact the developers.

PEDIATRIC EVALUATION OF DISABILITY INVENTORY (PEDI)

Developers

Stephen M. Haley, Wendy J. Coster, Larry H. Ludlow, Jane T. Haltiwanger, and Peter J. Andrellos, PEDI Research Group, Department of Rehabilitation Medicine, New England Medical Center Hospital, 75K/R, 750 Washington Street, Boston, Massachusetts 02111-1901; Fax: 617-956-5353

Purpose

The PEDI (Version 1) is a measure of functional performance and caregiver assistance in the domains of self-care, mobility, and social function in children with chronic illness and disabilities, ages 6 months to 7.5 years.[1]

Description

The PEDI is a judgment-based standardized structured interview or questionnaire for parents or clinicians/educators of young children with a variety of disabilities. The PEDI measures both the capability and performance of functional skills of children ages 6 months to 7.5 years. The PEDI is also expected to be useful in children older than 7.5 years if functional skills are considered delayed. The PEDI is divided into three scales: Functional Skills, Caregiver Assistance, and Modifications. Each scale addresses the content domains of self-care, mobility, and social function. Scales can be collectively or independently administered. Summary scores can be calculated from the Functional Skills and Caregiver Assistance Scales. These scores can be transformed into standard scores or scaled scores. Standard scores can be used for norm referencing with respect to chronologic age. Scaled scores can be used to provide an indication of performance along a continuum from 0 to 100, with higher scores representing greater functional performance and less caregiver assistance.

Conceptual/Theoretical Basis of Construct Being Measured

The authors of the manual define functional skills as the "essential activities required in the child's nat-ural environments of home and school."[1] Disability and function were defined based on the World Health Organization's International Classification of Impairments, Disabilities and Handicaps[2] and on the Nagi model.[3] Capability is conceptualized as skills in which the child has demonstrated mastery and competence.[1] Performance is related to the amount of assistance required to complete daily functional activities.[1]

Groups Tested with This Measure

The authors report that the PEDI is most appropriate for children with physical or combined physical and cognitive disabilities. The PEDI has also been used in clinical trials with children who are either candidates for or have undergone hemidecorticectomy,[4] who are undergoing selective dorsal rhizotomy,[5–8] and with osteogenesis imperfecta,[9,10] as well as orthopedic and other neurologic groups.[11]

Language

English

Application/Administration

Methods of administration include structured interviews with parents, observations by professionals or caregivers familiar with the child, or professional judgment based on knowledge of the child's capabilities.[1] Respondents are asked to report on the child's typical performance. The time required to administer the PEDI ranges from 20 minutes to 1 hour depending on the child's age and disability and the mode of administration selected. The PEDI should be completed in a quiet, private room. It is recommended that the administrator have experience in working with children and an understanding of normal development. Training includes review of the manual, a trial of scoring case examples in the manual, and watching other trained persons administer the scales. Equipment needed for the PEDI is the test manual, score form, and a computer. A software program for data entry, scoring, and generation of individual summary score profiles is available. Summary scores cannot be calculated if items are omitted.

Typical Reliability Estimates

Internal Consistency
- Cronbach' s alpha = 0.95 to 0.99 from the normative sample[1]

Interrater
- Inter-interviewer: ICC = 0.96 to 0.99 for the normative standardization sample[1] and 0.84 to 1.00 for the clinical standardization sample[1]
- Parent versus clinician: ICC = 0.20 to 0.93 for the Functional Skills scale and 0.15 to 0.95 for the Caregiver Assistance scale[12]

Test–Retest
- ICC: 0.67 to 1.00 on the Functional Skills scale and 0.63 to 0.98 on the Caregiver Assistance scale

Typical Validity Estimates

Content
Content validity was examined using 31 experts in pediatric rehabilitation who provided quantitative ratings and specific feedback on the appropriateness of items.[13] In addition, Rasch modeling was used in content specification and scale validation, summary score development, and goodness of fit between individual child profiles and the overall hierarchical structure intended for each scale.[13]

Criterion
No gold standard exists for the construct being measured.

Construct—Cross-sectional

Convergent
- BDIST: r = 0.62 to 0.92, in similar content domains[1,14,15]
- Wee Functional Independence Measure: r = 0.80 to 0.97 in similar domains[1,15]
- Gross Motor Function Measure: r = 0.75 to 0.85[16]
- Peabody Developmental Motor Scales (n = 25): r = 0.24 to 0.95[12]

Known Groups. Statistical significance of values not available, but in the normative sample (n = 412), subgroupings of infants, preschoolers, and school-age children demonstrated a progression of mean scores as age increased, lending support to the assumption that performance of hierarchical functional tasks is age dependent.[1]

Between normative group (n = 412) and clinical samples (n = 102) of children with varied levels of disability, the summary scores were used to pre-dict groupings. The PEDI was able to discriminate between groups at the $p < 0.001$ level, except for a few scores at the 6-month to 2-year age level.[1]

Discriminant. Not available

Construct—Longitudinal/Sensitivity to Change

Convergent. Not available

Known Group. In children with mild to moderate traumatic injuries who were expected to make considerable recovery, the PEDI was able to detect recovery of function from baseline to the 5- or 6-month follow-up on both the normative standard scores and scaled scores (paired t-tests, $p < 0.001$ to 0.031).[1]

Discriminant. Not available

Interpretability

General Population Values (Customary or Normative Values)
Standardization of the PEDI[1] was done on 412 children without disabilities, and data are available in the manual.

Typical Responsiveness Estimates

Individual Patient. Not available. However, there is some suggestion that the PEDI can detect statistically significant changes in mobility, self-care, and social functional skills in children after selective dorsal rhizotomy surgery for up to 12 months postoperatively.[7,8]

Between Group. Not available

References

1. Haley SM, Coster WJ, Ludlow LH, Haltiwanger JT, Andrellos PJ. **Pediatric Evaluation of Disability Inventory (PEDI). Version 1.0. Boston (MA): New England Medical Center Hospitals; 1992.**
2. World Health Organization. International classification of impairments, disabilities and handicaps. Geneva: World Health Organization; 1980.
3. Nagi SZ. Disability concepts revisited: implications for prevention. In: Disability in America: toward a national agenda for prevention. In: Pope AM, Tarlov AR, editors. Washington (DC): National Academy Press; 1991.
4. Graveline C, Young NL, Hwang P. Disability evaluation in children with hemidecorticectomy: use of the Activity Scales for Kids and the Pediatric Evaluation of Disability Inventory. J Child Neurol 2000;15:7–14.
5. Nordmark E, Jarnlo G-B, Hagglund G. Comparison of the Gross Motor Function Measure and Pediatric Evaluation of Disability Inventory in assessing motor function in children undergoing selective dorsal rhizotomy. Dev Med Child Neurol 2000;42:245–52.
6. Steinbok P. Outcomes after selective dorsal rhizotomy for spastic cerebral palsy. Childs Nerv Syst 2001;17:1–18.

7. Dudgeon BJ, Libby AK, McLaughlin JF, Hays RM, Bjornson KF, Roberts TS. Prospective measurement of functional changes after selective dorsal rhizotomy. Arch Phys Med Rehabil 1994;75:46–53.

8. Bloom KK, Nazar GB. Functional assessment following selective posterior rhizotomy in spastic cerebral palsy. Childs Nerv Syst 1994;10:84–6.

9. Engelbert RH, Gulmans VA, Uiterwaal CS, Helders PJ. Osteogenesis imperfecta in childhood: perceived competence in relation to impairment and disability. Arch Phys Med Rehabil 2001;82:943–8.

10. Engelbert RH, Custers JWH, van der Net J, van der Graaf Y, Beemer FA, Helders PJM. Functional outcome in osteogenesis imperfecta: disability profiles using the PEDI. Pediatr Phys Ther 1997;9:18–22.

11. Haley SM, Dumas HM, Ludlow LH. Variation by diagnostic and practice pattern groups in the mobility outcomes of inpatient rehabilitation programs for children and youth. Phys Ther 2001;81:1425–36.

12. Nichols DS, Case-Smith J. Reliability and validity of the Pediatric Evaluation of Disability Inventory. Pediatr Phys Ther 1996;8:15–24.

13. Haley SM, Coster WJ, Faas RM. A content validity study of the Pediatric Evaluation of Disability Inventory. Pediatr Phys Ther 1991;3:177–84.

14. Feldman AB, Haley SM, Coryell J. Concurrent and construct validity of the Pediatric Evaluation of Disability Inventory. Phys Ther 1990;70:602–10.

15. Schultz CJ. Concurrent validity of the Pediatric Evaluation of Disability Inventory [thesis]. Medford (MA): Tufts University; 1992.

16. Wright FV, Boschen KA. The Pediatric Evaluation of Disability Inventory (PEDI): validation of a new functional assessment outcome instrument. Can J Rehabil 1993;7:41–2.

17. Reid DT, Boschen KA, Wright V. Critique of the Pediatric Evaluation of Disability Inventory (PEDI). Phys Occup Ther Pediatr 1993;13:57–87.

18. Haley SM, Coster WJ. Response to Reid DT et al.'s critique of the Pediatric Evaluation of Disability Inventory. Phys Occup Ther Pediatr 1993;13:89–93.

19. Hey LA, Kasser J, Rosenthal R, et al. Feasibility and discriminant validity of a parent self-administered version of the Pediatric Evaluation of Disability Inventory. Dev Med Child Neurol 1992;34(9 Suppl 66):19.

20. Haley SM. The Pediatric Evaluation of Disability Inventory (PEDI). J Rehabil Outcomes Measurement 1997;1:61–9.

21. Young NL, Wright JG. Measuring pediatric physical function. J Pediatr Orthop 1995;15:244–53.

22. Haley SM, Ludlow LH, Coster WJ. Pediatric Evaluation of Disability Inventory: clinical interpretation of summary scores using Rasch rating scale methodology. Phys Med Rehabil Clin North Am 1993;4:529–40.

23. Nordmark E, Jarnlo G-B, Hagglund G. The American Pediatric Evaluation of Disability Inventory (PEDI). Applicability of PEDI in Sweden for children aged 2.0-6.9 years. Scand J Rehabil Med 1999;31:95–100.

24. Coster WJ, Haley SM, Baryza MJ. Functional performance of young children after traumatic brain injury: a 6-month follow-up study. Am J Occup Ther 1994;48:211–8.

To obtain this measure, contact the developers.

QUEBEC BACK PAIN DISABILITY SCALE

Developers

Jacek A. Kopec,* John M. Esdaile,* Michal Abrahamowicz,* Lucien Abenhaim,† Sharon Wood-Dauphinee,‡ Donna L. Lamping,§ and J. Ivan Williams.‖ Affiliated with: *Department of Epidemiology and Biostatistics and Division of Clinical Epidemiology, Department of Medicine, Montreal General Hospital, McGill University, Montreal, Quebec; †Clinical Epidemiology Centre, Jewish General Hospital, Montreal, Quebec; ‡School of Physical and Occupational Therapy, McGill University, Montreal, Quebec; §Department of Public Health and Policy, London School of Hygiene and Tropical Medicine, London, United Kingdom; and ‖Institute of Clinical Evaluative Sciences, Sunnybrook Health Science Centre, North York, Ontario

Purpose

To measure functional disability associated with back pain.[1,2] The objective was to construct a scale that was based on a sound conceptual model of disability; acceptable to clients, clinicians, and researchers; comprehensive; empirically valid; informative over a wide range of disability levels; reliable; and sensitive to change. The scale can be recommended as an outcome in clinical trials, for monitoring the progress of clients participating in treatment or rehabilitation programs, and for comparing different groups of back pain clients.[1]

Description

The Quebec Back Pain Disability Scale (QBPDS) is a self-administered measure of functional disability associated with back pain. It contains 20 items scored on a 0 to 5 Likert scale. Each item asks about the level of difficulty associated with a particular activity, with the response categories ranging from "not difficult at all" to "unable." The scale provides an overall disability score, ranging from 0 (no disability) to 100 (maximum disability), by simple summation of the scores for each item.[1]

Conceptual/Theoretical Basis of Construct Being Measured

The authors adopted the World Health Organization's definition of disability as "any restriction or lack of ability to perform an activity in a manner or within the range considered normal for a human being."[2] They developed a core list of 25 elementary activities that appeared to determine the ability to perform a wide range of more complex tasks and behaviors. For each elementary activity, the authors developed items assessing the amount of difficulty in simple daily activities. The concept of difficulty was attractive from a theoretical point of view and was considered the most useful measure of disability by back pain experts.[2] The items pertain to six subdomains of activity: bed/rest, sitting/standing, ambulation, movement, bending/stooping, and handling large/heavy objects.[1]

Groups Tested with This Measure

Subjects in the original validation study were ambulatory clients with back pain.[1,2] Clients with neck pain only were excluded. Duration of back pain was less than 6 weeks in 19.8% and more than 1 year in 43.8%; pain radiated to one or both legs in 67.8%, and 12% had prior back surgery. The Dutch version of the QBPDS has been validated in patients with chronic low back pain in general practice.[3] In addition, the QBPDS has been used in workers compensated for low back pain[4] and in women with pelvic pain since pregnancy.

Languages

The QBPDS is available in English, French, Dutch, and German. The measure was originally developed in English.[1,2] It has been translated, culturally adapted, and validated in French[1,2] and Dutch.[3] The measure has been translated and culturally adapted but not formally validated in German (MAPI Institute, personal communication).

Application/Administration

The QBPDS is a self-administered questionnaire that can be completed in 3 to 5 minutes. No training or equipment is needed. The overall score ranges from 0 to 100 (without standardization) and is calculated by adding the item scores, for which a calculator may be helpful. Missing data are handled by adjusting the maximum score (based on the number of items answered), dividing the sum of item scores by the adjusted maximum score, and multiplying by 100 to obtain a score on a 0 to 100 scale. (The questionnaire and instructions for scoring are available from the authors.)

Typical Reliability Estimates

Internal Consistency
Cronbach's alpha = 0.95 to 0.96[1,3]

Interrater
Not applicable

Test–Retest
ICC = 0.90 to 0.92[1,3]

Typical Validity Estimates

Content
The items were developed from the literature, interviews with clients, focus groups, and expert opinion. Factor analysis and statistical techniques based on item response theory were applied to evaluate the items. Based on these analyses, as well as other statistical and clinical criteria, 20 items were selected for the final scale.[1,2]

Criterion
No gold standard exists for the concept being measured.

Construct—Cross-sectional

Convergent
- Correlation with the Roland-Morris Questionnaire (RMQ): $r = 0.77$,[1] $r = 0.80$[3]
- Correlation with the Oswestry Low Back Pain Disability Questionnaire: $r = 0.80$[1]
- Correlation with the 36-Item Short-Form Health Survey (SF-36) Physical Function: $r = 0.72$[1]
- Correlation with pain: $r = 0.54$,[1] $r = 0.74$[3]

Known Groups. Mean scores are significantly different according to radiation of pain, previous surgery or hospitalization, use of medication, work absence, or workers' compensation.[1]

Discriminant. Not available

Construct—Longitudinal/Sensitivity to Change

Convergent
- Correlation of QBPDS change score with RMQ change score: $r = 0.60$[3]
- Correlation of QBPDS change score with pain severity change: $r = 0.53$[3]
- Correlation of QBPDS change score with "course of complaints": $r = 0.35$[3]
- Correlation of change scores with a 15-point scale of global change: $r = 0.42$[1]
- Ability to detect change in patients self-rated as "better" (paired *t*-test, n = 84): $t_{83} = 8.40$[1]
- Standardized response mean for subjects self-rated as "better": SRM = 0.92[1]

Known Groups. Comparison between clients' self-rated change as better versus worse: Norman S = 0.19 ($F_{1,54} = 7.76$)[1]

Discriminant. Not available

Other. In multiple regression: significant independent effects of age ($t = 2.01$), sex ($t = 2.8$), leg pain ($t = 3.03$), and previous surgery ($t = 2.62$)[1]

Interpretability

General Population Values
(Customary or Normative Values)
- Score distribution in the original validation study[1]: mean score = 47.0, SD = 24.4, symmetric distribution, median score between 40 and 50, 25th percentile 20 to 30, 75th percentile 60 to 70
- Typical between-group differences (cross-sectional)[1]: radiation of pain versus no radiation: d = 12.6 points; previous surgery versus no surgery: d = 13.7 points; current use of medication versus no use: d = 18.4 points; absence from work versus no absence: d = 19.1 points. Adjusted differences in multiple regression: leg pain d = 9.6 points, previous surgery d = 11.6 points.

Typical Responsiveness Estimates

Individual Patients
- Mean change in patients self-rated as "better": 15.3 points[1]
- Mean change in patients self-rated as "no change": 1.9 points (nonsignificant improvement)[1]
- Distribution of differences in stable patients (method 1)[3]: mean difference = 0.36 points, SD of differences = 8.48 points

- 95% of the difference scores dispersed up to 16 points above and under the mean difference
- Standard error of measurement from the formula $SEM = sd \sqrt{1 - ICC}$, using data from Kopec et al[1]: SEM = 6.9 points

Between Groups

- Mean change in a trial of "coordination of primary care" (CORE): 20.9 points improvement in the intervention arm compared with a 9.1-point improvement in the usual care arm ($p = 0.01$) (ie, about 12 points difference in change scores)[4]
- Amount of change that best distinguishes between clients who have improved and those remaining stable: approximately 15 points[5]

References

1. Kopec JA, Esdaile JM, Abrahamowicz M, Abenhaim L, Wood-Dauphinee S, Lamping DL, et al. The Quebec Back Pain Disability Scale: measurement properties. Spine 1995;20:341–52.
2. Kopec JA, Esdaile JM, Abrahamowicz M, Abenhaim L, Wood-Dauphinee S, Lamping DL, et al. The Quebec Back Pain Disability Scale: conceptualization and development. J Clin Epidemiol 1996;49:151–61.
3. Schoppink LE, van Tulder MW, Koes BW, Beurskens SAJHM, de Bie RA. Reliability and validity of the Dutch adaptation of the Quebec Back Pain Disability Scale. Phys Ther 1996;76:268–75.
4. Rossignol M, Abenhaim L, Seguin P, Neveu A, Collet J-P, Ducruet T, et al. Coordination of primary health care for back pain. A randomized controlled trial. Spine 2000;25:251–8.
5. Fritz JM, Irrgang JJ. A comparison of a modified Oswestry Low Back Pain Disability Questionnaire and the Quebec Back Pain Disability Scale. Phys Ther 2001;81:776–88.

To obtain this measure, contact the developers, or it can be found in reference 1.

REINTEGRATION TO NORMAL LIVING (RNL) INDEX

Developers

Sharon L. Wood-Dauphinee, M. A. Opzoomer, J. Ivan Williams, B. Marchand, and W. O. Spitzer.[1,2]

Purpose

This evaluative instrument is an outcome measure to assess how well individuals return to normal living patterns following incapacitating disease or injury.

Description

The RNL Index is made up of 11 declarative statements (eg, I move around my community as I feel necessary), including the following domains: indoor, community, and distance mobility; self-care; daily activity (work and school), recreational and social activities; general coping skills; family role(s); personal relationships; and presentation of self to others. Each domain is accompanied by a visual analogue scale (VAS 0 to 10) or a 3- or 4-point categorical scale. The analogue scale is anchored by the statements "does not describe my situation" and "fully describes my situation." The categorical scales have interim response descriptors "partially describes my situation" (3 points) or "somewhat describes my situation" and "mostly describes my situation" (4 points). The items add up to a total score. When scored on the VASs, the sum is algebraically converted to be out of 100; otherwise, scores range from 11 to 33 (3 points) or 11 to 44 (4 points). There are two subscales: Daily Activity (mobility, participation in work, social and recreational activities) and Perception of Self (comfort with relationships and coping skills). Higher scores denote better reintegration, but some investigators have reversed the scoring to reflect the amount of disability.[3]

Conceptual/Theoretical Basis of Construct Being Measured

The RNL Index was based on a dictionary definition of integration. Reintegration was conceptualized as meaning the reorganization of physical, psycholog-ical, and social characteristics so that an individual can resume well-adjusted living after incapacitating illness or trauma.[1,2] The emphasis of the RNL focuses on the perceptions of the individual and on his/her autonomy rather than what is generally considered "normal" from a societal perspective. "The ability to function, to do what one wants to do or feels one has to do, not that one must be free of symptoms, disability or help in the form of human assistance or mechanical devices. Symptoms and disability can be tolerated as long as the individual can accomplish what one wishes to do to his own satisfaction."[2]

Groups Tested with This Measure

People with malignant tumors, degenerative heart disease, central nervous system disorders, arthritis, fractures, and amputations[1,2]; stroke[3,4]; spinal cord injury[5]; lower limb amputations[6]; traumatic brain injury[7-9]; rheumatoid arthritis[10]; subarachnoid hemorrhage[11]; hip fracture[4]; and physical disability[12]; and community-dwelling elderly.[13] In addition, the measure has been used in people who have ostomies or lower extremity sarcomas as well as in the elderly who have ruptured and unruptured cerebral aneurysms.

Languages

The RNL was developed in Canadian English and Canadian French.[1,2] No important differences between language groups were identified.

Application/Administration

The RNL can be interviewer administered (face to face or over the telephone), self-completed, or completed by a proxy.[1,2,4,7] The time to administer depends on mode and subjects but is always less than 10 minutes.

Typical Reliability Estimates

Internal Consistency

Cronbach's alpha for patient sample = 0.90, for significant others = 0.92, and for health professionals = 0.95. Corrected item to total correlations ranged from 0.39 to 0.75 for patients, 0.61 to 0.87 for significant others, and 0.70 to 0.90 for health professionals.[2] Cronbach's alpha for community-living elderly sample = 0.76 to 0.90.[13]

Interrater

Significant other to patient correlations, $r = 0.62$ and 0.69; health professional to patient correlations, $r = 0.39$ and 0.43.[2] Problems in RNL domains were more likely reported by proxy than patients in both face-to-face and telephone interviews.[4] At admission to a treatment program, patients' and proxies' scores did not differ significantly: at discharge and follow-up, they differed significantly ($U = 0$, $p < 0.001$).[7]

Test–Retest

- Community-dwelling elderly: $r = 0.83$. By age group: 75 to 79 years, $r = 0.82$; 80 to 84 years, $r = 0.93$; 85+ years, $r = 0.76$[13]
- Adults with traumatic brain injury: for patients, $r = 0.12$; for significant others, $r = 0.79$[7]

Typical Validity Estimates

Content

Content validity was deemed present owing to the method of development. It included literature reviews, incorporation of experiences of investigators, and applications of open- and close-ended questionnaires given to patients with myocardial infarction, cancer, and other chronic diseases; health professionals (physicians, social workers, physical and occupational therapists, psychologists); significant others of patients; and clergy and other lay people.[1,2]

Criterion

No gold (or even silver) standard was found.

Construct—Cross-sectional

Convergent. In those with mild traumatic brain damage, a significant association was found with discharge disposition in the post hospital phase.[9] Among lower limb amputees, the RNL and its Daily Activities subscale correlated in the expected direction and moderately with most of the items in the subscale related to physical performance of the Prosthetic Profile of the Amputee Questionnaire. It failed to correlate significantly with items related to use of the prosthesis[6] ($r = 0.36$ to 0.56). In those with long-standing spinal cord injury, the multiple regression analysis of the RNL reported significant beta coefficients with the Functional Independence Measure (FIM) (0.34), the Yale Scale Score (0.99), the CES-D

(0.87), living conditions (9.02), relationships (7.39), sexual life (6.96), and age (0.27).[5] With people with rheumatoid arthritis, scores on the RNL were significantly correlated with disease duration, number of affected joints, the FIM, the Lee Index (pain, fatigue, and stiffness), and the American Rheumatism Association Classification ($r = 0.31$ to 0.83).[10] In community-dwelling individuals with a disability, RNL scores were related to the Canadian Occupational Performance Measure (multiple regression model) and to the Satisfaction with Performance Scaled Questionnaire ($r = 0.72$).[12] In clients with cancer, RNL scores were marginally related to work status and disease status but were not related to family status, living arrangements, or the presence of problems in living during the first year after the diagnosis and treatment for cancer.[2] Further, they were significantly associated with the Quality of Life (QL) Index ($r = 0.68$) and a measure of psychological well-being (r ranged from 0.32 to 0.41).[2]

Known Groups. When people at 3 months and 1 year post-stroke were divided by levels of impairment (mild-moderate-severe according to Adam's Scale), by the presence or absence of depression (Zung scale), by levels of physical disability (independent-moderately dependent-dependent-FIM), and by levels of cognitive disability (independent-moderately dependent-dependent-FIM), RNL scores for these known groups demonstrated expected gradients and were significantly different as analyzed by analysis of variance. The differences between categories in these analyses ranged from 12 to 62%.[3] When people at a mean of 4.4 years post-traumatic brain injury were divided by baseline severity scores into mild, moderate, and severe categories, mean RNL scores by group were not significantly different.[8] However, when people with mild traumatic brain injury were divided according to definite post-traumatic stress, possible post-traumatic stress, and no post-traumatic stress, RNL scores were significantly different across the groups.[9] The RNL failed to significantly differentiate those with paraplegia and those with tetraplegia (mean scores = 81.8 [14.5] and 78.4 [14.5] in a long-term follow-up.[5]

Discriminant. Not available

Construct—Longitudinal/Sensitivity to Change

Convergent. When patients with a new diagnosis of cancer or myocardial infarction and their significant others were interviewed shortly after discharge from the acute care institution and 3 months later on the RNL and the Quality of Life indices, the change scores correlated significantly (patients' $r = 0.56$ and significant others' $r = 0.36$).[2]

Known Groups and *Discriminant* are not available.

Other Validity Coefficients

Convergent/Discriminant. In an elderly community-based population, the RNL demonstrated stronger positive correlations with instrumental activities of daily living and perceived health and stronger negative correlations with living alone and number of both bed days and chronic conditions than with gender as hypothesized. There was an unpredicted negative correlation between age and RNL.[13]

Interpretability

General Population Values
(Customary or Normative Values)

A distribution of RNL scores at a follow-up evaluation was proposed for individuals who had sustained a subarachnoid hemorrhage in terms of problems related to reintegration. Those scoring between 0 and 59 reported severe impairment, those scoring 60 to 79 had moderate impairment, those scoring 80 to 99 had mild impairment, and those scoring 100 had no impairment. It is unclear how this distribution was generated.

Typical Responsiveness Estimates

Individual Patient. In clients (myocardial infarction and cancer) who were newly diagnosed, hospitalized, treated and discharged from hospital, and followed up at 3 months, a preliminary evaluation of responsiveness by considering change scores in items showed that most patients changed at this level.[2] A similar preliminary evaluation of changes in group scores on subscales for these same patients showed some evidence of change in the overall index and in the Daily Functioning subscale but not in the Perception of Self subscale.[2]

Between Group. Clients receiving occupational therapy treatments and their significant others reported improvement on RNL scores from admission to discharge (effect size $d = 0.71$) and from discharge to follow-up (effect size $d = 0.61$).[7]

References

1. Wood-Dauphinee S, Williams JI. Reintegration to normal living as a proxy to quality of life. J Chron Dis 1987;40:491–9.
2. **Wood-Dauphinee SL, Opzoomer MA, Williams JI, Marchand B, Spitzer WO. Assessment of global function: the Reintegration to Normal Living Index. Arch Phys Med Rehabil 1988;69:583–90.**
3. Clarke PA, Black SE, Badley EM, Lawrence JM, Williams JL. Handicap in stroke survivors. Disabil Rehabil 1999;21:116–23.
4. Korner-Bitensky N, Wood-Dauphinee S, Siemiatcky J, Shapiro S, Becker R. Health related information post discharge: telephone versus face-to-face interviewing. Arch Phys Med Rehabil 1994;75:1287–96.
5. Daverat P, Petit H, Kemoun G, Dartigues JF, Barat M. The long term outcome in 149 patients with spinal cord injury. Paraplegia 1995;33:665–8.
6. Gauthier-Gagnon C, Grise M-C. Prosthetic Profile of the Amputee Questionnaire: validity and reliability. Arch Phys Med Rehabil 1994;75:1309–14.
7. Trombly CA, Radomsky MV, Davis ES. Achievement of self identified goals by adults with traumatic brain injury: phase I. Am J Occup Ther 1998;52:810–8.
8. Dawson DR, Levine B, Schwartz M, Stuss DT. Quality of life following traumatic brain injury. Brain Cogn 2000;44:35–9.
9. Friedland JF, Dawson DR. Function after motor vehicle accidents: a prospective study of mild head injury and post traumatic stress. J Nerv Ment Dis 2001;189:426–34.
10. Calmels P, Pereira A, Domenach M, Pallot-Prades B, Alexandre C, Minaire P. Functional ability and quality of life in rheumatoid arthritis: evaluation using the Functional Independence Measure and the Reintegration to Normal Living Index. Rev Rhumat 1994;61:723–31.
11. Carter BS, Buckley D, Ferraro R, Rordorf G, Ogilvy CS. Factors associated with reintegration to normal living after subarachnoid hemorrhage. Neurosurgery 2000;46:1326–33.
12. McColl MA, Paterson M, Davies D, Doubt L, Law M. Validity and utility of the Canadian Occupational Performance Measure. Can J Occup Ther 2000;67:22–33.
13. Steiner A, Raube K, Stuck AE, Aronow HU, Draper, Rubenstein LZ, et al. Measuring psychological aspects of well-being in older community residents: performance of four short scales. Gerontologist 1996;36:54–62.

This measure can be found on the accompanying CD-ROM. Prior to using the measure, you are strongly advised to contact the developers for administration and scoring guidelines and revisions to the measure not available at time of publication.

Rivermead Motor Assessment (RMA)

Developers

Nadina Lincoln and D. Leadbitter in 1979.[1] Correspondence to Dr. Nadina B. Lincoln, Reader in Psychology, School of Psychology, University of Nottingham, University Park, Nottingham, NG7 2RD, UK; e-mail: nbl@psychology.nottingham.ac.uk

Purpose

The RMA assesses the motor performance of people who have suffered a stroke and was developed for clinical and research use.[1,2] When it was developed, there were no short, reliable, valid, and scoreable systems for assessing movement.

Description

The RMA, a performance measure, consists of test items in three sections that are ordered hierarchically, that is, the first items are easier and become increasingly difficult toward the end of the evaluation. When a client fails one item, it is assumed that all subsequent items will also be failed, so not all items in the scale need to be administered.[3] The three sections test total body movements (gross function), leg and trunk movements, and arm movements.[2] Clients are assessed on each item on the scale, which is scored 0 or 1, depending on whether the client does the activity according to the specific instructions.[1]

Conceptual/Theoretical Basis of Construct Being Measured

The RMA is based on the assumption that stroke clients follow a consistent pattern of recovery. A cumulative model known as Guttman scaling, in which the activities assessed are ordered hierarchically according to their difficulty, was developed.[1] Guttman scaling is described as one way of demonstrating that activities in a scale belong together.[4] The mathematical procedure of Guttman scaling is said to be used "to examine the consistency of the hierarchy."[2]

Groups Tested with This Measure

Acute and chronic stroke clients

Language

English (United Kingdom)

Application/Administration

Clients are assessed by a physical therapist. The items are scored as pass or fail, and the client may have up to three trials to succeed. When three consecutive items are failed, the test stops, reducing the time to administer the test for lower-performing subjects.[1] The ambulatory client with a recovering upper extremity takes approximately 45 minutes to assess; more severely disabled patients take less time.[1]

Typical Reliability Estimates

Internal Consistency
Not available

Interrater
Seven raters evaluated seven stroke clients by viewing videotaped assessments. Analysis of variance (ANOVA) of the scores obtained indicated that, for all three subscales, variability between clients was higher than the variability between raters (F tests from ANOVA are reported but no ICCs). On the gross function and leg and trunk subscales, there were no significant differences on average scores for all clients across all raters. For the arm subscale, there was a significant difference across raters attributed to only one of the six raters. Revised scoring instructions were therefore produced for the arm scale, but further testing has not been forthcoming.[1]

Test–Retest
Stroke clients (4-week interval): $r = 0.66$, 0.93, and 0.88 for the gross function, leg and trunk, and arm subscales, respectively.[1] Chronic stroke clients[5]: no significant difference was found between patients' reporting and viewed performance. Over the four assessment periods, subjects were ranked with a high degree of consistency. Kendall's coefficient of concordance (W) on the total scores was good (W = 0.80; $\chi^2 = 60.9$; df = 57). The kappa value for the total score (treating each score as a categorical value, 1, 2, 3, 4, etc, depending on how many items were passed) was 0.23, indicating only poor agreement, across assessments. However, this kappa value was equivalent to a z score of 4.5; $p < 0.001$, indicating that this degree of agreement was much greater than chance. The kappa values for individual items across the four assessments were quite consistent (range of k from 0.33 to 0.38) but, again, in the "poor" classification. (Kappa values can be artificial-

ly low if many subjects achieve the same value because chance agreement is then very high.)

Typical Validity Estimates

Content
Content validity with Guttman scaling is evaluated on the extent to which total scores predict the number of consecutive items passed. Critical values for two indices, coefficient of reproducibility (CR) and coefficient of scalability (CS), were all exceeded in a study of 51 stroke clients, confirming the existence of a valid Guttman scale, which is both cumulative and unidimensional.[1]

Criterion
No gold standard exists for the construct being measured.

Construct
The concept of scalability—a hierarchy of abilities—was evaluated by one study on acute stroke clients[2] and one on nonacute stroke patients.[3] Fifty-one acute stroke clients were evaluated at 1, 3, and 6 weeks post stroke. The CS and CR for two of the subscales, gross function and arm, at all three time periods, met the critical values for a hierarchical scale. However, these critical values were not met for the subscale referring to leg and trunk function, indicating that, early on after stroke, these items are not hierarchically achieved.[2]

Construct—Longitudinal/Sensitivity to Change
In assessments of 51 acute stroke clients done at 1, 3, and 6 weeks post stroke, the proportion passing one item of the gross function subscale increased from 80 to 100% over this time period.[2] Similarly, the proportion passing 10 items (of a possible 13) increased from 5 to 50%. However, the scalability was not perfect as the proportion of persons able to climb stairs (the seventh most difficult item) was less than the proportion of persons able to walk 10 m unaided (the eighth most difficult item). The leg and trunk subscale was even less consistent.

In nonacute stroke clients,[3] the item ordering and changes over time were not consistent with a hierarchical scale. This was confirmed by a 1997 study of 206 stroke clients evaluated 6 and 12 months after discharge. Only the gross function subscale approached the critical values for CR and CS. The trunk and leg subscale was particularly poor as many subjects failed items judged to be easy and yet passed more difficult items. This was attributed to a change in treatment approach occurring since the first development of the scale in the 1970s.

Interpretability

General Population Values (Customary or Normative Values)
Not available

Typical Responsiveness Estimates

Individual Patient. A difference of 3 points in the RMA was the actual limit of reliability. Therefore, a total score difference of plus or minus 3 is likely to mean a clinically relevant change in functional level.[5]

Between Group. Not available

Comments
Lincoln and Leadbitter recommend that, when the scale is used with an older population, account should be taken of items failed owing to age rather than as a result of stroke. In addition, account must be taken of any additional disability the patient may present with, for example an amputation, and the principle of stopping after three consecutive errors should not be applied.[1] According to Streiner and Norman,[6] this type of scaling is better suited to behaviors that are developmentally determined (eg, crawling, standing, walking, running), for which mastery of one behavior virtually guarantees mastery of the lower-order behaviors. Guttman scaling may not be appropriate to assess function in the hemiplegic stroke client. It is not appropriate in assessing the kind of loss in function owing to focal lesions that arise in stroke clients, in whom impairment of some function may be unrelated to impairment of other functions.[7]

References

1. Lincoln NB, Leadbitter D. Assessment of motor function in stroke patients. Physiotherapy 1979;65:48–51.
2. Adams SA, Ashburn A, Pickering RM, Taylor D. The scalability of the Rivermead Motor Assessment in acute stroke patients. Clin Rehabil 1997;11:42–51.
3. Adams SA, Pickering RM, Ashburn A, Lincoln NB. The scalability of the Rivermead Motor Assessment in nonacute stroke patients. Clin Rehabil 1997;11:52–9.
4. Barer D, Nouri F. Measurement of activities of daily living. Clin Rehabil 1989;3:179–87.
5. Collen FM, Wade DT, Bradshaw CM. Mobility after stroke: reliability of measures of impairment and disability. Int Disabil Stud 1990;12:6–9.
6. Streiner DL, Norman GR. Health measurement scales: a practical guide to their development and use. Oxford: Oxford University Press; 1989.

To obtain this measure, contact the developers.

ROLAND-MORRIS QUESTIONNAIRE

Developers

M. Roland and R. Morris,[1] mroland@man.ac.uk

Purpose

To assess functional status and pain-related disability status in clients with low back pain.

Description

The Roland-Morris Questionnaire (RMQ) (also known as St. Thomas) is a 24-item self-report condition-specific functional status measure intended for clients with low back pain. Items were selected from the 136-item Sickness Impact Profile, a generic health status measure. The phrase "because of my back or back pain" was added to each item. Items are scored "1" if endorsed by a client and "0" if left blank. Thus, RMQ scores can vary from 0, the highest functional state, to 24, the lowest functional state.

Conceptual/Theoretical Basis of Construct Being Measured

None reported.

Groups Tested with This Measure

Clients with acute, subacute, and chronic back pain and various conservative, surgical, and behavioral intervention groups.

Languages

English, French (Canadian),[2] German,[3] Swedish,[3] Dutch,[3] Romanian,[3] Spanish,[3] Italian,[3] and Polish[3]

Application/Administration

This is a self-report measure in which clients circle the relevant responses. Most clients can complete the questions in 3 to 5 minutes.

Typical Reliability Estimates

Internal Consistency
- Coefficient alpha values: 0.87 to 0.92[4,5]

Interrater
Not applicable

Test–Retest
- ICC: 0.79 to 0.91[2,6]

Typical Validity Estimates

Content
No reference to content validity in the literature.

Criterion
No gold standard exists for the attribute being assessed.

Construct—Cross-sectional

Convergent
- Correlations with other condition-specific measures for persons with low back pain: $r = 0.75$ to 0.82[2,5,7]

Known Groups. Capable of discriminating among persons with different levels of impairment ($F_{1,141} = 18.18$), work status ($F_{2,146} = 19.86$), and location of pain ($F_{2,149} = 10.31$).[6]

Discriminant. Not available

Construct—Longitudinal/Sensitivity to Change

Convergent
- Change score correlations with the change scores of other condition-specific measures for persons with low back pain: $r = 0.64$ to 0.82[2,5,7]
- Correlation with prognostic rating of change: $r = 0.56$.[5]

Known Groups
- Dichotomized retrospective global rating of change: Norman's $S_{repeat} = 0.35$ ($p < 0.05$); receiver operating characteristic curve: area $= 0.79$ to 0.93[7–10]

Discriminant. Not available

Interpretability

General Population Values (Customary or Normative Values)
Not available

Typical Responsiveness Estimates

Individual Patient. Confidence in a measured score: 90% CI = ±3 RMQ points. Error is specific to a patient's score.[4] True change estimates: 90% of stable patients display a difference of less than 5 RMQ points on retest: $MDC_{90} = 5$ points. Error is specific to a patient's change score.[4] Minimal clinically important difference: MCID = 5 RMQ change points for the entire scale. MCID has been shown to be dependent on a patient's functional status level.[8,9]

Between Group. 2 to 3 RMQ points[3]

Comments

More is known about the measurement properties of the RMQ than any other functional status measure for clients with low back pain. Point estimates from head-to-head comparison studies suggest that the RMQ is more adept at detecting change than the Oswestry and Quebec measures.[2,10]

References

1. Roland M, Morris R. A study of the natural history of back pain. Part I: development of a reliable and sensitive measure of disability in low-back pain. Spine 1983;8:141–4.

2. Kopec JA, Esdaile JM, Abrahamowicz M, Abenhaim L, Wood-Dauphinee S, Lamping DL, et al. The Quebec Back Pain Disability Scale: measurement properties. Spine 1995;20:341–52.

3. Roland M, Fairbank J. The Roland-Morris Disability Questionnaire and the Oswestry Disability Questionnaire. Spine 2000;24:3115–24.

4. Stratford PW, Binkley J, Solomon P, Finch E, Gill C, Moreland J. Defining the minimal level of detectable change for the Roland-Morris Questionnaire. Phys Ther 1996;76:359–65.

5. Stratford PW, Binkley JM, Riddle DL. Development and initial validation of the Back Pain Functional Scale. Spine 2000; 25:2095–102.

6. Stratford PW, Binkley JM. A comparison study of the Back Pain Functional Scale and Roland-Morris Questionnaire. J Rheumatol 2000;27:1928–36.

7. Stratford PW, Binkley JM. Measurement properties of the RM-18 a modified version of the Roland-Morris disability scale. Spine 1997;22:2416–21.

8. Stratford PW, Binkley JM, Riddle DL. Sensitivity to change of the Roland-Morris back pain questionnaire: Part 1. Phys Ther 1998;78:1186–96.

9. Riddle DL, Stratford PW, Binkley JM. Sensitivity to change of the Roland-Morris back pain questionnaire: Part II. Phys Ther 1998;78:1197–207.

10. Beurskens AJHM, de Vet HCW, Koke AJA. Responsiveness of functional status in low back pain: a comparison of different instruments. Pain 1996;65:71–6.

To obtain this measure, contact the developers, or it can be found in reference 1.

SA-SIP30
(STROKE-ADAPTED SICKNESS IMPACT PROFILE)

Developers

A. van Straten, R. J. de Haan, M. Limburg, J. Schuling, P. M. Bossuyt, B. A. M. van den Bos. Correspondence to A. van Straten, PhD, Trimbos Institute, PO Box 725, 3500 AS Utrecht, Netherlands; e-mail: astraten@trimbos.nl.

Purpose

The purpose of the SA-SIP30 is to assess quality of life (QOL) in clients having sustained a stroke.[1]

Description

The new stroke-adapted 30-item measure was adapted from the original Sickness Impact Profile (SIP136). It is a 30-item questionnaire that can be administered through interview or self-administered.[2] All responses are "yes" or "no." It comprises eight domains: Body Care and Movement, Social Interaction, Mobility, Communication, Emotional Behavior, Household Management, Alertness Behavior, and Ambulation. It measures observable behavior, and the scoring of items, subscales, dimensions, and total score is the same as for the original SIP136 version. The scores are presented as a percentage of maximal dysfunction, ranging from 0 to 100%, with higher scores indicating less desirable health outcomes.[3]

Conceptual/Theoretical Basis of Construct Being Measured

Quality of life is said to lie beyond the disease-handicap continuum,[4] and there is general agreement that the effects of treatment should be measured in terms of quality and quantity of survival.[5] Three aspects of functioning, physical, social, and emotional, are generally referred to as QOL.[1] The SIP is one of the most widely used measures to assess QOL. The SA-SIP30 was constructed to overcome the major disadvantage of the SIP, its length.[1] According to the developers, the original SIP and the stroke-adapted 30-item version of the SIP mainly measure aspects of disability instead of health-related QOL; both SIP versions provide more clini-

cal information than the frequently used disability measures, and in stroke outcome research, the SA-SIP30 should be preferred over the original SIP.[3]

Groups Tested with This Measure

Communicative stroke clients at 6 months post stroke[3]

Language

English

Application/Administration

The SA-SIP30 can be administered through interview or self-administered. There is no evidence of suitability for use with proxies.[2] The average completion time has not been reported.

Typical Reliability Estimates

Internal Consistency

Cronbach's alpha for the total SA-SIP30 (0.85), the psychological dimension (0.78), and the physical dimension (0.82). On a subscale level, the alpha coefficients were sufficient with the exception of the subscales Emotional Behavior (0.57) and Ambulation (0.54). The theoretically estimated Spearman-Brown coefficients were higher than the alphas found in the original SIP136.[1]

Interrater

Not reported (see original version).

Test–Retest

Not reported (see original version).

Typical Validity Estimates

Content

1. *Exclusion of the least relevant items.* Using a multistep, statistical process, the items that were judged to be least relevant for stroke clients within each subscale were excluded; items with a very skewed response pattern were dropped, and items applying to less than 10% of all clients were removed. The relevance of the remaining items within each subscale was subsequently assessed statistically with linear regression analysis with a forward selection

strategy, using the F statistic with $p = 0.5$ as the criteria level for selection. For each subscale, the item selection was stopped when the items included in the regression model explained 80% of the score variation of the concerned original total subscale.[1]

2. *Excluding the least relevant subscales.* A stepwise linear regression procedure with forward inclusion was performed to explain the variation of the total original SIP136 score with the (shortened) subscales. The selection of relevant subscales was stopped when adding another subscale into the model did not result in an increase in the percentage of explained variance of more than 1%.[1]

3. *Excluding unreliable items.* The last step focused on the exclusion of items that did not contribute to the homogeneity of the subscales, provided that three items remained in each subscale.[1]

Criterion
No gold standard exists for the construct being measured.

Construct—Cross-sectional
A principal component analysis confirmed a physical dimension and a psychosocial dimension. Twenty percent of the SA-SIP30-explained score variance could be ascribed to the physical dimension and 11% to the psychosocial dimension.[1]

Convergent. The SA-SIP30 total score could explain 91% of the variation on the original SIP136 total scores. Furthermore, 87% of the original physical dimension scores could be explained by the SA-SIP30 and 88% of the psychosocial dimension scores. For the different subscales, the percentages of explained variance ranged from 69 (Social Interaction) to 84% (Emotional Behavior). The Spearman rank correlation coefficient between the SA-SIP30 and the SIP136 total scores was 0.96 ($p < 0.01$).[1]

Known Groups. The SA-SIP30 was unable to distinguish between clients with supratentorial and infratentorial strokes ($p = 0.67$). The SA-SIP30 is able to distinguish clients with lacunar infarctions from those with cortical or subcortical lesions;

clients with lacunar infarcts reported better functional health than those with cortical or subcortical lesions on the total SA-SIP30 ($p < 0.01$), its psychosocial dimension ($p < 0.01$), and all subscales with the exception of Emotional Behavior ($p = 0.49$) and Mobility ($p = 0.07$).[1]

Discriminant. Not available

Construct—Longitudinal/Sensitivity to Change
Not available

Interpretability

General Population Values (Customary or Normative Values)
In general, clients with an SA-SIP30 of > 33 were unable to live independently; experienced at least some problems in mobility, self-care, and in performing their main activity; and valued their health related QOL as poor. The psychosocial dimension scores remain largely unexplained; no cutoff values could be demonstrated.[3]

Typical Responsiveness Estimates
Not available

Comments
The items of the SA-SIP30, like the original SIP136, are worded in the negative sense, which is contrary to the philosophy of rehabilitation: "glass half full versus glass half empty."

References
1. van Straten A, de Haan RJ, Limburg M, Schuling J, Bossuyt PM, van den Bos GAM. A stroke-adapted 30-item version of the Sickness Impact Profile to assess quality of life (SA-SIP30). Stroke 1997;28:2155–61.
2. Buck D, Jacoby A, Massey A, Ford G. Evaluation of measures used to assess quality of life after stroke. Stroke 2000;31:2004–10.
3. van Straten A, de Haan RJ, Limburg M, van den Bos GAM. Clinical meaning of the Stroke-Adapted Sickness Impact Profile-30 and the Sickness Impact Profile-136. Stroke 2000;31:2610–5.
4. Tennant A, Geddes JML, Fear J, Hillman M, Chamberlain MA. Outcome following stroke. Disabil Rehabil 1997;19:278–84.
5. Fallowfield L. The quality of life: the missing measurement in health care. London: Souvenir Press; 1990.

To obtain this measure, contact the developers, or it can be found in reference 1.

SF-36® (Medical Outcomes Study 36-Item Short-Form Health Survey)

Developers

John E. Ware Jr, Cathy D. Sherbourne, Ron D. Hays, Anita Stewart, Sandy Berry, and Barbara Gandek; www.sf-36.com, www.qlmed.org/mot

Purpose

This evaluative scale was designed as an indicator of perceived health status for use in general and specific populations. It has been useful in comparing the relative burden of diseases, evaluating the effectiveness of different treatments, and identifying "at-risk" individuals.

Description

A 36-item survey that includes eight multi-item scales measuring physical functioning (PF) (10 items), role limitations owing to physical health problems (RP) (4 items), bodily pain (BP) (2 items), general health perceptions (GH) (5 items), vitality (VT) (4 items), social functioning (SF) (2 items), role limitations owing to emotional problems (RE) (3 items), and mental health (MH) (5 items). There is also a single transition item that indicates perceived change in health. Response choices range from two-level to six-level scales. The scores on all subscales range from 0 to 100, with higher scores indicating better health states. A physical and a mental health component can be derived from the items. These two subcomponents have been standardized to have a mean of 50 and a standard deviation of 10. Version 2.0 of the SF-36, introduced in 1996 to improve several aspects of the standard version 1.0, includes a five-level response choice in place of the two-level response choices for items in the two role functioning scales and six-level response choices for the MH and the VT items. There is also an acute version of the SF-36 that uses a 1-week recall period and is useful when the effects of treatment are expected to occur rapidly.

Conceptual/Theoretical Basis of Construct Being Measured

Most items were adapted from the measures that were used in the Rand Health Insurance Experiment surveys and the Medical Outcomes Study (MOS).

The centrality of the individual's point of view in monitoring the quality of medical care outcomes was an underlying concept in the development of the SF-36. Although the creation of a brief scale was desirable, it also needed to be comprehensive, representing both physical and mental health dimensions. From the more than 40 concepts and scales studied in the MOS, a subset of eight health concepts was selected.[1–4]

Groups Tested with This Measure

General populations, elderly individuals. It has been used to estimate disease burden in more than 130 diseases and conditions[2,5,6] (see also the SF-36 Website).

Languages

More than 50 languages, including Canadian English and Canadian French.[7] The International Quality of Life Assessment (IQOLA) Project has been designed to translate and adapt the SF-36 and to validate, norm, and document the new translations as required for their use in international studies of health outcomes.[8] The IQOLA Website (www.iqola.org) provides information about the project, and the e-mail contact is <info@iqola.org>. Information about the availability of SF-36 translations can be accessed on the SF-36 Website, and some translations are available for purchase at that site.

Application/Administration

The SF-36 can be self-administered by persons aged 14 years or older or administered by trained interviewers either in person or by telephone. It takes 5 to 10 minutes to complete; elderly people may require up to 20 minutes. Standard SF-36 scoring is most commonly used. Subscale scores can also be calculated manually using a series of steps.[1,4] As a first step, all items are oriented so that a higher score represents better health. Two items, GH rating (item 1) and BP (item 7), require recalibration to meet the assumption of equal intervals. For item 1, the recommended scoring is as follows: excellent = 5.0, very good = 4.4, good = 3.4, fair = 2.0, poor = 1.0. For item 7, none = 6.0, very mild = 5.4, mild = 4.2, moderate = 3.1, severe = 2.2, and very severe = 1.0. Scores for item 8 take account of the answers to item

TABLE 1 Reliability Estimates for SF-36

Sample	Internal Consistency (Cronbach's α)	Test–Retest
Sample from MOS with chronic medical and psychiatric conditions (n = 1,014)[9]	0.78 to 0.93	
General practice patients (n = 1,582)[10]	0.73 to 0.96	
General practice patients (n = 187); 2-week interval[10]		r = 0.60 to 0.81
Individuals over 65 years of age (n = 8,117)[11]	> 0.79 for all subscales	
Chronic stroke (n = 90)[12]	> 0.60 for all subscales	
Chronic stroke (n = 849)[13]	0.80 to 0.96	
Chronic stroke (n = 106); 3-week interval[13]		ICCs = 0.30 (MH) to 0.81 (GH, BP)
Multiple sclerosis (n = 150)[14]	0.77 to 0.94	
Arthritis (n = 1,016)[15]	0.75 (BP) to 0.91 (PF)	
Rheumatoid arthritis (n = 233); 2-week interval[16]		ICCs = 0.76 to 0.93
Asthma (n = 142)[17]	0.64 (RE) to 0.86 (PF)	

MOS = Medical Outcomes Study; MH = mental health; GH = general health; BP = bodily pain; PF = physical functioning; RE = role limitations related to emotional problems.

7: if no pain is recorded on either item, then item 8 is scored 6.0. If item 8 is answered not at all but item 7 is greater than none, then item 8 is scored 5. For the remaining categories of item 8, a little bit = 4, moderately = 3, quite a bit = 2, and extremely = 1. If less than 50% of the items in each subscale are missing, a mean of the nonmissing items is substituted. Scores for items on each scale are added to give subscale scores. Finally, the raw scores are transformed to a 0 to 100 scale using the following formula: transformed scale = [(actual raw score – lowest possible raw score)/possible raw score range] x 100. A computerized algorithm for scoring the subscales and the mental and physical summary scores is available. Information about an on-line automated scoring service is available at www.qmetric.com. Version 2.0 scoring uses norm-based scoring algorithms for all eight subscales (T-score transformations with mean, 50 ± 10 [SD]), which has made the SF-36 summary measures much easier to interpret.

Typical Reliability Estimates

Internal Consistency
See Table 1.

Interrater
Examined in the context of proxy/subject in a study with 38 chronic stroke survivors and their caregivers (spouses, daughters, and siblings), ICCs ranged from 0.15 (RE) to 0.67 (PF).[18]

Test–Retest
See Table 1.

Typical Validity Estimates

Content
Systematic comparisons of the content of the SF-36 with that of other generic health surveys indicate that it includes eight of the most frequently measured health concepts. Multiple indicators of behavioral function, perceived well-being, social and role disability, and evaluations of health in general were chosen to measure the physical and mental health dimensions.[1–4] Detailed information about content validity can be found in the SF-36 manuals.[1,19]

Criterion

Concurrent. Although not criteria in the sense of being "gold standards," comparisons of scale scores with ability to work, symptoms, use of care, and a range of criteria for the MH scale suggested significant and consistent associations with the validation criteria.[1] For example, hospitalization rate during the past 3 months was nearly 10 times higher for those who evaluated their health as "poor" compared with "excellent."

Predictive. Evaluated among 877 chronically ill persons who were 65 years or older participating in the MOS,[20] the GH scale differentiated the most with respect to mortality: the death rate for patients in the lowest quartile was nearly three times that in the highest quartile. The PF scale was also highly predictive of mortality. Further, those individuals in the lowest quartile of the subscales measuring physical health were twice as likely to be hospitalized over a 2-year period than were those in the highest quartile.

Construct—Cross-sectional

Factor analytic methods were used to evaluate the construct validity of the SF-36 in relation to a two-factor physical and mental model of health across populations.[19] Principal component analyses performed in 23 subgroups of MOS patients differing in demographic characteristics and medical conditions strongly supported the two-dimensional model of health.

Convergent/Discriminant. As hypothesized, the correlation between comparable dimensions on the SF-36 and other measures, for example, the physi-

cal subscales of the SF-36 and other physical scales, was higher than the correlations between less comparable dimensions, for example, the physical functioning and emotional scales (Table 2).

Known Groups. In validity testing of the SF-36 subscales on MOS data, four mutually exclusive groups were formed: (1) minor uncomplicated chronic medical conditions (n = 638), (2) serious complicated chronic medical conditions (n = 168), (3) psychiatric conditions (n = 163), and (4) both serious and psychiatric conditions (n = 45). Hypotheses were supported in that the means on the physical subscales were lower in those with serious medical conditions than in the group with minor medical conditions, whereas the mental subscales were similar between these groups and much higher than the group with psychiatric conditions. The group with both physical and psychiatric conditions scored low on both physical and mental subscales. The MH scale best distinguished between patients with-

TABLE 2 Correlations Between SF-36 Scales and Other Measures

Scales	PF	RP	BP	GH	VT	SF	RE	MH	Population
Nottingham Health Profile									Patients from
Physical Morbidity	−0.52		−0.45		−0.36	−0.35		−0.19	general
Social Isolation	−0.20		−0.18		−0.36	−0.41		−0.47	practices
Pain	−0.47		−0.55		−0.33	−0.35		−0.21	(UK)[10]
Emotional Reactions	−0.18		−0.28		−0.55	−0.53		−0.67	
Energy	−0.37		−0.37		−0.68	−0.51		−0.47	
EuroQoL									Stroke[21]
Mobility	0.57	0.38	0.40	0.39	0.40	0.47	0.27	0.10	
Self-care	0.65	0.33	0.35	0.39	0.43	0.53	0.24	0.10	
Activities	0.63	0.39	0.33	0.43	0.45	0.54	0.32	0.06	
Pain	0.39	0.36	0.66	0.44	0.39	0.43	0.29	0.12	
Psychological	0.34	0.29	0.37	0.44	0.41	0.41	0.43	0.21	
Overall HRQL	0.51	0.40	0.49	0.66	0.60	0.56	0.33	0.08	
Utility	0.64	0.39	0.53	0.54	0.54	0.63	0.37	0.17	
FIM (Motor Domain)	0.68					0.34	0.04		Multiple
Expanded Disability Scale	0.82		−0.07			0.29			sclerosis[14]
General Health Questionnaire						−0.56		0.59	
Patient-assessed disease activity	−0.40	−0.51	−0.67	−0.41	−0.42	−0.50	−0.35	−0.29	Rheumatoid
Health Assessment Questionnaire	−0.89	−0.53	−0.57	−0.50	−0.50	−0.65	−0.35	−0.30	arthritis[16]
VAS-Pain	−0.56	−0.61	−0.80	−0.49	−0.52	−0.61	−0.36	−0.36	
Hospital Depression and Anxiety Questionnaire	−0.44	−0.47	−0.48	−0.65	−0.67	−0.60	−0.62	−0.80	

PF = physical functioning; RP = role limitations owing to physical health problems; BP = bodily pain; GH = general health; VT = vitality; SF = social functioning; RE = role limitations owing to emotional problems; MH = mental health; HRQL = health-related quality of life; FIM = Functional Independence Measure; VAS = visual analogue scale.

in the psychiatric group who differed only in the severity of their disorder.

The means on three physical subscales (PF, SF, and RP) were significantly lower in patients with more severe multiple sclerosis than in the group with less impairment.[14] All subscales and the summary scores were lower for those having a SCI with upper body difficulty (mental component scale [MCS] = 53.8; physical component scale [PCS] = 24.4) than for those with a SCI without an upper body difficulty (MCS = 58.8, PCS = 35.2). The subscales and summary scores were able to differentiate those with a severe work disability from those without a severe work disability.[22] In a cohort of 90 long-term stroke clients dichotomized into groups with self-care and mental health dependencies and those without these disabilities, the mean scores for all eight subscales were significantly lower in the dependent groups than in the independent groups.[12] In individuals with cervical spine disorders (n = 146), classified as not working related to their neck disorder or work not affected,[23] both the mean PCS and MCS scores were lower in those who were off work (33 ± 7, 43 ± 14) than in the group without work alterations (37 ± 7, 47 ± 11). In a pooled sample of 1,106 patients with arthritis, the SF-36 scales and summary measures most highly correlated with physical health were best in detecting cross-sectional differences among severity groups across all severity indicators. The BP scale was the most accurate in distinguishing among patients who differed in arthritis severity followed by the PF scale, the RP scale, and the PCS.[24]

Construct—Longitudinal/Sensitivity to Change

Convergent. The associations between changes in arthritis-specific measures and the SF-36 over a 2-week interval showed the correlations to be strongest between arthritis severity and SF-36 scales most related to physical health, in particular the BP and RP subscales.[24]

Known Groups. Relative validity (RV) coefficients, indicating a measure's validity in relation to the best measure, are higher for a measure that yields a larger difference between comparison groups and/or estimates group differences with less error.[17] In clients with arthritis, the physical subscales were most sensitive to longitudinal change.[24] The BP scale was most responsive (RV median – 1.00) to changes in arthritis severity followed by the PCS scale (RV median = 0.70), the RP scale (RV median = 0.50), and the PF scale (RV median = 0.43). Per-

sons with asthma participating in a clinical trial (n = 142) were assessed at baseline, prior to the intervention or placebo, and again at 8 weeks.[17] One or more of the SF-36 scales discriminated significantly between groups in all nine comparisons. The PF and the RP were consistently more valid than the other subscales (RV = 0.17 and 0.58, respectively) and were the only two generic subscales that discriminated between groups of patients defined in terms of changes in forced expiratory volume in 1 second (RV = 0.26 to 0.58). The PCS discriminated significantly between groups in all nine comparisons (RV = 0.19 to 0.61).

In 81 patients undergoing hip replacement at 3 months after surgery, 89% reported improvements.[25] The SF-36 was more responsive than an activities of daily living and a handicap scale, and the largest changes were seen on the BP (effect size = 1.2 at 3 months and 1.5 at 6 to 12 months), PF (1.1, 1.3), and RP (0.8, 1.2) scales. The SF-36 and the Sickness Impact Profile (SIP) were administered to 54 patients undergoing hip replacement.[26] The SIP exhibited more of a ceiling effect than did the SF-36 and was less responsive at 3 months postoperatively. Although both scales exhibited standardized response means (SRMs) of a large effect, the SF-36 was more responsive (PF: 1.26 compared to 0.88 on the physical index of the SIP).

On discharge from a program of rehabilitation therapy for those with cervical spine disorders (n = 69), both the MCS and the PCS were able to detect change over time, but only the PCS was able to differentiate between those who had met their goals and those who did not.[23] In individuals with multiple sclerosis, 44 patients who received 3 weeks of inpatient rehabilitation therapy showed small effect sizes for the SF-36 dimensions, ranging from 0.01 to 0.30, whereas those on other measures, including the Functional Independence Measure and the General Health Questionnaire, were moderate in magnitude (0.56, 0.51). Emotional role limitations and pain demonstrated the largest effect sizes (0.27 to 0.30).[14]

Standardized response means were calculated for the SF-36 subscales in a group of the 233 patients with rheumatoid arthritis who reported improvement over 3 months.[16] The BP subscale showed the largest change (SRM > 0.8), the PF and VT subscales exhibited moderate change (0.5 to 0.8), and the remaining subscales showed a small to moderate change (0.2 to 0.5).

Discriminant. Not available

TABLE 3 SF-36 Subscale Scores in Several Populations

Sample	PF	RP	BP	GH	VT	SF	RE	MH
Canadian norms[28]	85.8 (20.0)	82.1 (33.2)	75.6 (23.0)	77.0 (17.7)	65.8 (18.0)	86.2 (19.8)	84.0 (31.7)	77.5 (15.3)
Hypertension[1]	73.4 (26.4)	62.0 (39.4)	72.3 (24.4)	63.3 (19.7)	58.3 (21.4)	86.7 (20.7)	76.7 (35.7)	77.9 (17.4)
Back pain and hypertension[1]	66.3 (28.6)	46.7 (40.5)	59.3 (24.6)	58.5 (21.6)	52.3 (22.7)	81.5 (24.4)	70.9 (30.0)	74.9 (18.6)
Osteoarthritis and hypertension[1]	57.4 (29.2)	38.2 (39.4)	55.0 (26.3)	59.0 (21.4)	49.5 (22.1)	79.7 (27.1)	74.8 (37.4)	78.0 (19.0)

PF = physical functioning; RP = role limitations owing to physical health problems; BP = bodily pain; GH = general health; VT = vitality; SF = social functioning; RE = role limitations owing to emotional problems; MH = mental health.

Interpretability

General Population Values
(Customary or Normative Values)

Age- and sex-adjusted population norms exist for several countries and the Canadian norms and values for several common conditions are presented in Table 3.

Typical Responsiveness Estimates

Not available

Comments

Some SF-36 subscales have been shown to have 10 to 20% less precision than the long-form MOS measures that the SF-36 scales were constructed to reproduce. This disadvantage is weighed against the fact that some of these long-form measures place a much greater burden on the respondent. Although it has been demonstrated that the eight subscales and the two summary scales rarely miss a noteworthy difference in physical or mental health status in group comparisons, this reduction in precision should be taken into account in planning clinical studies.[2]

As with all health status scales, the interpretation of individual patient scores must take into account the amount of "noise" in the scores they yield. A much higher standard of score reliability is required for measures interpreted at the individual level as opposed to average scores for large groups of patients. For this reason, to date, there is limited available evidence to support the application of the SF-36 in monitoring individual patients over time.[19]

Information is lacking on the use of the SF-36 in noncommunity-based individuals, in particular hospitalized individuals. Several studies tested the SF-36 with those institutionalized in nursing homes and reported that face validity was quite weak, as evidenced by the large numbers of items that were not relevant to the group.[27] Further, in its use among elderly respondents (age range 65 to 103 years) at ambulatory health settings,[29] 43% were unable to self-complete the questionnaire owing to visual problems, writing difficulties, or a general unfamiliarity with completing questionnaires. They found that some role functioning items were not applicable to their situations, and the item "I expect my health to get worse" was seen as very negative.

References

1. **Ware JE, Snow KK, Kosinski M, Gandek B. SF-36 Health Survey: manual and interpretation guide. Boston (MA): The Health Institute, New England Medical Center; 1993.**
2. **Ware JE. SF-36 Health Survey update. Spine 2000;25:3130–9.**
3. **Ware JE, Sherbourne CD. The MOS 36-Item Short-Form Health Survey (SF-36): I. Conceptual framework and item selection. Med Care 1992;30:473–81.**
4. McDowell I, Newell C. Measuring health: a guide to rating scales and questionnaires. 2nd ed. New York: Oxford University Press; 1996.
5. Shiely J-C, Bayliss MS, Keller SD, Tsai C, Ware JE. SF-36 Health Survey annotated bibliography: first edition (1988–1995). Boston (MA): The Health Institute, New England Medical Center; 1996.
6. Tsai C, Bayliss MS, Ware JE. SF-36 Health Survey annotated bibliography: 1996 supplement. Boston (MA): The Health Assessment Laboratory, New England Medical Center; 1997.
7. Wood-Dauphinee S, Gauthier L, Gandek B, Magnan L, Pierre U. Readying a US measure of health status, the SF-36, for use in Canada. Clin Invest Med 1997;20:224–38.
8. Gandek B, Ware JE. Special Issue: Translating Functional Health and Well-being: International Quality of Life Assessment (IQOLA) project studies of the SF-36 survey. J Clin Epidemiol 1998;51:903–1214.
9. McHorney CA, Ware JE, Lu JFR, Sherbourne CD. The MOS 36-Item Short-Form Health Survey (SF-36): III. Tests of data quality, scaling assumptions, and reliability across diverse patient groups. Med Care 1994;32:40–66.
10. Brazier JE, Harper R, Jones NMB, Oçathain A, Thomas KJ, Usherwood T. Validating the SF-36 health survey questionnaire: new outcome measure for primary care. BMJ 1992;305:160–4.

11. Walters SJ, Munro JF, Brazier JE. Using the SF-36 with older adults: a cross-sectional community-based survey. Age Ageing 2001;30:337–43.

12. Anderson C, Laubscher S, Burns R. Validation of the Short Form 36 (SF-36) Health Survey questionnaire among stroke patients. Stroke 1996;27:1812–6.

13. Dorman P, Slattery J, Farrell B, Dennis M, Sandercock P. Qualitative comparison of the reliability of health status assessments with the EuroQol and SF-36 questionnaires after stroke. Stroke 1998;29:63–8.

14. Freeman JA, Hobart JC, Langdon DW, Thompson AJ. Clinical appropriateness: a key factor in outcome measure selection: the 36-Item Short Form Health Survey in multiple sclerosis. J Neurol Neurosurg Psychiatry 2000;68:150–6.

15. Kosinski M, Keller SD, Hatoum HT, Kong SX, Ware JE. The SF-36 Health Survey as a generic outcome measure in clinical trials of patients with osteoarthritis and rheumatoid arthritis: tests of data quality, scaling assumptions, and score reliability. Med Care 1999;37:M10–22.

16. Ruta DA, Hurst NP, Kind P, Hunter M, Stubbings A. Measuring health status in British patients with rheumatoid arthritis: reliability, validity and responsiveness of the Short-Form 36-Item Health Survey (SF-36). Br J Rheumatol 1998;37:425–36.

17. Ware JE, Kemp JP, Buchner DA, Singer AF, Nolop KB, Goss TF. The responsiveness of disease-specific and generic health measures to changes in the severity of asthma among adults. Qual Life Res 1998;7:235–44.

18. Segal ME, Schall RR. Determining functional/health status and its relation to disability in stroke survivors. Stroke 1994;25:2391–7.

19. Ware JE, Kosinski M, Keller SD. SF-36 physical and mental summary scales: a user's manual. Boston (MA): The Health Institute, New England Medical Center; 1994.

20. McHorney CA. Measuring and monitoring general health status in elderly persons: practical and methodological issues in using the SF-36 Health Survey. Gerontologist 1996;36:571–83.

21. Dorman PJ, Dennis M, Sandercock P. How do scores on the EuroQol relate to scores in the SF-36 after stroke? Stroke 1999;30:2146–51.

22. Andresen EM, Fouts BS, Romeis JC, Brownson CA. Performance of health-related quality-of-life instruments in a spinal cord injured population. Arch Phys Med Rehabil 1999;80:877–84.

23. Riddle DL, Stratford PW. Use of generic versus region-specific functional status measures on patients with cervical spine disorders. Phys Ther 1998;78:951–63.

24. Kosinski M, Keller SD, Ware JE, Hatoum HT, Kong SX. The SF-36 Health Survey as a generic outcome measure in clinical trials of patients with osteoarthritis and rheumatoid arthritis. Relative validity of scales in relation to clinical measures of arthritis severity. Med Care 1999;37:M23–39.

25. Harwood RH, Ebrahim S. A comparison of the responsiveness of the Nottingham Extended Activities of Daily Living Scale, London Handicap Scale and SF-36. Disabil Rehabil 2000;22:786–93.

26. Stucki G, Liang MH, Phillips C, Katz JN. The Short-Form-36 is preferable to the SIP as a generic health status measure in patients undergoing elective total hip arthroplasty. Arthritis Care Res 1995;8:174–81.

27. Andresen EM, Gravitt GW, Aydelotte ME, Podgorski CA. Limitations of the SF-36 in a sample of nursing home residents. Age Ageing 1999;28:562–6.

28. Hopman W, Towheed T, Anastassiades T. Canadian normative data for the SF-36 Health Survey. Can Med Assoc J 2000;163: 265–71.

29. Hayes V, Morris J, Wolfe C, Morgan M. The SF-36 Health Survey questionnaire: is it suited for use with older adults? Age Ageing 1995;24:120–5.

This measure or ordering information can be found at the Website address included in this review.

SF-12®
(12-Item Short-Form Health Survey)

Developers

John E. Ware, Jr, Mark Kosinski, and Susan D. Keller; www.sf-36.com, www.qlmed.org/mot

Purpose

This evaluative scale is a multipurpose short-form generic measure of health status. It was developed to be a much shorter, yet valid, alternative to the SF-36 for use in large surveys of general and specific populations and large longitudinal studies of health outcomes.

Description

The 12 items in the SF-12 are a subset of those in the SF-36. Items from each of the eight concepts represented in the SF-36 Health Survey are included in the SF-12: physical functioning (2 items), role limitations owing to physical health problems (2 items), bodily pain (1 item), general health perceptions (1 item), vitality (1 item), social functioning (1 item), role limitations owing to emotional problems (2 items), and mental health (2 items). Response choices range from two-level to six-level response scales. Physical (PCS-12) and Mental (MCS-12) Component Summary scales are derived from the items. These two subcomponents are transformed to have a mean of 50 and a standard deviation of 10 in the US population. The SF-12 has a standard version with a 4-week recall period and an acute version that uses a 1-week recall period.[1,2]

Conceptual/Theoretical Basis of Construct Being Measured

The development of the two summary measures from the SF-36, which capture about 85% of the reliable variance in the eight SF-36 subscales, led to the idea that it might be possible to construct a shorter health survey that would reproduce the SF-36 physical (PCS-36) and mental (MCS-36) summary measures with fewer items.[1,3] Because the number of items in a survey is a function of the number of health dimensions for which separate scores are to be estimated, fewer questions are needed to cal-

culate two summary scores than to calculate eight scale scores. In those applications for which two summary scores are sufficient, a shorter survey may prove to be valid and practical enough for more widespread use.[1,2]

Groups Tested with This Measure

The data from two studies, The National Survey of Functional Health Status, a cross-sectional survey used to gather norms for the SF-36, and the Medical Outcomes Study, a study of adult patients with chronic conditions, were used in the construction of the SF-12 and the preliminary tests of reliability and validity.[1,2] The SF-12 has subsequently been tested on general populations and clients with heart disease, stroke, arthritis, and psychiatric disorders.

Languages

The translation work has been under the auspices of the International Quality of Life Project Assessment (IQOLA).[4] Data from general population surveys in Denmark, France, Germany, Italy, the Netherlands, Norway, Spain, Sweden, and the United Kingdom were analyzed to cross-validate the selection of questionnaire items for the SF-12. To date, there are no published data on the psychometric performance of the SF-12 in Canadian French and Canadian English. The IQOLA Website (www.iqola.org) provides further information about the project, and the e-mail contact is <info@iqola.org>.

Application/Administration

The survey can be self-administered by persons aged 14 years or older or administered by trained interviewers either in person or by telephone. It takes about 2 minutes to complete. The PCS-12 and MCS-12 are scored using norm-based methods. Physical and mental regression weights and a constant for both measures come from the general US population.[1,2] The advantages of the standardization and norm-based scoring are that the results for one can be meaningfully compared with the other and their scores have a direct interpretation in relation to the distribution of scores in the general US pop-

TABLE 1 Reliability Estimates for SF-12

Sample	Internal Consistency (Cronbach's α)	Test–Retest
Sample from US population (n = 232); 2-week interval[2,5]		0.89 (PCS-12)
		0.76 (MCS-12)
General practice patients (UK) (n = 187); 2-week interval[2,6]		0.86 (PCS-12)
		0.77 (MCS-12)
Severe mental illness (n = 77); 1-week interval[7]		0.73 (PCS-12)
		0.80 (MCS-12)
Stroke and heart disease (n = 1,831)[8]	0.84 (PCS-12)	
	0.81 (MCS-12)	

ulation. SF-12 algorithms have been made available to computer software vendors. Information about an on-line automated scoring service is available at <www.qmetric.com>.

Typical Reliability Estimates

Internal Consistency
See Table 1.

Interrater
Not available for the interviewer-administered application

Test-Retest
See Table 1.

Typical Validity Estimates

Content
The SF-12 items and improved scoring algorithms reproduced at least 90% of the variance in the PCS-36 and MCS-36 in both general and patient populations and produced the profile of the eight SF-36 health concepts sufficiently for large sample studies.[1]

Criterion

Concurrent. Tests of criterion validity have used the SF-36 as the gold standard. In these comparisons, the PCS-12 and the MCS-12 scores were calculated from the subset of SF-12 items embedded within the SF-36. Conclusions about the reliability and validity vary little between studies in which the SF-12 items were embedded with the other SF-36 items in comparison with the SF-12 items administered alone (Table 2).[1]

The correlations between the PCS-12 and PCS-36 have been very high (range $r = 0.94$ to 0.97), as have the correlations between the MCS-12 and the MCS-36 (range $r = 0.94$ to 0.98).[10,11]

Predictive. Not available

Construct—Cross-sectional

Convergent/Discriminant
- The EuroQoL-5D visual analogue scores were positively correlated with both component scores ($r = 0.55$ for PCS-12 and $r = 0.41$ for MCS-12).

Table 2 Comparison of SF-36 and SF-12 Mean Values for Different Samples

Sample	PCS-36	PCS-12	MCS-36	MCS-12
General US population (SD)[1]	50.1 (9.9)	50.1 (9.5)	50.0 (10.0)	50.0 (9.6)
Hypertension[1] mean (SE)	45.6 (0.4)	46.5 (0.4)	53.3 (0.3)	53.0 (0.4)
Clinical depression[1] mean (SE)	47.9 (0.7)	47.9 (0.7)	33.4 (0.8)	34.4 (0.7)
Stroke (SD)[9]	44.2 (11.3)	43.7 (10.3)	54.8 (9.7)	53.3 (9.7)
Parkinson's disease (SD)[10]	21.7 (12.0)	23.3 (11.9)	28.8 (11.9)	29.0 (11.5)
Congestive heart failure (SD)[10]	31.1 (12.7)	31.5 (12.2)	39.0 (13.4)	38.4 (12.5)
Multiple sclerosis (SD)[11]	36.1 (12.5)	36.2 (12.4)	48.0 (10.7)	45.9 (10.4)

TABLE 3 Effect Sizes for SF-12 and SF-36 Summary Scores in Randomized Trials[13]

Sample	PCS-12	PCS-36	MCS-12	MCS-36
Congestive heart failure (n = 61); 1-month interval	−0.01	0.04	0.10	0.11
Sleep apnea (n = 63); 1-month interval	0.61	0.58	0.77	0.81
Hernia open surgery arm (n = 69); 10-day interval	−2.14	−2.00	−1.17	−1.13
Hernia open surgery arm (n = 66); 10-day interval	−0.83	−0.77	−0.66	−0.67

- In clients with multiple sclerosis,[11] the measure of functional disability was correlated with both the PCS-36 ($r = -0.63$) and the PCS-12 ($r = -0.55$), whereas the correlations between the physical summary scales and a measure of mood disturbance were weaker ($r = -0.29$). However, this measure of mood disturbance was more highly correlated with the MCS-12 ($r = -0.44$) and the MCS-36 ($r = -0.42$).

- In persons with severe mental illnesses,[7] the MCS-12 was more highly correlated with the mental health indexes (correlations ranged from 0.11 to 0.49) than the physical health indexes (0.10 to 0.20). Similarly, the PCS-12 was more highly correlated with the physical health indexes (0.17 to 0.31) than with the mental health indexes (0.01 to 0.18).

Known Groups. Using the Medical Outcomes Study data, clients were categorized into four groups differing in physical and/or mental health. As hypothesized, in tests of physical differences, the MCS-12 yielded very low relative validity coefficients compared to the best SF-36 scale. Similarly, in tests of validity involving groups differing in mental health, the PCS-12 yielded very low relative validity coefficients.[1,2] In a sample of adult Americans, significantly lower mean PCS-12 scores were observed for respondents reporting specific chronic conditions including diabetes, hypertension, heart disease, arthritis, chronic obstructive pulmonary disease, and asthma.[12] Although the MCS-12 score was not different between those with and without the above conditions, it was significantly lower in those reporting depressive feelings. Hypotheses involving known groups has also been supported in a sample of individuals with stroke and heart disease[8] and severe mental illness.[7]

Construct—Longitudinal/Sensitivity to Change

Convergent. See Table 3.

Known Groups. The SF-12, the EuroQoL, and two asthma-specific measures were administered to asthma patients at baseline (n = 235) and 6 months later (n = 134).[14] Disease-specific instruments were the most responsive to self-reported asthma transition, whereas the PCS-12 demonstrated a standardized response mean of a small to moderate size (0.35) and the MCS-12 was not responsive (0.03).

In a follow-up of those who recovered from clinical depression over a 2-year period in the Medical Outcomes Study, the MCS-12 (0.91) and the MCS-36 (1.38) measures were better than the physical summary measures in detecting an improvement.[1]

Discriminant. Not available

Interpretability

General Population Values (Customary or Normative Values)
See Table 2.

Typical Responsiveness Estimates
Not available

Comments

Although the shorter SF-12 form improves efficiency and lowers cost, there are limitations. The SF-12 reproduces the eight-scale profile with fewer levels than the SF-36 scales and yields less precise scores, as would be expected for single-item and two-item scales.[15] Therefore, if the detail about health that is available through the eight-scale profile is required, the SF-36 is the preferred measure.

References

1. Ware JE Jr, Kosinski M, Keller SD. SF-12: how to score the SF-12 physical and mental health summary scales. 2nd ed. Boston (MA): The Health Institute, New England Medical Center; 1995.

2. Ware JE Jr, Kosinski M, Keller SD. A 12-item short-form health survey. Construction of scales and preliminary tests of reliability and validity. Med Care 1996;34:220–33.

3. Ware JE Jr, Kosinski M, Keller SD. SF-36 physical and mental health summary scales: a user's manual. Boston (MA): The Health Institute, New England Medical Center; 1994.

4. Gandek B, Ware JE Jr, Aaronson NK, Apolone G, Bjorner JB, Brazier JE, et al. Cross-validation of item selection and scoring for the SF-12 Health Survey in nine countries: results from the IQOLA Project. J Clin Epidemiol 1998;51:1171–8.

5. McHorney CA, Kosinski M, Ware JE Jr. Comparisons of the costs and quality of norms for the SF-36 health survey collected by mail versus telephone interviews: Results from a national survey. Med Care 1994;32:551.

6. Brazier JE, Harper R, Jones N, Ocathain A, Thomas K, Usherwood T. Validating the SF-36 health survey questionnaire: new outcome measure for primary care. BMJ 1992;305:160–4.

7. Salyers MP, Bosworth HB, Swanson JW, Lamb-Pagone J, Osher FC. Reliability and validity of the SF-12 Health Survey among people with severe mental illness. Med Care 2000;38:1141–50.

8. Lim LL, Fisher JD. Use of the 12-Item Short Form (SF-12) Health Survey in an Australian heart and stroke population. Qual Life Res 1999;8:1–8.

9. Pickard AS, Johnson JA, Penn A, Lau F, Noseworthy T. Replicability of SF-36 summary scores by the SF-12 in stroke patients. Stroke 1999;30:1213–7.

10. Jenkinson C, Layte R. Development and testing of the UK SF-12. J Health Serv Res Policy 1997;2:14–8.

11. Nortvedt MW, Riise T, Myhr K, Nyland HI. Performance of the SF-36, SF-12, and RAND-36 summary scales in a multiple sclerosis population. Med Care 2000;38:1022–8.

12. Johnson JA, Coons SJ. Comparison of the EQ-5D and SF-12 in an adult US sample. Qual Life Res 1998;7:155–66.

13. Jenkinson C, Layte R, Jenkinson D, Lawrence K, Petersen S, Paice C. A shorter form health survey: can the SF-12 replicate results from the SF-36 in longitudinal studies? Journal of Public Health Medicine 1997;19:179–86.

14. Garratt AM, Hutchinson A, Russell I. Patient-assessed measures of health outcome in asthma: a comparison of four approaches. Respir Med 2000;94:597–606.

15. Riddle DL, Lee KT, Stratford PW. Use of SF-36 and SF-12 health status measures: a quantitative comparison for groups versus individual patients. Med Care 2001;39:867–78.

This measure or ordering information can be found at the Website address included in this review.

SIP (Sickness Impact Profile)

Developers

Marilyn Bergner, Ruth Bobbitt, Shirley Kressel, William Pollard, Betty Gilson, and Joanne Morris.[1] Address: Medical Outcomes Trust, Inc., 20 Park Plaza, Suite 1014, Boston, Massachusetts 02116; e-mail: info@outcomes-trust.org.

Purpose

The SIP provides a broad measure of client-perceived, health-related dysfunction based on how illness changes daily activities and behaviors. The SIP is an appropriate outcome measure for use in assessing health care services for clinicians, researchers, and third-party payers.

Description

The SIP is a generic questionnaire that can be interview or self-administered. It consists of 136 statements that describe activities of daily living. These statements are grouped and scored in 12 categories; 3 of the categories can be further combined into the Physical Dimension and 4 into the Psychosocial Dimension. The other categories are classified as independent categories. Scores for each of the categories, the two dimensions, and the overall SIP can be derived. A shorter SIP68 contains 68 items grouped into 6 categories.[2] Scores for each category and dimension range between 0 and 100. A higher score indicates a greater level of dysfunction.

Conceptual/Theoretical Basis of Construct Being Measured

The SIP is based on observable behaviors that reflect illness-related dysfunction from minimal to maximal dysfunction.[1] Its development was prompted by the need to have a quantitative measure of functional performance because much of medical care resulted in improved function rather than an outright "cure."

Groups Tested with This Measure

The SIP has been validated in clients with chronic obstructive pulmonary disease (COPD),[3,4] total hip replacement,[5] chronic low back pain,[6] rheumatoid arthritis, hip replacement, hyperthyroidism,[7] asthma,[8] congestive heart failure,[6] ankylosing spondyli-tis, spinal cord injury, back and neck complaints, cancer, stroke, and Crohn's disease.[6] The 68-item SIP has been validated in clients with rheumatoid arthritis, ankylosing spondylitis, spinal cord injury, Crohn's disease, and cancer.[6]

Languages

English. The SIP has been culturally adapted for use in the United Kingdom and is known as the Functional Limitations Profile (FLP). Language and scale weights were modified.[9] Some validation has been performed for translations into French,[10] Spanish,[11] Dutch,[12] and Swedish.[13] The SIP has also been translated into German, Danish, and Norwegian.[14]

Application/Administration

The SIP can be interviewer administered, interviewer delivered/self-administered, or mail delivered/self-administered. The client is instructed to answer affirmatively (or check) only those statements that describe them "today" and are related to their health. Each item is weighted based on the level of implied dysfunction. Interview administration ranges from 20 to 30 minutes. The SIP is scored manually after its administration by summing the weighted values of the checked scored items, dividing this score by the total possible score, and multiplying by 100. No special equipment is required. Interviewers should receive standardized training as outlined in the SIP administration training manual. Although validity can be maintained by omitting categories of statements, the developers of the SIP state that all statements within a particular category should be administered to each client.

Typical Reliability Estimates

Internal Consistency

- Cronbach's alpha = 0.94, 0.94, and 0.81 for the interviewer-administered, interviewer-delivered/self-administered, and mail-delivered/self-administered questionnaires, respectively[7]
- 0.94 overall, 0.91 for the dimensions, and 0.60 to 0.90 for the categories[15]

Interrater

Not available for interviewer-administered questionnaire

Test–Retest

- ICC = 0.75 to 0.97 in rehabilitation medicine out- and inpatients, speech pathology clients, outpatients with chronic health problems, and a group of enrollees from a prepaid health plan who were well at the time[7] and individuals with arthritis[16]

Typical Validity Estimates

Content

Over 1,100 items were collected from clients, caregivers, and health care professionals in varied practice areas. Statements were sorted, redundant items were deleted, and discriminating statements related to similar activities were clarified.

Criterion

No gold standard exists.

Construct—Cross-sectional

Convergent

- Self-assessment of dysfunction: $r = 0.52$ to 0.69[7]
- Self-assessment of sickness: $r = 0.54$ to 0.63[7]
- Index of disability: $r = 0.55$ to 0.61[7]
- Clinicians' assessment of dysfunction and sickness: $r = 0.50$ and 0.40[7]
- Other questionnaires (SF-36, Functional Status Questionnaire, shortened Arthritis Impact Measurement Scales, and Modified Health Assessment Questionnaire): $r = 0.63$ to 0.82[5]

Known Groups. In clients with hyperthyroidism, total hip replacement, and rheumatoid arthritis,[17] the differentiation of cluster of SIP category scores was distinct for each client group and was consistent with clinical observations.

Discriminant

- In COPD, 6-Minute Walk Test: $r = -0.64$
- Forced vital capacity (FVC), forced expiratory volume in 1 second (FEV$_1$), and peak expiratory flow rate: significant correlation with total or dimension scores[18]
- In COPD, the SIP did not show significant deterioration in total score (higher score) when FEV$_1$, FVC, and partial pressure of arterial carbon dioxide (PaCO$_2$) significantly deteriorated.[3]

Construct—Longitudinal/Sensitivity to Change

Convergent. Correlation between change scores of the 136-item SIP and the 68-item SIP for the following conditions: rheumatoid arthritis ($r = 0.75$ to 0.90), ankylosing spondylitis ($r = 0.59$ to 0.94), spinal cord injury ($r = 0.69$ to 0.94), Crohn's disease ($r = 0.77$ to 0.94), and cancer ($r = 0.77$ to 0.94).[6]

Known Groups and *Discriminant* are not available.

Interpretability

General Population Values (Customary or Normative Values)

Not available

Typical Responsiveness Estimates

Not available

References

1. **Bergner M. The Sickness Impact Profile: conceptual formulation and methodology for the development of a health status measure. Int J Health Serv 1976;6:393–415.**
2. de Bruin AF, Diederiks JPM, de Witte LP, Stevens FCJ, Philipsen H. The development of a short generic version of the Sickness Impact Profile. J Clin Epidemiol 1994;47:407–18.
3. Lacasse Y, Wong E, Guyatt G, Goldstein R. Health status measurement instruments in chronic obstructive pulmonary disease. Can Respir J 1997;4:152–64.
4. Curtis JR, Deyo RA, Hudson LD. Health-related quality of life among patients with chronic obstructive pulmonary disease. Thorax 1994;49:162–70.
5. Katz JN, Larson MG, Phillips CB, Fossel AN, Liang MH. Comparative measurement sensitivity of short and longer health status instruments. Med Care 1992;30:917–25.
6. de Bruin AF, Diederiks JPM, de Witte LP, Steven FCJ, Philipsen H. Assessing the responsiveness of a functional status measure: the Sickness Impact Profile versus the SIP68. J Clin Epidemiol 1997;50:529–40.
7. **Bergner M, Bobbitt RA, Carter WB, Gilson B. The Sickness Impact Profile: development and final revision of a health status measure. Med Care 1981;19:787–805.**
8. Juniper EF. Assessing health-related quality of life in asthma. Can Respir J 1997;4:145–51.
9. Coons SJ, Rao S, Keininger DL, Hays RD. A comparative review of generic quality-of-life instruments. Pharmacoeconomics 2000;14:1713–35.
10. Chwalow AJ, Lurie A, Bean K, Parent du Chatelet I, Venot A, Dusser D, et al. A French version of the Sickness Impact Profile (SIP): stages in the cross cultural validation of a generic quality of life scale. Fundam Clin Pharmacol 1992;6:319–26.
11. Esteva M, Gonzalez N, Ruiz M. Reliability and validity of a Spanish version of the Sickness Impact Profile [abstract]. Arthritis Rheum 1992;35 Suppl 9:S219.
12. Jacobs HM, Luttik A, Touw-Otten FW, Kastein M, de Melker RA. Measuring impact of sickness in patients with nonspecific abdominal complaints in a Dutch family practice setting. Med Care 1992;30:244–51.
13. Sullivan M, Ahlmen M, Archenholtz B, Svensson G. Measuring health in rheumatic disorders by means of a Swedish version of the Sickness Impact Profile. Results from a population study. Scand J Rheumatol 1986;15:193–200.

14. Deyo RA, Inui TS, Leininger JD, Overman SS. Measuring functional outcomes in chronic disease: a comparison of traditional scales and self-administered health status questionnaire in patients with rheumatoid arthritis. Med Care 1983;21:180–92.

15. de Bruin AF, de Witte LP, Stevens F, Diederiks JPM. Sickness Impact Profile: the state of the art of a generic functional status measure. Soc Sci Med 1992;35:1003–14.

16. Anderson RT, Aaronson NK, Bullinger M, McBee WL. A review of the progress towards developing health-related quality of life instruments for international clinical studies and outcomes research. Pharmacoeconomics 1996;10:336–55.

17. Pollard WE, Bobbitt RA, Bergner M, Gilson BS. The Sickness Impact Profile: validation of a health status measure. Med Care 1976;14:146–55.

18. Jones PW, Baveystock CM, Littlejohns P. Relationships between general health measured with the Sickness Impact Profile and respiratory symptoms, physiological measures, and mood in patients with chronic airflow limitation. Am Rev Respir Dis 1989;140:1538–43.

To obtain this measure, contact the developers.

St. George's Respiratory Questionnaire (SGRQ)

Developers

Paul W. Jones, F. H. Quirk, C. M. Baveystock, and P. Littlejohns.[1,2] Contact: Dr. Paul W. Jones, Division of Physiological Medicine, St. George's Hospital Medical School, Cramer Terrace, London SW 17 ORF, UK; e-mail: pjones@sghms.ac.uk

Purpose

To assess health-related quality of life (HRQL) in adults with mild to severe chronic obstructive pulmonary disease (COPD), asthma,[1,2] and bronchiectasis.[3] Developed to evaluate clinical change over time.

Description

The SGRQ is a self-report condition-specific HRQL measure intended for clients with COPD, asthma, and/or bronchiectasis. Fifty items (with a total of 76 responses) are divided into three components: symptoms (frequency and duration over the last year), activity (physical activities that cause or are limited by breathlessness "these days"), and impacts (psychosocial disturbances owing to lung disease, such as stigmatization and employment issues). The symptoms component contains items on a 4- or 5-point Likert scale. A true/false response format is provided for items in the other two components. Each item has an empirically derived weight that provides an estimate of the level of distress associated with the symptom or state described in the question. These weights are used to calculate a score for each section and a total score. The score is obtained by adding up the item weights that correspond to each response, dividing the summed weights by the maximum possible score, and expressing the result as a percentage. Component and total scores range from 0 to 100%, with 0% indicating no impact on HRQL and 100% the worst possible score.

Conceptual/Theoretical Basis of Construct Being Measured

The developers provide a limited description of how they define "quality of life." They suggest that the SGRQ measures the effects of airways disease on "patients' lives, health, and perceived well-being."[1]

Groups Tested with This Measure

The SGRQ has been validated in groups of people with COPD,[1,2] asthma,[1,2] and bronchiectasis.[3] In addition, it has recently been validated in lung transplant candidates and recipients.[4] This measure has also been used with patients with idiopathic pulmonary fibrosis and acute respiratory distress syndrome.

Languages

The original version of the SGRQ is available in British English.[1,2] It has been translated, culturally adapted, and validated in American English,[5] French,[6] Spanish, and Swedish. It is also available in Danish, Dutch, German, Greek, Italian, Norwegian, Portuguese, and Thai (contact Dr. Jones for information regarding translations).

Application/Administration

The SGRQ is a self-administered questionnaire, but if literacy is an issue, it can be used in a face-to-face interview. Patients respond by placing a checkmark in the circle next to the relevant responses. Most patients can complete the questionnaire in 10 to 15 minutes. Clinicians or researchers can score this measure in less than 5 minutes with the use of a calculator or computer.

Typical Reliability Estimates

Internal Consistency

Cronbach's alpha: (a) COPD: 0.76 to 0.77[7]; (b) bronchiectasis: 0.90 (symptoms), 0.89 (activity), 0.92 (impacts)[3]; (c) lung transplant candidates and recipients: 0.77 (symptoms), 0.91 (activity), 0.93 (impacts), 0.95 (total)[4]

Interrater

Not applicable

Test–Retest

ICC: 0.91 (asthma),[1,2] 0.92 (COPD),[1,2] 0.97 (bronchiectasis)[3]

Typical Validity Estimates

Content

No reference to content validity in the literature.

Criterion

No gold standard exists for the attribute being assessed (HRQL).

Construct—Cross-sectional

Convergent. *Total Score*
- COPD: Chronic Respiratory Disease Questionnaire (CRQ): $r = -0.73$[7]
- COPD/asthma: Sickness Impact Profile (SIP) total score: $r = 0.71$[1]

Component Scores
COPD/Asthma
- SGRQ symptoms versus Medical Respiratory Council (MRC) cough: $r = 0.59$
- SGRQ activity versus 6-Minute Walk Test: $r = 0.59$
- SGRQ activity versus SIP physical: $r = 0.61$
- SGRQ impact versus SIP psychosocial: $r = 0.65$[2]

Bronchiectasis
- SGRQ activity versus 36-Item Short-Form Health Survey (SF-36) questionnaire physical component summary: $r = -0.70$[3]
- SGRQ impact versus SF-36 mental component summary: $r = -0.41$[3]

Lung Transplant Candidates and Recipients
- SGRQ activity versus SF-36 physical function: $r = -0.83$[4]
- SGRQ impact versus SF-36 role-emotional: $r = -0.65$[4]

Discriminant
- COPD/asthma: SGRQ symptoms versus SIP psychosocial: $r = 0.26$[2]

Known Groups. In patients with bronchiectasis, the total SGRQ score has been shown capable of discriminating among persons with different rates of infection ($F_{2,108} = 17.8$) and different levels of respiratory symptoms including wheeze ($F_{2, 108} = 13.7$) and dyspnea ($F_{4,106} = 32.9$).[3] The total score has also been shown capable of discriminating between lung transplant candidates and recipients: (ANOVA, $p < 0.001$).[4]

Construct—Longitudinal/Sensitivity to Change

Convergent. *Total SGRQ Score*
- COPD/asthma: change in total SIP score: $r = 0.32$[2]
- COPD: change in CRQ: $r = -0.53$[8]
- Bronchiectasis: change in SF-36 physical component summary: $r = -0.35$; change in fatigue physical: $r = 0.31$; change in MRC wheeze: $r = 0.26$; change in shuttle test: $r = -0.28$; change in MRC dyspnea scale: $r = 0.38$[3]

Known Groups. Not available

Discriminant
- COPD/asthma: change in FEV_1: $r = 0.22$; change in FVC: $r = 0.26$[2]

Interpretability

General Population Values (Customary or Normative Values)
Not available

Typical Responsiveness Estimates

Individual Patient. Not available

Between Group. Minimal clinically important difference (total score): 4 points[1] (–4 indicates improvement). A change of –8 points indicates moderate treatment effects and –12 points indicates large treatment effects.[9]

References

1. Jones PW, Quirk FH, Baveystock CM. The St. George's Respiratory Questionnaire. Respir Med 1991;85 Suppl B:25–31.

2. Jones PW, Quirk FH, Baveystock CM, Littlejohns P. A self-complete measure of health status for chronic airflow limitation: the St. George's Respiratory Questionnaire. Am Rev Respir Dis 1992;145:1321–7.

3. Wilson CB, Jones PW, O'Leary CJ, Cole PJ, Wilson R. Validation of the St. George's Respiratory Questionnaire in bronchiectasis. Am J Respir Crit Care Med 1997;156:536–41.

4. Bjourtuft SK, Lund MB, Kongshaug K, Geiran O, Boe J. Health-related quality of life in lung transplant candidates and recipients. Respiration 2000;67:159–65.

5. Barr JT, Schumacher GE, Freeman S, Lemoine M, Bakst AW, Jones PW. American translation, modification and validation of the St. George's Respiratory Questionnaire. Clin Ther 2000;22:1121–45.

6. Bouchet C, Guillemin F, Thi THH, Cornett A, Briancon S. Validity of a disease specific quality of life instrument, the St. George's Respiratory Questionnaire, in patients with chronic respiratory disease. Rev Mal Respir 1996;13:43–6.

7. Rutten-van Molken M, Roos G, Van Noord JA. An empirical comparison of the St George's Respiratory Questionnaire (SGRQ) and the Chronic Respiratory Questionnaire (CRQ) in a clinical trial setting. Thorax 1999;54:995–1003.

8. Guyatt GH, Feeney DH, Patrick DL. Measuring health-related quality of life. Ann Intern Med 1993;118:622–9.

9. Jones PW and the Nedocromil Sodium Quality of Life Study Group. Quality of life, symptoms and pulmonary function in asthma: long term treatment with nedocromil sodium examined in a controlled multicentre trial. Eur Respir J 1994;7:55–62.

10. Finnerty JP, Keeping I, Bullough I, Jones J. The effectiveness of outpatient pulmonary rehabilitation in chronic lung disease: a randomized controlled trial. Chest 2001;119:1705–10.

To obtain this measure, contact the developers.

STREAM (STROKE REHABILITATION ASSESSMENT OF MOVEMENT)

Developers

N. Mayo, N. Korner Bitensky, R. Cabot, I. Danys, K. Daley, and S. Wood-Dauphinee, Jewish Rehabilitation Hospital, Montreal, Quebec

Purpose

An evaluative instrument to assess motor recovery as reflected through the re-emergence of voluntary limb movement and recovery of basic mobility post stroke.[1]

Description

The STREAM is a performance-based measure and includes 30 items divided among three main subscales: 10 items that assess voluntary motor ability of the upper extremity, 10 items that assess voluntary motor ability of the lower extremity, and 10 items for basic mobility. A 3-point ordinal scale is used for scoring voluntary movement of the limbs and a 4-point ordinal scale for basic mobility. The scoring also includes the letters a, b, and c to assess the quality of movement, although this is not reflected in the final score. The final score for each subscale and the total STREAM is out of 100.[1]

Conceptual/Theoretical Basis of Construct Being Measured

Motor recovery is influenced by several factors such as side and size of the lesion, age, comorbid conditions, motivation, communication, cognition, and pain and is manifested by the re-emergence of voluntary movement and restoration of basic mobility. The STREAM is intended to measure these fundamental building blocks that reflect motor recovery. It is related hierarchically to other measures of impairments and disabilities in that it is intended to measure basic motor ability—one step beyond the level of primary impairments and one step before functional mobility and measures of activities of daily living.[1]

Groups Tested with This Measure

Individuals in the acute phase of recovery from stroke, across the entire spectrum of severity: mild, moderate, and severe.[1–4]

Languages

Canadian English and Canadian French[1]

Application/Administration

The STREAM takes approximately 15 to 20 minutes to administer, and equipment required is a sturdy stool, a support surface (eg, bed), and stairs with railings. Instructions should be given verbally, demonstrated, and repeated to the client as necessary. The client is permitted three attempts for each item, and the best performance is recorded. An item should be excluded (scored an X) if movement is limited by marked restriction of passive range or pain. The STREAM can be used in clinical, research, and community settings.[1]

Typical Reliability Estimates

Internal Consistency

Assessed on 26 individuals with stroke.[3] Coefficient alpha for the three subscales and the total STREAM score were 0.97 to 0.98.

Interrater

Twenty experienced physiotherapists were trained and interrater and test–retest reliability were assessed through videotaped assessments using generalized correlation coefficients (a more generalized ICC); values for subscales and total score were 0.98 to 0.995).[5]

Test–Retest

Generalized correlation coefficients were 0.96 for the upper extremity and 0.99 for the other subscales and the total score.[5]

Typical Validity Estimates

Content

Items in the original STREAM were adapted from clinical experience and from existing published assessments. Further content validation was carried out through the recommendations of two consensus panels, the first consisting of 10 physical therapists from hospital acute care, in- and outpatient rehabilitation, and long-term care and the second consisting of nine physical therapists suggested by the first panel. The task of the first panel was to revise

TABLE 1 Relationship of STREAM Scores with Discharge Destination

Classification based on STREAM Scores	Home n (%)	Not Home n (%)	χ^2 (2 df)
0–60 (n = 20)	2 (10)	18 (90)	20 ($p < 0.0001$)
61–95 (n = 29)	16 (55)	13 (45)	
96–100 (n = 14)	12 (86)	2 (14)	

and supplement items included in the original version of the STREAM and that of the second panel was to revise the decisions made by the first panel and to further modify the STREAM if necessary. The procedures followed during the consensus panel meetings closely approximated the "nominal group process." The panels produced an intermediate test version of the STREAM compromising 43 items. The internal consistency of this 43-item STREAM was evaluated using scores on STREAM for 26 individuals with stroke who demonstrated the full range of motor ability. Interitem and item-to-total correlations were derived for each item. The interrater agreement on scoring individual items was evaluated using a sample of 20 individuals undergoing rehabilitation following stroke and pairs of raters. Item reduction was carried out based on a priori criteria for acceptable values of kappa statistics for interrater agreement and correlations for internal consistency analysis. This item reduction process resulted in the final 30-item version of the STREAM with three subscales.[1]

Criterion

Concurrent. Not available

Predictive. All tests of validity on the STREAM were performed on 63 individuals with a wide range of stroke severities.[2] The relationship of STREAM scores during the first week post stroke with discharge destination at 3 months post stroke is shown in Table 1.[2]

The relationship of STREAM scores during the first week post stroke with gait speed and Barthel Index scores at 3 months post stroke was also examined. Groups of individuals who differed by 1 SD on the STREAM would differ in gait speed by 0.22 m/s and on the Barthel Index by 8 points.[2]

Construct—Cross-sectional

Convergent and Discriminant

Table 2 shows the Pearson correlations of the subscale STREAM scores with other measures of impairment and disability at three points in time post stroke (n = 63).[2]

TABLE 2 Pearson Correlations of STREAM Scores with Other Measures

STREAM Subscale	Time Post Stroke	Box and Block Affected UE	Box and Block Unaffected UE	Barthel Index	Balance Scale	TUG Ability	Gait Speed
UE	1 wk	0.78	0.31	0.67	0.57	0.69	0.56
	5 wk	0.79	0.36	0.66	0.61	0.49	0.53
	3 mo	0.76	0.31	0.67	0.53	0.60	0.64
LE	Initial	0.53	0.40	0.71	0.73	0.75	0.74
	5 wk	0.64	0.29	0.59	0.55	0.59	0.55
	3 mo	0.70	0.30	0.63	0.55	0.51	0.65
Mobility	Initial	0.66	0.55	0.84	0.88	0.85	0.83
	5 wk	0.69	0.40	0.75	0.71	0.57	0.65
	3 mo	0.66	0.40	0.82	0.78	0.62	0.76

All correlations significant at the $p = 0.0001$ level except for the unaffected arm of the Box and Block at all three evaluations ($p < 0.025$).
UE = upper extremity; LE = lower extremity; TUG = Timed Up and Go.

TABLE 3 Mean STREAM Scores (CI)

Classification of Barthel Index Scores*	First Week Post Stroke	5 Weeks	3 Months
Good (61–100)	88.14 (84–92)	91.7 (88–95)	91.6 (88–95)
n	42	52	59
Fair (41–60)	59.5 (41–77)	62.8 (35–90)	60.8 (−35–156)
n	8	7	3
Poor (0–40)	40.4 (24–57)	58.7 (11–107)	47.8
n	13	4	1

*Significance test between the three Barthel Index classifications performed using analysis of variance, $p < 0.05$ except between the fair and the poor group at 5 weeks and all mean comparisons at 3 months ($p > 0.05$).
CI = 95% confidence interval.

Known Groups. The STREAM was able to distinguish between three groups classified based on Barthel Index (Table 3) and Balance Scale scores (Table 4).[2]

Construct—Longitudinal/Sensitivity to Change

In a study that assessed the impact of stroke on various measures of impairment and disability during the first week post stroke and 5 weeks later, the standardized response mean (SRM) for the STREAM was 0.89 (0.67 to 1.09). For the entire study population, the STREAM had a comparable SRM to the Timed Up and Go (SRM = 0.88) but a lower one compared with the Barthel Index (SRM = 0.99), the Berg Balance Scale (SRM = 1.04), and 5-m walk comfortable gait speed (SRM = 1.22). Among individuals with severe stroke, the STREAM, in addition to the Berg Balance Scale and the Barthel Index, was more responsive compared to gait speed, and the opposite was true among individuals with a mild or moderate stroke.[4]

Other Validity Coefficients

Differences in STREAM scores for individuals with stroke participating in a randomized clinical trial:

1. A randomized clinical trial compared two groups; an intervention group that consisted of subjects who were discharged early from the acute care hospital with home rehabilitation versus a usual care group. A proportional odds ratio from an ordinal regression was reported that reflected the impact of the intervention on STREAM scores. Four weeks after the intervention, this odds ratio was 1.66; 3 months after the intervention, it was 1.91. This indicated that subjects in the intervention group were 66% and 91% more likely to be in a higher STREAM category as compared to the usual care group, at 1 month and 3 months post intervention, respectively.[3]

2. This study assessed the impact of body weight support (BWS) on functional outcomes post stroke through a randomized clinical trial. In this study, an initial version of the STREAM was used that consisted of 25 items; the maximum score was 55, with higher scores signaling better function. After a 6-week training period, the

TABLE 4 Mean STREAM Scores (CI)

Classification of Balance Scores*	First Week Post Stroke	5 Weeks	3 Months
Good (41–56)	91.3 (88–95)	93.5 (90–97)	94.7 (92–97)
n	30	45	49
Fair (21–40)	77.9 (68–87)	71.5 (55–88)	70.1 (56–86)
n	15	10	14
Poor (0–20)	44.3 (31–58)	64.5 (38–92)	—
n	18	8	0

*Significance test between the three Balance Scale classifications performed using analysis of variance, $p < 0.05$ except between the fair and the poor group at 5 weeks ($p > 0.05$).
CI = 95% confidence interval.

BWS group had a significantly higher mean score of 37.2 (se = ± 2.1) on the STREAM compared with the no BWS group, which had a mean score of 29.4 (se = ± 3.1).[6]

Interpretability

See Known Groups above.

General Population Values
Customary or Normative Values)

Studies that have used this measure have reported scores that range from 75 (± 21) for individuals with stroke prior to discharge from the acute care hospital to 85.7 (± 11) for individuals with stroke who required rehabilitation services post discharge.[2,3]

Typical Responsiveness Estimates

Not available

References

1. Daley K, Mayo N, Wood-Dauphinee S, Danys I, Cabot R. **Verification of the Stroke Rehabilitation Assessment of Movement (STREAM). Physiother Can 1997;49:269–78.**

2. Ahmed S, Mayo NE, Higgins J, Salbach N, Finch L, Wood-Dauphinee S. **Validity of the Stroke Rehabilitation Assessment of Movement (STREAM). Submitted.**

3. Mayo NE, Wood-Dauphinee S, Cote R, Gayton D, Carlton J, Buttery J, et al. There's no place like home: an evaluation of early supported discharge for stroke. Stroke 2000;31:1016–23.

4. Salbach NM, Mayo NE, Richards C, Finch L, Higgins J, Ahmed S. Responsiveness of gait speed and other clinical measures in acute stroke. Arch Phys Med Rehabil 2001;82:1204–12.

5. Daley K, Mayo N, Wood-Dauphinee S. Reliability of scores on the Stroke Rehabilitation Assessment of Movement (STREAM) measure. Phys Ther 1999;79:8–19.

6. Visintin M, Barbeau H, Korner-Bitensky N, Mayo NE. A new approach to retrain gait in stroke patients through body weight support and treadmill stimulation. Stroke 1998;29:1122–8.

This measure can be found on the accompanying CD-ROM. Prior to using the measure, you are strongly advised to contact the developers for administration and scoring guidelines and revisions to the measure not available at time of publication.

STROKE IMPACT SCALE (SIS)

Developers

P. W. Duncan and colleagues at the Center of Aging, University of Kansas Medical Center, 3901 Rainbow Boulevard, Kansas City, KS 66160-7117; e-mail: pduncan@kumc.edu; Website: www2.kumc.edu/coa

Purpose

The SIS is a disease-specific evaluative instrument that measures the impact of stroke in multiple domains, including physical, emotional, memory/thinking, communication, and social participation, with a proxy version to capture the impact of stroke on those persons unable to respond.[1-3]

Description

The SIS (Version 3.0) is a 59-item scale assessing eight domains: strength, hand function, mobility, activities of daily living (ADL) (combined ADL and instrumental activities of daily living [IADL]), emotion, memory, communication, and social participation. Version 3.0 was developed from the earlier second version containing 64 items in eight domains.[2] The eight domains can be collapsed into five, with the first four domains combining into a composite physical function domain, or they can be scored individually; all other domains must be scored as individual domains.[1] The items in each domain are ordered hierarchically from the least to most difficult based on clinical perception of difficulty and Rasch analysis.[2] A final question assesses the person's global perception of the amount of recovery since the onset of stroke on a visual analogue scale from 0 (no recovery) to 100 (full recovery).

A shortened version, the SIS-16, containing items that evaluate physical function, is also available.[4] Proxy versions of the SIS and SIS-16 to improve the generalizability of the measure to those clients with cognitive and language disabilities are in the development stage and are available on the Website.[3]

Conceptual/Theoretical Basis of Construct Being Measured

Developed as a comprehensive measure of health outcomes post-stroke to cover the aspects within a person's life for which the existing instruments did not or inadequately measured changes in mild or moderately affected stroke survivors. It was developed from the perspective of the patient, caregivers, and stroke health care professionals to measure multidimensional important consequences of stroke.[5] The SIS incorporates the World Health Organization model of disability and participation, assessing more than the physical aspects of stroke such as emotion, memory, and communication. It reduces the burden of multiple instruments used in assessing outcome post-stroke.[1]

Groups Tested with This Measure

Version 3.0 was tested on survivors of ischemic or hemorrhagic stroke ranging in severity from mild to severe, as defined by the National Institutes of Health Stroke Scale (scores from 2 to 20).[2] Version 2.0 was tested on mild and moderate stroke (Orpington scores < 3.2 and 3.2 to 5.2, respectively).[1] The SIS proxy versions were tested in patients recruited as part of a stroke registry.[3]

Languages

Rigorous translation methodology was used to produce 14 cross-cultural and valid language versions: Danish, Dutch (Belgium), English (Australia/New Zealand, United Kingdom, United States), French (Belgium, Canada, France), German (Austria, Germany), Italian, Norwegian, Portuguese, Spanish, and Swedish. For translated versions, interested individuals should contact Katrin Conway or Isabelle Mear, MAPI Research Institute Cultural Adaptation Department, 27 rue de la Villette, 69003 Lyon, France; Fax: +33 4 72 13 66 68; e-mail: kconway@mapi.fr or imear@mapi.fr.

Application/Administration

A face-to-face interviewer-administered instrument that takes 15 to 20 minutes to conduct. Performance is self-reported on a 5-point scale, with scores for strength ranging from "no strength" to "a lot of strength," for memory, communication, ADL/IADL, mobility, composite physical function, and hand function; the scores range from "extremely difficult/cannot do" to "not difficult at all," and for emotion and participation, the scores range from "none of the time" to "all of the time." Total scores for each domain are calculated on a continuous scale from 0, indicating a poor outcome, to 100, indicating the best outcome. Domain scores can be calculated either manually or by computer using the Access programs from the Website, which also produce a summary report per person. Algorithms to deal with missing responses for a particular subject are also provided.[1] The proxy version should be administered if the patient is unable to follow a three-step command for any reason (cognitive ability or language problems).[3] Proxies are considered as those individuals who have known the patient for at least 1 year and see the patient at least once a week. Instructions for scoring and administering all of the instruments (SIS, SIS-16, and their proxy versions) are available on the Website, along with videotapes for the administration of the measures.

Typical Reliability Estimates

Internal Consistency
Cronbach's alpha = 0 .93 to 1.00.[2]

Interrater
Not available

Test–Retest
Version 2.0 ICCs = 0.70 to 0.92 across seven of the eight domains. The emotion domain was unreliable, with an ICC of 0.57. Not available for version 3.0.

Other
The strength of the agreement between clients and proxies for the SIS and SIS-16 as measured by ICCs ranged from 0.50 (memory domain) to 0.84 (SIS-16). The proxies consistently underestimated the scores of the clients.[3]

Typical Validity Estimates

Content
Validity was established through its development from focus groups that included stroke survivors, caregivers, and health care professionals who were experts in stroke.

Criterion

Concurrent. Not applicable; see convergent validity.

Predictive. Not available

Construct—Cross-sectional
After removal of five items from four domains in Version 2.0,[2] the fit (mean square value < 1.3) of each item in each domain confirmed the unidimensionality of each domain. Thus, the items in each domain now only measure the construct of that domain. Additionally, a Rasch analysis testing of the ordering of the items in each domain by difficulty matched the theoretical ordering, confirming construct validity.

Convergent. A correlational analysis compared each of the domains to established standardized measures (Table 1).[1]

Additionally, multiple regression analysis revealed that the physical function, emotion, and participation domains were significant components of the person's global evaluation, explaining 45% of the recovery. The SIS, SIS-16, and SIS proxy versions were compared to the Folstein Mini-Mental State Examination, Barthel Index, Lawton IADL, and Motricity scale (Rankin) with correlations all above 0.67, except for the proxy SIS memory domain (0.37).

Known Groups. For each of the domains except memory, persons with mild strokes had on average significantly higher scores than those with moderate strokes, with the 3-month and 6-month scores higher than the 1-month scores.[1] Six of the eight domains in version 2.0 discriminated ($p < 0.02$) the four levels of the Rankin index (0/1, 2, 3, 4) at 6 months post stroke; memory and emotion could not distinguish different levels.[1]

The SIS, SIS-16, and SIS proxy versions were equally capable of distinguishing four Rankin categories (0/1, 2, 3, 4/5) in 287 patients and their proxies. The scores were significantly different across all Rankin categories for all domains, including memory and emotion.[3] Each domain is capable of reliably distinguishing different strata of persons within that domain. Strength and memory discriminate three levels (high, average, low), ADL/IADL and mobility three to four levels (high, above average, below average, low), and the composite physical domain four levels. The domains of ADL/IADL, mobility, and the combined physical function are capable of capturing a wide range of disabilities (separation indices of 27.57, 34.14, and 23.03, respectively). However, community, emotion, and hand function domains perform more poorly

TABLE 1 Correlations of SIS Domain Scores with Other Measures

Domain	Established Measure	Pearson Correlation
Strength	NIH, FM total	−0.59, 0.79
Hand function	FM upper extremity motor	0.81
Mobility	FIM, BI, Duke Mobility, SF-36 physical function (Q3)	0.83, 0.82, 0.83, 0.84
ADL/IADL	BI, FIM motor, IADL	0.84, 0.84, 0.82
Memory	Folstein MMSE	0.58
Communication	FIM Social/Cognition, NIH language	0.53, −0.44
Emotion	Geriatric Depression Scale, SF-36 mental health	−0.77, 0.74
Participation	SF-36 physical role, SF-36 emotional role, SF-36 social function	0.45, 0.28, 0.70
Composite physical function	BI, FIM motor, SF-36 physical function (Q3), IADL	0.76, 0.79, 0.75, 0.73
Percent recovery	BI, IADL, SF-36 physical function, FIM motor, FIM cog-social, SF-36 mental health, SF-36 social function, NIH, FM	0.58, 0.47, 0.52, 0.57, 0.34, 0.40, 0.43, 0.50, 0.43

NIH = National Institutes of Health; FM = Fugl-Meyer Assessment of Sensorimotor Recovery After Stroke; FIM = Functional Independence Measure; BI = Barthel Index; SF-36 = 36-Item Short-Form Health Survey; IADL = instrumental activities of daily living; MMSE = Mini-Mental State Examination.

because of the narrower range of difficulty across the items and distinguish two levels (high and low).[2] The memory, communication, and emotion domains will only detect those stroke survivors with major limitations, whereas the hand function domain items are too difficult and only capture those with minor difficulties. The specific separation ability of each domain requires further testing.

Discriminant. Not available

Construct—Longitudinal/Sensitivity to Change

Convergent. Not available

Known Groups. Severity and time post stroke affected the sensitivity of each domain. The sensitivity assessed by a *t* statistic was adequate in minor strokes from 1 to 3 months and from 1 to 6 months post-stroke but not from 3 to 6 months. Among persons with stroke of moderate severity, sensitivity was adequate across the three time points for all domains. An exception was at 3 to 6 months post-stroke, when the sensitivity in the domains of hand function, strength, communication, memory, and emotion was low.[1]

Discriminant. Not available

Interpretability

General Population Values (Customary or Normative Values)
The mean patient self-reported scores with their standard deviations for each domain are included in Table 2. Proxy values were quite similar.[3]

Typical Responsiveness Estimates
A 10- to 15-point change in a domain score may represent a clinically significant change. The developers based this on the ICCs' within-subject standard deviation range of 6 to 15 points seen in test–retesting. However, further validation of the clinical meaningful change is needed.

Other
A floor effect exists in the hand function domain, with 40.2% of moderate stroke survivors unable to perform in this domain. A ceiling effect exists in the communication domain, with 35.0% of mild stroke survivors scoring the top score.[1]

TABLE 2 Mean SIS Scores

SIS Domain	Rankin 0/1 Mean (SD)	Rankin 2 Mean (SD)	Rankin 3 Mean (SD)	Rankin 4/5 Mean (SD)
Patient				
Strength	76.9 (16.7)	67.0 (14.8)	59.0 (20.0)	39.2 (20.4)
Memory	85.7 (13.0)	80.2 (15.7)	68.8 (21.5)	75.0 (22.3)
Emotion	83.4 (15.6)	76.7 (15.9)	70.1 (18.1)	64.4 (18.2)
Communication	90.2 (11.7)	83.5 (15.0)	70.6 (25.0)	78.0 (17.8)
ADL/IADL	88.8 (10.3)	73.6 (14.8)	57.0 (16.4)	38.9 (18.1)
Mobility	77.4 (15.8)	65.9 (16.0)	58.9 (17.7)	31.2 (18.3)
Hand function	86.0 (17.0)	66.4 (25.2)	45.2 (29.6)	14.2 (20.3)
Participation	80.0 (19.4)	60.6 (20.4)	49.2 (23.7)	41.1 (23.4)
SIS-16 physical	84.3 (10.8)	71.5 (14.0)	59.6 (15.4)	36.8 (15.9)

ADL = activities of daily living; IADL = instrumental activities of daily living.

References

1. Duncan PW, Wallace D, Lai SM, Johnson D, Embretson S, Laster LJ. The Stroke Impact Scale Version 2.0 Evaluation of Reliability, Validity, and Sensitivity to Change. Stroke 1999;30: 2131–40.

2. Duncan PW, Lai SM, Perara S, and the GAIN Americas Investigators. Rasch Analysis of a new stroke specific outcome scale: The Stroke Impact Scale. Submitted.

3. Duncan PW, Lai SM, Tyler D, Perera S, Reker DM, Studenski S. Evaluation of proxy responses to the Stroke Impact Scale. In Press

4. Duncan PW, Lai SM, Bode RK, Perera S, and the GAIN Americas Investigators. Stroke Impact Scale-16 (SIS-16): A brief instrument for assessing physical function in stroke patients. In Press

5. Duncan PW, Wallace D, Studenski S, Lai SM, Johnson D. Conceptualization of a new stroke specific outcome measure: The Stroke Impact Scale. Topics in Stroke Rehabilitation 2001; 8:19–33.

This measure or ordering information can be found at the Website address included in this review.

TEMPA (Test d'Évaluation des Membres Supérieurs des Personnes Agées)

Developers

Johanne Desrosiers, Réjean Hébert, and Élisabeth Dutil

Purpose

To evaluate upper extremity performance, mainly of older people with impairments or disabilities.

Description

The TEMPA is a performance-based test composed of nine standardized tasks representing daily activities: five tasks are bilateral (open a jar and take a spoonful of coffee; unlock a lock and open a pill container; write on an envelope and stick on a stamp; tie a scarf around one's neck; shuffle and deal playing cards) and four are unilateral (pick up and move a jar; pick up a pitcher and pour water into a glass; handle coins; pick up and move small objects), for a total of 13 different items.[1] All of the test material is placed in precise, predetermined positions on a set of shelves designed to ensure a high level of standardization in performing the tasks.

Conceptual/Theoretical Basis of Construct Being Measured

A theoretical framework of important sensorimotor skills for upper extremity performance was developed from the literature review. Upper extremity performance was defined as the integration and mutual interaction of sensorimotor parameters (motor coordination, gross and fine dexterity, strength, endurance, range of motion, sensibility) in daily activities.

Groups Tested with This Measure

Clients with various upper extremity disabilities and people without upper extremity disabilities.

Languages

French and English

Application/Administration

The time to administer the entire test varies according to the person (about 20 minutes). The examiner scores the performance according to three measurement criteria: speed of execution, functional rating, and task analysis.[1] All tasks should be done as quickly as possible. For speed of execution, each task is timed to the nearest tenth of a second, beginning as soon as the subject's hands leave the table and ending the moment the task is completed. Functional rating refers to the subject's independence on each task; it is measured using a four-level scale: 0 = the task is successfully completed, without hesitation or difficulty; −1 = some difficulty with the task; −2 = great difficulty in completing the entire task; and −3 = the individual could not complete the task, even when assistance was offered. The task analysis section quantifies the difficulties experienced by the subject according to five dimensions related to upper extremity sensorimotor skills: strength, range of motion, precision of gross movements, prehensions, and precision of fine movements. Equipment needed is available from the manufacturer and distributor (Les équipements adaptés Physipro, Sherbrooke, Québec).

Typical Reliability Estimates

Internal Consistency
Not available

Interrater
Cohen's weighted kappas and ICCs were moderate to strong (0.75 to 1.0).[2]

Test–Retest
Cohen's weighted kappas and ICCs were moderate to strong (0.70 to 1.0).[2]

Typical Validity Estimates

Content
The development of the TEMPA was based on a literature review of sensorimotor skills and consultations with expert clinicians.

Criterion
No gold standard exists for the construct being measured.

Construct—Cross-sectional

Convergent. Tested with 104 subjects aged 60 to 94 years[3] by estimating the correlation between the

TEMPA and two clinical tests measuring similar concepts, namely the Action Research Arm Test[4] and the Box and Block Test[5] (r = 0.90 to 0.95 and 0.73 to 0.78, respectively, depending on the task). Also, the TEMPA is strongly correlated with an activities of daily living test (r = 0.69 to 0.71, depending on the task).[3]

Known Groups and *Discriminant* are not available.

Construct—Longitudinal/Sensitivity to Change
Not available

Other
In a clinical trial of arm ability training among 74 individuals with upper extremity paresis, 45 with stroke, and 15 with traumatic brain injury (TBI), the intervention groups improved significantly on the task time. Prior to intervention, the average task time was approximately 230 seconds. After therapy, there was an 18% reduction in the time for the group treated with the advanced arm training.[7] The 10% difference was considered clinically meaningful by the authors. The training efficacy was similar for both stroke and TBI.

Interpretability

General Population Values
(Customary or Normative Values)
Normative data of the maximum speed of execution were developed with 360 healthy subjects randomly recruited by age and sex strata (60 to 69, 70 to 79, and 80 and over).[6] Normative values were also developed in the summer of 2001 with people aged 45 to 59 years (not yet published).

Only values for time to execute tasks are available, and the times depended on age and gender. For example, the task with the shortest time of exe- cution was picking up and moving a jar with the right hand, and the times, for women, ranged from 1.5 to 1.8 seconds across age groups. For men, across-group times ranged from 1.5 to 1.7 seconds. The task with the longest execution time was shuffling and dealing playing cards. The values for women (across age group) ranged from 14.7 to 19.1 seconds, and for men, the corresponding values ranged from 15.0 to 19.0 seconds, for age group, respectively. The time needed to pick up a pitcher and pour water into a glass ranged from 7.2 to 9.3 seconds across age group, and for men, the range was 7.4 to 9.0 seconds.[6]

Typical Responsiveness Estimates
Not available

References

1. Desrosiers J, Hébert R, Dutil É. TEMPA. Manuel d'administration [administration manual]. Sherbrooke (PQ): Centre de recherche en gérontologie et gériatrie; 1993.
2. Desrosiers J, Hébert R, Dutil É, Bravo G. Development and reliability of an upper extremity function test for the elderly: the TEMPA. Can J Occup Ther 1993;60:9–16.
3. Desrosiers J, Hébert R, Dutil É, Bravo G, Mercier L. Validity of a measurement instrument for upper extremity performance: the TEMPA. Occup Ther J Res 1994;14:267–81.
4. Cromwell FS. Occupational therapists' manual for basic skills assessment: primary prevocational evaluation. Pasadena (CA): Fair Oaks Printing; 1965. p. 29–31
5. Lyle RC. A performance test for assessment of upper limb function in physical rehabilitation treatment and research. Int J Rehabil Res 1981;4:483–92.
6. Desrosiers J, Hébert R, Bravo G, Dutil É. Upper extremity performance test for the elderly (TEMPA): normative data and correlates with sensorimotor parameters. Arch Phys Med Rehabil 1995;76:1125–9.

To obtain this measure, contact the developers. Equipment needed is available from Les équipements adaptés Physipro, Sherbrooke, QC, Canada.

TEST OF INFANT MOTOR PERFORMANCE (TIMP)

Developers

Suzann K. Campbell, G. L. Girolami, T. H. A. Kolobe, E. T. Osten, and M. Lenke.[1] Contact Suzann Campbell: e-mail SKC@uic.edu; Fax: 312-996-4583. Further information: www.thetimp.com

Purpose

The TIMP is a functional motor performance instrument that can be used in both research and clinical practice to (1) identify infants under the age of 4 months with delayed motor development (corrected for prematurity if necessary), (2) measure change in typically developing infants with precision over 2-week periods of time, (3) develop intervention goals for infants with delayed motor development, (4) measure change resulting from interventions, and (5) educate parents about infant motor development. Research on the TIMP also provides evidence that scores at 3 months of age can be used to predict infant motor development at 12 months of age.[2]

Description

The 59 items on Version 3 of the TIMP provide a comprehensive assessment of developing head and trunk control (31 Elicited Items rated on 5- to 7-point scales) as well as spontaneous selective control of arms and legs (28 dichotomous Observed Items) for infants over the period from 32 weeks postconceptional age through 4 months post term. The TIMP can be used with both full-term and prematurely born infants. Total raw scores range from 0 to 170, with high scores reflecting more optimal performance.

Conceptual/Theoretical Basis of Construct Being Measured

TIMP items were created to assess functional motor performance for infants of all ages in both special care nursery settings and community-based early intervention programs. Items were designed to (1) measure the postural and selective control of movement needed for functional performance in daily life interactions with caregivers and (2) discriminate between infants with typical development and those who are delayed or have movement dysfunction. Conceived as a functional motor performance examination, the TIMP does not emphasize the testing of reflexes, muscle tone, or physiologic responses. In keeping with systems theories of motor development, the Elicited Items of the TIMP present infants with a variety of tasks to which they are expected to respond with appropriate postural alignment or movement. Problems to be solved by the infant include organization of responses to interesting visual and auditory spectacles or placement in a variety of positions in space, including prone, supine, side-lying, and supported sitting and standing.

Groups Tested with This Measure

Full-term infants and infants born prematurely, both high and low risk for poor motor outcome based on perinatal medical conditions.

Languages

English. Research has been conducted on white, black (African and African American), and Latino/a (primarily Mexican and Puerto Rican) infants in the United States.[1]

Application/Administration

Initial observation of spontaneous activity in the infant allows scoring of 28 Observed Items. Thirty-one Elicited Items involve placing the infant in a variety of positions in space or recording motor responses to interesting sights and sounds. The TIMP requires an average of 30 minutes to administer and score (time ranges from about 18 to 42 minutes, depending on infant ability and behavior and the experience of the tester). Equipment required includes a rattle, red ball, and squeak toy. To use the TIMP safely, physical therapists or occupational therapists must have experience in the safe handling of fragile infants. Using the TIMP requires a minimum of 8 to 10 hours learning the content of the items and a month or more of frequent testing of infants at a variety of ages. A CD-ROM self-instructional package for learning to administer and score the TIMP is available from the test developers.

Typical Reliability Estimates

Internal Consistency

Based on Rasch psychometric analysis of 1,723 tests from infants of varying ages and medical risk factors, the TIMP items demonstrated an item separation index of 21.37, indicating the ability of items to measure at least 21 different levels of performance and a reliability of 1.00 with a model error of 0.48 (Suzann K. Campbell, personal communication, 2001). Item point biserial correlations ranged from –0.10 to 0.78, with 29 of 59 greater than 0.50. A future test revision will involve deleting some items that appear to fit poorly the construct of functional motor performance.

Interrater

Based on multiple regression analysis, there were no significant differences between testers trained by the developers[3]; the ICC was 0.95 in research by independent investigators.[4]

Test–Retest

0.89 based on testing repeated over a 3-day period in 106 infants of varying age and medical risk.[3]

Typical Validity Estimates

Content

Ninety-eight percent of TIMP Elicited Items are similar to demands for movement placed on infants by caregivers in interactions such as bathing, dressing, and play.[5]

Criterion

Concurrent. No gold standard for construct being measured.

Predictive. At 3 months corrected age (CA), a cutoff on the TIMP of –0.5 SD from the mean had sensitivity of 0.92, specificity of 0.76, positive predictive validity of 0.39, and negative predictive validity of 0.98 for prediction of Alberta Infant Motor Scale (AIMS) performance above/below the 5th percentile in 82 infants at 12 months CA.[2]

Construct—Cross-sectional

Convergent. 0.64 with the AIMS in 90 infants at 3 months CA.[6]

Known Groups. In multiple regression analysis, infants with larger numbers of medical conditions in the perinatal period performed significantly less well than same-age healthier peers; no significant differences between groups based on race/ethnicity were

found.[1] See also the description of longitudinal analysis that follows.

Discriminant. Not available

Construct—Longitudinal/Sensitivity to Change

Convergent. Not available

Known Groups. Longitudinal growth curves from weekly testing up to 4 months CA of infants with a variety of risk factors differed significantly.[7] Full-term infants and low-risk preterm infants were indistinguishable, but both groups performed significantly better than three groups of high-risk infants (infants born weighing < 1,500 g, those with bronchopulmonary dysplasia, those with brain insult). Infants with brain insults (perinatal asphyxia, periventricular leukomalacia, grade III or IV intraventricular hemorrhage) performed significantly worse than all other infants both in absolute terms and in slope of development across time as they fell further behind the other groups. Black infants (African or African American) performed slightly better than white or Latino/a infants.

Discriminant. Not available

Interpretability

General Population Values (Customary or Normative Values)

Age standards for performance from 32 weeks postconceptional age through 13 weeks post term were obtained from testing approximately 150 infants (black, white, Latino/a) from the Chicago metropolitan area.[8] Data for the development of age standards are being collected in 1,200 infants of all races/ethnicities in 10 regions of the United States; the results are expected to be available for the TIMP Version 4 in 2003 (Suzann K. Campbell, personal communication, 2001).

Typical Responsiveness Estimates

Individual Patient. Anecdotal case reports illustrate use of the TIMP to document delay and to plan individual treatment, but estimates of change with intervention are not available.[8]

Between Group. The initial research version of the TIMP (then called the Supplemental Motor Test) was sensitive to the effects of a neurodevelopmental treatment program provided to infants of 34 to 35 weeks postconceptional age in a special care nursery setting.[9] Estimates of amount of change are not available. Version 3 of the TIMP at 4 months CA was responsive to the effects on randomly assigned prematurely born infants with poor initial TIMP scores of a home physical therapy program provided by parents on hospital discharge.[10]

References

1. Campbell SK, Kolobe THA, Osten ET, Lenke M, Girolami GL. Construct validity of the Test of Infant Motor Performance. Phys Ther 1995;75:585–96.

2. Campbell SK, Kolobe THA, Wright B, Linacre JM. Predictive validity of the Test of Infant Motor Performance with the Alberta Infant Motor Scale. Dev Med Child Neurol. In press.

3. Campbell SK. Test-retest reliability of the Test of Infant Motor Performance. Pediatr Phys Ther 1999;11:60–6.

4. Lekskulchai R, Cole J. The relationship between the scarf ratio and subsequent motor performance in infants born preterm. Pediatr Phys Ther 2000;12:150–7.

5. Murney ME, Campbell SK. The ecological relevance of the Test of Infant Motor Performance Elicited Scale items. Phys Ther 1998;78:479–89.

6. Campbell SK, Kolobe THA. Concurrent validity of the Test of Infant Motor Performance with the Alberta Infant Motor Scale. Pediatr Phys Ther 2000;12:1–8.

7. Campbell SK, Hedeker D. Discriminative validity of the Test of Infant Motor Performance. J Pediatr 2001;139:546–51.

8. Campbell SK. The infant at risk for developmental disability. In: Campbell SK, editor. Decision making in pediatric neurologic physical therapy. Philadelphia (PA): Churchill Livingstone; 1999. p. 260–332.

9. Girolami G, Campbell SK. Efficacy of a Neuro-Developmental Treatment program to improve motor control of preterm infants. Pediatr Phys Ther 1994;6:175–84.

10. Lekskulchai R, Cole J. Effect of a developmental program on motor performance in infants born preterm. Aust J Physiother 2001;47:169–76.

This measure or ordering information can be found at the Website address included in this review, or contact the developers.

TIMED-STANDS TEST

Developers

Maryellen Csuka and Daniel J. McCarty, Department of Medicine, Medical College of Wisconsin, Milwaukee, Wisconsin

Purpose

To measure lower extremity muscle strength.

Description

A performance-based measure that records the time needed for an individual to stand 10 times from a standard chair in seconds. A shorter time indicates better performance.

Conceptual/Theoretical Basis of Construct Being Measured

None reported.

Groups Tested with This Measure

Healthy males and females,[1] clients with classic polymyositis or dermatomyositis[1] and rheumatoid arthritis (RA),[2] and outpatients (OPs) from pulmonary, cardiology, metabolic, and walk-in evaluation clinics.[2]

Language

English

Application/Administration

A straight-back chair 44.5 cm high and 38 cm deep is used. The time required to complete 10 full stands from a sitting position is recorded with a stopwatch to the nearest tenth of a second. One practice stand is performed for positioning and learning of the task. Subjects are encouraged to perform the task as quickly as possible. All stands are performed either barefooted or with low-heeled shoes. Simultaneous use of the upper extremities is not permitted.

Typical Reliability Estimates

Internal Consistency
Not applicable

Interrater
Not available

Test–Retest
Mean coefficient of variation: 6.8% (SD 3.4) in 12 healthy subjects three times in succession.[1] $r = 0.88$ in 16 patients with stable RA twice over 10 weeks by multiple examiners.[2]

Typical Validity Estimates

Content
No reference to content validity in the literature.

Criterion
No gold standard exists for the construct being measured.

Construct—Cross-sectional

Convergent
- 50′ walking time: $r = 0.66$, $p < 0.000$ in clients with RA; $r = 0.46$, $p = 0.000$ in OPs[2]
- Lower extremity manual muscle strength: $r = 0.47$, $p = 0.000$ in clients with RA; $r = 0.60$, $p = 0.000$ in OPs[2]

Known Groups. Outpatients completed the test in shorter time than clients with RA (t-test, $p = 0.001$).[2] Outpatients with fewer comorbidities completed the test in shorter time than those with more comorbidities (analysis of variance [ANOVA], $p = 0.000$).[2] No relation to degree of comorbidity in clients with RA (ANOVA, $p = 0.27$).[2] Rheumatoid arthritis clients with low disease activity (= sum of joint count, observer global assessment, self-reported physical activity, pain, and 50′ walking time) completed the test in shorter time than those with high disease activity (ANOVA, $p = 0.002$).[2]

Discriminant. Not available

Construct—Longitudinal/Sensitivity to Change
Not available

Other Validity Coefficients
- Height: multiple regression, $p > 0.05$ in healthy men and women[1]
- Weight: multiple regression, $p > 0.05$ in healthy men[1]
- Weight (age adjusted): multiple regression, $p < 0.05$; increase in $r^2 = 0.03$ in healthy women[1]
- Height/weight ratio: multiple regression, $p > 0.05$ in healthy men and women[1]

- Age: $r = 0.88$ and $r = 0.71$ (no p values provided) in healthy men and women, respectively[1]
- Age: $r = 0.22$, $p = 0.06$ in OPs (mean age 61, SD 7.2)[2]
- Age: $r = 0.07$, $p = 0.54$ in clients with RA (mean age 62, SD 9.6)[2]
- Pain: $r = 0.36$, $p = 0.004$ in clients with RA[2]
- Tender joint count: $r = 0.33$, $p = 0.005$ in clients with RA[2]
- Observer's global assessment of lower extremity arthritis activity: $r = 0.40$, $p = 0.001$ in clients with RA[2]
- Self-reported arthritis impact on physical function: $r = 0.31$, $p = 0.09$; mobility: $r = 0.30$, $p = 0.01$; activities of daily living: $r = 0.16$, $p = 0.19$; dexterity: $r = 0.26$, $p = 0.02$; physical activity: $r = 0.33$, $p = 0.004$ ($p < 0.005$ was considered statistically significant owing to multiple comparisons); household activities: $r = 0.22$, $p = 0.07$; and pain: $r = 0.36$, $p = 0.02$ in clients with RA[2]

Interpretability

General Population Values
(Customary or Normative Values)
- Prediction equations[1]: ($R^2 - 0.50$ age)
- Women: time (seconds) = $7.6 + 0.17 \times$ age
- Men: time (seconds) = $4.9 + 0.19 \times$ age

Age- and sex-predicted mean times and the upper limits (90% prediction region) for healthy men and women 20 to 85 years of age are available.[1]

Typical Responsiveness Estimates
Not available

Comments

An overview of modified sit-to-stand tests is available.[3] Modified versions of the original Timed-Stands Test have been suggested as valid and reliable for renal transplant candidates[4] and older adults.[5] There are no data to support this measure's ability to detect change in individuals or groups; therefore, it needs to be used as an outcome measure with caution until this measurement property has been tested.

References

1. Csuka M, McCartty DJ. Simple method for measurement of lower extremity muscle strength. Am J Med 1985;78:77–81.
2. Newcomer KL, Krug HE, Mahowald ML. Validity and reliability of the Timed-Stands Test for patients with rheumatoid arthritis and other chronic diseases. J Rheumatol 1993;20:21–7.
3. Bohannon RW. Sit-to-stand test for measuring performance of lower-extremity muscles. Percept Mot Skills 1995;80:163–6.
4. Bohannon RW, Smith J, Hull D, Palmeri D, Barnhard R. Deficits in lower extremity muscle and gait performance among renal transplant candidates. Arch Phys Med Rehabil 1995;76:547–51.
5. Jones CJ, Rikli RE, Beam WC. A 30-s chair-stand test as a measure of lower body strength in community-residing older adults. Res Q Exerc Sport 1999,70.113–9.

To obtain this measure, contact the developers, or it can be found in reference 1.

TUG (TIMED UP AND GO)

Developer

Diane Podsiadlo, CLSCNDG, 2525 Boulevard Cavendish, Bureau 110, Montreal, Quebec H4B 2Y4; Fax: 514-485-6406

Purpose

To measure mobility, balance, and locomotor performance in elderly people with balance disturbances.[1,2]

Description

Originally developed by Mathias et al (Get-up and Go Test),[3] this performance measure was designed to easily evaluate the risk of falls using balance and basic functional mobility. A categorical scale is used ranging from 1 to 5, where 1 indicates "normal function" and 5 indicates "severe abnormal functional" mobility. Scores greater than 3 indicate that clients are at risk for falling, requiring further attention. In 1991, the scale's scoring system was modified to incorporate time as the measuring component to assess general balance and function.[4] The scale was modified to address the imprecision of the intermediate scores on the original version that had poor interrater reliability.[4]

Groups Tested with This Measure

People with Parkinson's disease (PD)[2]; elderly people with or without cognitive impairment[5]; people with lower limb amputations,[1] total joint arthroplasty,[6] cerebral vascular accidents,[6] and hip fracture[4,6]; clients with rheumatoid and osteoarthritis[4]; and deconditioned elderly people.[4]

Conceptual/Theoretical Basis of Construct Being Measured

None reported.

Language

English

Application/Administration

The TUG requires that individuals wear comfortable/regular footwear and use their customary walking aid when performing the test. The client rises from a standard armchair (46 cm seat height to ground), walks 3 meters at a comfortable safe pace, turns, walks back to the chair, and sits down. Timing commences with the verbal instruction "go" and stops when the client returns to the seated position. A practice trial is recommended to familiarize the client with the test.[4] In PD clients, it has been suggested that the command "start" be used instead of the command "go," which may introduce error.[2] The TUG requires 1 to 2 minutes to administer. The score is the actual time required to accomplish the task and is measured using a standard stopwatch.[4,7] No training is required for the individual administering the test. Variation in seat type does not appear to make any difference in the test's outcome.[8]

Typical Reliability Estimates

Internal Consistency
Not applicable

Interrater
- ICC = 0.99[4]
- ICC = 0.98 in PD clients[2]
- ICC = 0.56 in cognitively impaired and 0.50 in unimpaired populations[5] (see Comments section).
- ICC = 0.96 in clients with transtibial and transfemoral unilateral amputation[1]
- Kendall coefficient = 0.85 for physiotherapists and 0.686 for senior doctors[3]

Test-Retest
Not available

Other
Intrarater:
- ICC = 0.99[4]
- ICC = 0.92[5]
- ICC = 0.93[1]

Typical Validity Estimates

Content
No reference to content validity in the literature.

Criterion
No gold standard available[1,4]

Construct—Cross-sectional

Convergent

- Groningen Activity Restriction Scale (GARS) and Sickness Impact Profile 68-item version (SIP68): $r = 0.39$ to 0.40.[1]
- Berg Balance Scale, Gait Speed, and Barthel Index: $r = -0.51$ to -0.72.[4] When the scores were log transformed, the correlation ranged from -0.61 (gait) to -0.81 (Berg Balance Scale).[4]
- Gait time (seconds): $r = 0.75$. Correlation with gait speed (m/s) or log-transformed gait speed was -0.55 and -0.61, respectively, in elderly orthopedic rehabilitation clients with total hip replacement, total knee arthroplasty, and hip fractures.[6]

Known Groups

- Cognitively unimpaired clients can perform the TUG faster than cognitively impaired clients; $p = 0.001$.[5]
- Discriminated between PD clients on levodopa and those not on levodopa when compared to individuals without PD (t[12.13] = 3.78, $p = 0.003$ not on levodopa and t[14.92] = 3.79, $p = 0.002$)[2]

Discriminant

- Correlation of TUG and Emotional Stability of SIP68: $r = -0.04$[1]

Construct—Longitudinal/Sensitivity to Change
Not available

Interpretability

Table 1 shows normative values for elderly volunteers residing in the community.[9]

Typical Responsiveness Estimates
Not available

Comments

- Tested in a frail elderly population, Podsiadlo et al reported guidelines for function[4]: < 10 seconds = freely independent; < 20 seconds = independent in basic tub or shower transfers and able to climb most stairs and go outside alone; > 30 seconds = dependent in most activities
- Interrater ICC of 0.50 and 0.56 can be questioned as the time interval was 112 ± 72.4 days[5]
- Whitney et al suggested that the advantage of the TUG is that it can be administered quickly, but a disadvantage is that only a few aspects of balance are tested.[7]
- Shumway-Cook et al reported that the TUG is a sensitive (87%), specific (87%) measure for identifying community-dwelling adults who are at risk for falls.[10]
- There are no data to support this measure's ability to detect change in individuals or groups; therefore, it needs to be used as an outcome measure with caution until this measurement property has been tested.

TABLE 1 Mean TUG Scores

Age (yr)	Without Cane		With Cane	
	Mean ± SD	Range	Mean ± SD	Range
65–69				
Males	9.93 ± 1.40	7.60–12.25	11.57 ± 1.31	9.84–15.15
Females	10.15 ± 2.91	5.94–22.97	14.19 ± 4.67	7.46–27.13
70–74				
Males	10.45 ± 1.85	8.25–14.50	12.23 ± 1.88	9.41–15.70
Females	10.37 ± 2.23	6.89–16.47	14.27 ± 5.22	7.00–33.34
75–79				
Males	10.48 ± 1.59	8.44–13.82	11.82 ± 5.22	9.18–16.81
Females	10.98 ± 2.68	6.69–15.91	15.29 ± 5.08	6.28–29.90

References

1. Schoppen T, Boonstra A, Groothoff JW, de Vries J, Goeken LN, Eisma WH. The Timed "Up and Go" test: reliability and validity in persons with unilateral lower limb amputation. Arch Phys Med Rehabil 1999;80:825–8.

2. Morris S, Morris ME, Iansek R. Reliability of measurements obtained with the Timed "Up & Go" Test in people with Parkinson disease. Phys Ther 2001;81:810–8.

3. Mathias S, Nayak US, Isaacs B. Balance in elderly patients: the "Get-Up and Go" Test. Arch Phys Med Rehabil 1986;67:387–9.

4. Podsiadlo D, Richardson S. The Timed "Up & Go": a test of basic functional mobility for frail elderly persons. J Am Geriatr Soc 1991;39:142–8.

5. Rockwood K, Awalt E, Carver D, MacKnight C. Feasibility and measurement properties of the Functional Reach and the Timed Up and Go Tests in the Canadian Study of Health and Aging. J Gerontol A Biol Sci Med Sci 2000;55A:M70–3.

6. Freter SH, Fruchter N. Relationship between Timed "Up and Go" and gait time in an elderly orthopaedic rehabilitation population. Clin Rehabil 2000;14:96–101.

7. Whitney SL, Poole JL, Cass SP. A review of balance instruments for older adults. Am J Occup Ther 1998;52:666–71.

8. Eekhof JA, De Bock GH, Schaapveld K, Springer MP. Short report: functional mobility assessment at home. Timed Up and Go Test using three different chairs. Can Fam Phys 2001;47:1205–7.

9. Thompson M, Medley A. Performance of community dwelling elderly on the Timed Up and Go Test. Phys Occup Ther Geriatr 1995;13:17–30.

10. Shumway-Cook A, Brauer S, Woollacott M. Predicting the probability for falls in community-dwelling older adults using the Timed Up & Go Test. Phys Ther 2000;80:896-903.

To obtain this measure, contact the developers, or it can be found in reference 4.

UPPER EXTREMITY FUNCTIONAL SCALE (UEFS)

Developers

G. Pransky, M. Feuerstein, J. Himmelstein, J. N. Katz, and M. Vickers-Lahti,[1] Occupational and Environmental Health Program, Department of Family and Community Medicine, University of Massachusetts Medical Center, Worcester, MA 10655-0309

Purpose

To assess the upper extremity functional status of clients with a variety of conditions and levels of severity. The UEFS is relevant to a working population.

Description

The UEFS is an eight-item self-report upper extremity functional status measure. Each item is scored 1 (no problem) to 10 (major problem, cannot do it at all). Total scores vary from 8 to 80.

Conceptual/Theoretical Basis of Construct Being Measured

None reported.

Groups Tested with This Measure

Clients with a spectrum of upper extremity conditions of varying duration.

Language

English

Application/Administration

The UEFS is self-administered, and most clients can complete the measure in less than 3 minutes.

Typical Reliability Estimates

Internal consistency
Coefficient alpha values: 0.83 to 0.93[1]

Interrater
Not applicable

Test–Retest
Type 2,1 intraclass correlation coefficient: 0.94[2]

Typical Validity Estimates

Content
Not reported

Criterion
No gold standard exists for the construct being measured.

Construct—Cross-sectional

Convergent
- Correlation with pain: 0.47 to 0.67
- Correlation with impairment measures: 0.27 to 0.44[1,2]
- Correlation with the Upper Extremity Functional Index: 0.82[2]

Known Groups. Discriminates between levels of work status (t_{71} = 2.97), duration of symptoms (t_{71} = 2.11), and Phalen's test (t_{86} = 2.17).

Discriminant. Not available

Construct—Longitudinal/Sensitivity to Change

Convergent
- Correlation of 0.32 to 0.50 with change in impairment measures and 0.58 with average change in pain[1]
- Correlation of 0.44 with pooled index of change and 0.37 with prognostic rating of change[2]

Known Groups and **Discriminant** are not available.

Other Validity Coefficients
SRM 0.81 for carpal tunnel, 1.33 for upper extremity disorders[1]

Interpretability

General Population Values (Customary or Normative Values)
Not available

Typical Responsiveness Estimates

Individual Patient. $SEM_{test-retest}$ = 4.1 UEFS points, MDC_{90} = 9.6 UEFS points

Between Group. Not available

References

1. **Pransky G, Feuerstein M, Himmelstein J, Katz JN, Vickers-Lahti M. Measuring functional outcomes in work-related upper extremity disorders. Development and validation of the Upper Extremity Function Scale. J Occup Environ Med 1997; 39:1195–202.**
2. Stratford PW, Binkley JM, Stratford DM. Development and initial validation of the Upper Extremity Functional Index. Physiother Can 2001;53:259–67.

To obtain this measure, contact the developers, or it can be found in reference 1.

VISUAL ANALOGUE SCALE (VAS)

Developers
Unknown

Purpose
Subjective measurement of pain intensity in clinical and experimental settings.

Description
The VAS is a self-report instrument that consists of a 10-cm (100-mm) straight line of either horizontal or vertical orientation. The line is anchored by two extremes of pain: "no pain" and "pain as bad as it could be."

Conceptual/Theoretical Basis of Construct Being Measured
None reported.

Groups Tested with This Measure
Individuals with acute pain[1-3] (emergency department, postsurgical), chronic pain,[4] rheumatoid arthritis,[5,6] cancer,[7] orthopedic,[8] and temporomandibular joint dysfunction.[9]

Languages
English, Portuguese,[6] Dutch[9]

Application/Administration
Clients are presented with a 10-cm line on a piece of paper and a pen. They are instructed to mark their perceived level of pain intensity on the line. The instrument is then scored by the clinician measuring, with a ruler, the distance in millimeters from the "no pain" anchor to the mark placed on the line by the client. The resulting measure represents the client's level of pain. Possible scores range from 0 to 100.

Typical Reliability Estimates

Internal Consistency
Not applicable

Interrater
Not applicable

Test–Retest
0.71 to 0.99[5-7]

Typical Validity Estimates

Content
No reference in the literature.

Criterion
No gold standard exists.

Construct—Cross-sectional

Convergent. Correlations with other measures of pain intensity (McGill Pain Questionnaire, numeric pain rating scale): 0.30 to 0.95[6,7]

Known Groups and *Discriminant* are not available.

Construct—Longitudinal/Sensitivity to Change
Not available

Other Validity Coefficients
Effect size = 1.34 ("usual" pain: VAS compared to numeric pain rating scale and a verbal rating scale of pain)[8]

Interpretability

General Population Values (Customary or Normative Values)
Score > 30 mm equal to or greater than "moderate" pain, score > 54 mm equal to or greater than "severe" pain.[3]

Typical Responsiveness Estimates

Individual Patient
- Confidence interval in measured score: 95% CI = ± 20 mm[9]
- Smallest detectable difference (minimal detectable change): ± 28 mm[9]

Between Group. Not available

Comments
Limitations to the use of the VAS have been reported with respect to elderly and less literate populations. Also, errors associated with administration in terms of reproducing the line (photocopying) and scoring the instrument (measuring the line) have been reported.

References

1. Berthier F, Potel G, Leconte P, Touze M, Baron D. Comparative study of methods measuring acute pain intensity in an ED. Am J Emerg Med 1998;16:132–6.

2. DeLoach LJ, Higgins MS, Caplin AB, Stiff JL. The visual analogue scale in the immediate postoperative period: intrasubject variability and correlation with a numeric scale. Anesth Analg 1998;86:102–6.

3. Collins SL, Moore A, McQuay HJ. The visual analogue scale: what is moderate pain in millimetres? Pain 1997;72:95–7.

4. Scott J, Huskisson EC. Graphic representation of pain. Pain 1976;2:175–84.

5. Scott J, Huskisson EC. Vertical or horizontal visual analogue scales. Ann Rheum Dis 1979;38:560.

6. Ferraz MB, Quaresma MR, Aquina LR, Atra E, Tugwell P, Goldsmith CH. Reliability of pain scales in the assessment of literate and illiterate patients with rheumatoid arthritis. J Rheumatol 1990;17:1022–4.

7. Ahles T, Ruckdeschel J, Blanchard E. Cancer-related pain-II: assessment with visual analogue scales. J Psychosom Res 1984; 28:121–4.

8. Bolton JE, Wilkinson RC. Responsiveness of pain scales: a comparison of three intensity measures in chiropractic patients. J Manipulative Physiol Ther 1998;21:1–7.

9. Kropmans TJB, Dijkstra PU, Stegenga B, Stewart R, de Bont LGM. Smallest detectable difference in outcome variables related to painful restriction of the temporomandibular joint. J Dent Res 1999;78:784–9.

This measure can be found in reference 4.

Walk Test (2-Minute) (2MWT)

Developers

R. J. A. Butland, J. Pang, E. R. Gross, A. A. Wood-cock, and D. M. Geddes[1] modified the 12-Minute Walk Test into shorter versions (mainly 2 and 6 minute). Affiliation: Brompton Hospital, London, England (from 1982).

Purpose

To assess exercise tolerance[1]; originally developed for individuals with chronic airflow limitation.

Description

The 2MWT is a performance-based test. Distance walked in 2 minutes is measured and reported in meters or feet. A greater distance indicates a better performance. It was originally modified from the 12-Minute Walk Test, which was based on a 12-minute running test by Cooper.[2]

Conceptual/Theoretical Basis of Construct Being Measured

None reported.

Groups Tested with This Measure

Individuals with chronic airflow limitation[1] and/or chronic heart failure,[3] individuals with chronic obstructive pulmonary disease (COPD),[4] children with cystic fibrosis,[5] frail elderly individuals,[6] individuals with lower limb amputation,[7] neurologically impaired adults undergoing rehabilitation,[8] and those with Parkinson's disease.[9]

Language

English

Application/Administration

This test is ideally conducted in an enclosed quiet corridor. Clients are instructed to walk from end to end, covering as much ground as possible in 2 minutes. Distance walked in 2 minutes is measured using a measuring wheel (also known as a trundle) or markings in the corridor. Rate of perceived exertion (using Borg Scale), oxygen saturation (using an oximeter), and heart rate can also be monitored throughout the test. Encouragement should be standardized with respect to type and timing. Training and learning effect must be considered (see below).

Typical Reliability Estimates

Internal Consistency

Not applicable.

Interrater

- ICC: 0.93 to 0.95 in frail elderly individuals[6]

Test–Retest

- ICC: 0.82 to 0.89 in frail elderly persons[6] and 0.97 in neurologically impaired adults undergoing rehabilitation[8]
- Training effect: No significant improvement on second testing in children with cystic fibrosis (no p value provided).[5] Training effect observed for the first two tests in individuals with chronic airflow limitation and/or heart failure ($p < 0.0001$).[3] The distance walked significantly increased over the first three trials in individuals with Parkinson's disease and a control group (p not reported).[9]
- Time of day: The time of day had no effect on distance (no p value provided)[3] in individuals with chronic airflow limitation and/or heart failure.

Other

Encouragement: Within-person SD (with encouragement) = 8.2 meters[3] in individuals with chronic airflow limitation and/or heart failure. Within-person SD (without encouragement) = 6.4 meters[3] in individuals with chronic airflow limitation and/or heart failure.

Typical Validity Estimates

Content

Some authors argue that 2 minutes of walking are not reflective of exercise capacity or requirements of daily living.[8]

Criterion

Concurrent

- VO_2/kg: $r = 0.55$ in elderly people with COPD[4]
- VO_{2max}: $r = 0.45$ in elderly people with COPD[4]
- 6-minute walk: $r = 0.96$ in individuals with chronic airflow limitation and/or heart failure[1] and $r = 0.95$ in elderly with COPD[4]
- 12-minute walk: $r = 0.94$ in elderly with COPD[4]

Predictive. Not available

Construct—Cross-sectional

Convergent

- Physical functioning subscale of the 36-Item Short-Form Health Survey (SF-36): $r = 0.22$ to 0.48 in clients with amputations[7]
- Houghton scale: $r = 0.49$ in clients with amputations[7]
- Rivermead Mobility Index: $r = 0.75$ in individuals with stable neurologic impairment[8]
- 10-meter timed walk: $r = -0.61$ in individuals with stable neurologic impairment[8]

Known Groups

- Individuals who do not use a mobility aid walked further than those with an aid in stable "neurologically" impaired patients ($p < 0.001$)[8]
- Individuals without leg sensory impairment walked further than those with sensory impairment in stable "neurologically" impaired patients ($p < 0.001$)[8]
- Greater distance walked in control group compared to individuals with Parkinson's disease (no p value provided)[9]

Discriminant. Not available

Construct—Longitudinal/Sensitivity to Change

Convergent

- Change in VO_2/kg: $r = 0.53$ in elderly people with COPD[4]
- Change in VO_{2max}: $r = 0.53$ in elderly people with COPD[4]

Known Groups. Not available

Discriminant

- Better correlation with VO_2/kg ($r = 0.55$) and VO_{2max} ($r = 0.45$) than spirometric values ($r = 0.04$ to 0.13) in elderly people with COPD[4]
- No correlation with mental composite score of SF-36 ($p > 0.4$) but correlation with the physical functioning subscale of SF-36 ($r = 0.22$ to 0.48, $p < 0.008$) in people with amputations[7]

Interpretability

Within-person SD/treatment effect = 0.90 in individuals with chronic airflow limitation and/or heart failure ($p < 0.0001$)[3]

General Population Values
(Customary or Normative Values)

Not available. Refer to general population values for the 6-Minute Walk Test.

Comments

The walk test reflects exercise capacity involving the lower extremities only. Although it was originally developed to measure exercise tolerance, other constructs were also thought to be reflected in this measure (eg, functional capacity or performance, walking ability, lower extremity function). The data to support criterion validity would depend on the construct being measured.

References

1. Butland RJA, Pang J, Gross FR, Woodcock AA, Geddes DM. Two-, six, and twelve-minute walking tests in respiratory disease. BMJ 1982;284:1607–8.
2. Cooper KH. A means of assessing maximal oxygen intake. Correlation between field and treadmill testing. JAMA 1968; 203:201–4.
3. Guyatt GH, Pugsley SO, Sullivan MJ, Thompson PJ, Berman LB, Jones NL, et al. Effect of encouragement on walking test performance. Thorax 1984;39:818–22.
4. Bernstein ML, Despars JA, Singh NP, Avalos K, Stansbury DW, Light RW. Reanalysis of the 12-minute walk in patients with chronic obstructive pulmonary disease. Chest 1994;105:163–7.
5. Upton CJ, Tyrrell JC, Hiller EJ. Two minute walking distance in cystic fibrosis. Arch Dis Child 1988;63:1444–8.
6. Connelly DM, Stevenson TJ, Vandervoort AA. Between- and within-rater reliability of walking tests in a frail elderly population. Physiother Can 1996;48:47–51.
7. Brooks D, Parsons J, Hunter JP, Devlin M, Walker J. The 2-Minute Walk Test as a measure of functional improvement in persons with lower limb amputation. Arch Phys Med Rehabil 2001;82: In press.
8. Rossier P, Wade DT. Validity and reliability comparison of 4 mobility measures in patients presenting with neurological impairment. Arch Phys Med Rehabil 2001;82:9–13.
9. Light KE, Behrrman AL, Thigben M, Triggs WJ. The 2-Minute Walk Test: a tool for evaluating endurance in clients with Parkinson's disease. Neurol Rep 1997;21:136–9.
10. Solway S, Brooks D, Lacasse Y, Thomas S. A qualitative systematic overview of the measurement properties of functional walk tests used in the cardiorespiratory domain. Chest 2001; 119:256–70.

This measure can be found in reference 1.

WALK TEST (6-MINUTE) (6MWT)

Description

The 6MWT is a performance-based test. Distance walked in 6 minutes is measured and reported in meters or feet. A greater distance indicates a better performance. The 6MWT was derived from the 12-Minute Walk Test by Butland and colleagues[1] (which was modified from Cooper's 12-Minute Run Test[2]), who were exploring the possibility of using walking tests of shorter duration.

Conceptual/Theoretical Basis of Construct Being Measured

No conceptual basis for exercise tolerance was cited in the literature.

Groups Tested with This Measure

Individuals with chronic obstructive pulmonary disease (COPD)[3] and/or heart failure,[3] peripheral arterial disease,[4–7] fibromyalgia,[8–11] cystic fibrosis,[12–14] pulmonary hypertension,[15–17] renal failure,[18] total hip arthroplasty,[19] Paget's disease of the bone,[20] sequelae of poliomyelitis,[21] and stroke[22–24]; elderly individuals[3,25–27]; individuals with pacemakers[3]; transplant candidates with end-stage lung disease[28,29]; individuals undergoing lung volume reduction surgery and pulmonary resection[3]; individuals receiving noninvasive mechanical home ventilation[30]; children with end-stage heart and lung disease[31]; and older healthy adults.[32–34]

Languages

No information available

Application/Administration

This test is ideally conducted in an enclosed, quiet corridor. Clients are instructed to walk from end to end, covering as much ground as possible in 6 min-utes. Individuals are told that they may rest if they become too short of breath or tired to continue but to resume walking when they are able to do so. At the end of the 6 minutes, the clients are told to stop. Distance walked and number and duration of rests in the 6 minutes are measured. Rating of perceived exertion, dyspnea, oxygen saturation, and heart rate can also be monitored. Encouragement should be standardized with respect to type and timing. In most populations, at least two practice walks should be administered before measurements are recorded (see below).

Typical Reliability Estimates

Internal Consistency
Not applicable

Interrater
Not available

Test–Retest
Among Individuals with Chronic Heart and Lung Disease
- ICC: 0.91 to 0.92[35]
- Significant increase in distance walked between first three trials[35,36]

Among Individuals with Heart Failure
- ICC: 0.82 to 0.96[37–41]
- Significant increase in distance walked between trial one and two but no significant increase on the third trial[42–44]

Among Individuals with COPD
- Significant increase in distance walked between first three trials[45]

Among Individuals with Fibromyalgia
- ICC: 0.73 to 0.98[9,11]
- Significant increase in distance walked between trial one and two but no significant increase on the third trial[8,9,11]

Among Older Adults and Elderly Individuals
- ICC: 0.93 to 0.95[26,33]

Among Individuals with Peripheral Arterial Disease
- ICC: 0.94[4]

Among Individuals with End-Stage Lung Disease Who Are Transplant Candidates
- ICC: 0.99[29]

Among Other Populations

- Significant increase in distance walked between trial one and two among individuals with late sequelae of poliomyelitis[21] and renal failure[18]
- No significant difference in distance walked with repeated trials among children with cystic fibrosis[13] or individuals with pacemakers[46]

Other

- Encouragement associated with a significant increase in distance walked among individuals with chronic heart and lung disease ($p < 0.02$)[47]

Typical Validity Estimates

Content

Patients with heart failure and pacemakers consider this test representative of daily physical activity.[46,48]

Criterion

Concurrent. *Among Individuals with COPD*

- VO_2: $r = 0.51$[49]
- VO_2/kg: $r = 0.67$[49]
- CO_2: $r = 0.40$[49]
- CO_2/kg: $r = 0.48$[49]
- VO_{2peak}: $r = 0.64$[50]
- W_{max}: $r = 0.81$[51]

Among Individuals with End-Stage Lung Disease Who Are Transplant Candidates

- VO_{2max}: $r = 0.73$[29]

Among Individuals with Heart Failure

- VO_{2max}: $r = 0.06$ to 0.90[38,39,41–44,52–56]
- Workload maximum: $r = 0.68$[41]

Among Individuals with Pacemakers

- Work capacity: $r = 0.74$[46]

Among Individuals with Pulmonary Hypertension

- VO_{2max}: $r = 0.70$[16]

Among Individuals with Fibromyalgia

- VO_{2peak} (mL/kg/min): $r =$ not significant to 0.66[10,11]

Among Individuals with Peripheral Arterial Disease

- VO_{2max}: $r = 0.37$[4]

Among Children with Cystic Fibrosis

- Workload maximum: $r = 0.76$[13]
- VO_{2max}: $r = 0.76$[13]

Among Children with End-Stage Heart and/or Lung Disease

- VO_{2max}: $r = 0.70$[31]
- Physical work capacity: $r = 0.64$[31]

Predictive. Length of hospitalization: $r = 0.32$ to 0.40 among individuals undergoing lung volume reduction surgery[57]

Construct—Cross-sectional

Convergent. *Among Individuals with COPD*

- Functional status questionnaire scores: $r = 0.36$ to 0.73[35,36,50,58–61]
- Physical activity measured with an accelerometer: $r = 0.60$ to 0.95[45,60]
- Self-rating of walking ability relative to other patients: $r = 0.59$[62]
- Dyspnea and perceived exertion ratings: $r = 0.30$ to 0.65[35,51,60,63,64]
- 2-Minute Walk Test: $r = 0.89$ to 0.95[1,49]
- 12-Minute Walk Test: $r = 0.96$ to 0.97[1,49]
- Shuttle Walk Test: $r = 0.68$[65]
- Cycle ergometry: $r = 0.57$ to 0.58[35,36]
- Quality of life scores: $r = 0.02$ to 0.64[50,51,58,60,66–68]
- Spirometry: $r = 0.05$ to 0.68[49–51,60,64,69]
- $PaCO_2$: $r = -0.31$[69]

Among Individuals with Heart Failure

- Upper and lower extremity strength: $r = 0.33$ to 0.41[55]
- Anaerobic threshold: $r = 0.46$ to 0.54[42,53]
- Ejection fraction: $r = 0.32$ to 0.34[11,53]
- Mean pulmonary artery pressure: $r = 0.33$[53]
- New York Heart Association (NYHA) functional classification: $r = 0.45$ to 0.58[36,41]
- Dyspnea ratings: $r = -0.50$ to 0.59[35]
- Cycle ergometery: $r = 0.42$ to 0.58[35,36]
- Peak expiratory flow: $r = 0.68$[53]
- Functional status questionnaires scores: $r = 0.37$ to 0.79[35–37]

Among Older Adults

- Age: $r = -0.51$[32]
- Height: $r = 0.54$[32]
- Quadriceps strength: $r = 0.62$[32]
- Measures of balance and function: $r = 0.52$ to 0.73[33]
- 36-Item Short-Form Health Survey (SF-36) physical function subscale: $r = 0.55$[33]
- SF-36 general health subscale: $r = 0.39$[33]

Among Individuals with Fibromyalgia

- Fibromyalgia Impact Questionnaire scores: $r = -0.20$ to -0.49[10,11]

Among Individuals with Peripheral Arterial Disease

- Energy expenditure of physical activity: $r = 0.63$[5]
- Walking impairment questionnaire $r = 0.56$[6]
- Measures of balance: $r = 0.20$ to 0.28[7]
- Ankle/Brachial Index: $r = 0.55$[4]

Among Individuals with Late Sequelae of Poliomyelitis
- Cardiorespiratory conditioning index: $r = 0.50$[21]
- Health and functional status scores: $r = 0.57$ to 0.67[21]

Among Individuals with Pulmonary Hypertension
- Cardiac output: $r = 0.48$[16]
- Total peripheral resistance: $r = -0.49$[16]

Among Individuals with Cystic Fibrosis
- Spirometry: $r =$ not significant to 0.49[12,13]
- Resting oxygen saturation: $r = 0.35$[12]

Among Individuals with Total Hip Arthroplasty
- SF-36 Physical Component Score: $r = 0.69$[19]
- Western Ontario McMaster Osteoarthritis (WOMAC) score: $r = 0.64$[19]

Among Individuals Receiving Noninvasive Home Mechanical Ventilation
- Oxygen Cost Diagram: $r = 0.65$[30]

Known Groups. *Among Individuals with Lung Disease*
- Capable of distinguishing between patients with COPD undergoing inpatient rehabilitation from those undergoing outpatient rehabilitation ($p < 0.001$)[58,59]
- Capable of distinguishing between bilateral lung transplant recipients and single lung transplant recipients ($p < 0.01$)[70]

Among Older Adults and Elderly Individuals
- Capable of distinguishing between elderly women with osteoporotic vertebral compression fractures and those without fracture[27]
- Capable of distinguishing between males and females[32]
- Capable of distinguishing active from inactive individuals ($p < 0.0001$)[33]

Among Individuals with Heart Failure
- Capable of distinguishing between NYHA classifications[41,44,48,71,72]
- Capable of distinguishing between individuals with and without heart failure[48,72]

Among Other Populations
- Capable of distinguishing individuals with Paget's disease of the bone from those without ($p < 0.001$)[20]
- Capable of distinguishing individuals with peripheral arterial disease from those without ($p < 0.001$)[7]
- Capable of distinguishing individuals with primary pulmonary hypertension from those without[16]
- Capable of distinguishing individuals with fibromyalgia from those without[8]

- Capable of distinguishing between pacemaker modes[73]

Discriminant. *Among Individuals with COPD*
- Mental health subscale of SF-36: $r = -0.10$[60]
- Measures of depression, mood, anxiety, self-esteem: not significant[69]
- Spirometry: conflicting results—see convergent validity

Among Children with End-Stage Heart and/or Lung Disease
- Spirometry: not significant[31]

Construct—Longitudinal/Sensitivity to Change Estimates

Convergent. *Among Individuals with COPD*
- Change in VO_{2max}: $r = 0.64$[49]
- Change in VCO_{2max}: $r = 0.49$[49]

Among Individuals with Heart Failure
- Change in Chronic Heart Questionnaire scores: $r = 0.47$ to 0.70[37]
- Change in global rating: $r = 0.78$[37]

Among Individuals with Fibromyalgia
- Change in Fibromyalgia Impact Questionnaire scores: $r =$ not significant to 0.59[10]
- Change in VO_{2peak}: not significant[10]

Among Individuals with Total Hip Arthroplasty
- Change in SF-36 physical component summary score: $r = 0.58$[19]
- Change in WOMAC: $r = 0.54$ to 0.57[19]

Among Individuals Receiving Noninvasive Home Mechanical Ventilation
- Change in Oxygen Cost Diagram: not significant[30]

Known Groups and **Discriminant** are not available.

Other Validity Coefficients

Thresholds ranging from 300 to 400 meters predictive of morbidity and mortality/survival among individuals with pulmonary hypertension,[15–17] individuals undergoing lung surgery,[74,75] individuals with COPD,[76] transplant candidates with end-stage lung disease,[28] and individuals with heart failure.[38,39,41,71] However, other investigators have found 6MWT not predictive of these events among individuals with heart failure.[42,52,56]

Although specific thresholds are not indicated, 6MWT distance has been suggested as being predictive of survival after pulmonary rehabilitation for individuals with COPD,[59] of death for individuals with cystic fibrosis awaiting transplantation[14] and those undergoing lung volume reduction surgery,[57,77] and of dropping out of an exercise program among frail elderly individuals.[25]

Among Individuals with Heart Failure
- Responsiveness coefficient: 1.73[37]

Among Individuals with Chronic Heart and Lung Disease
- Responsiveness index: 0.74[47]

Among the Elderly
- Responsiveness index: 0.60[26]

Among Individuals with Stroke
Data for responsiveness in stroke come from randomized trials that used the 6MWT as an outcome measure.[22–24] In a trial of the effectiveness of 6 weeks of treadmill training with body weight support involving 100 individuals,[22] the mean change in the distance walked in 6 minutes following the intervention was 102.8 meters (SD: 67.4) compared with 58.8 meters (SD: 72.2) for individuals in the control group. An 8-week home-based exercise program, which was piloted on 20 subjects, resulted in a change of 59.4 meters compared with 34.7 meters following usual care.[23] A 4-week exercise class to improve locomotor tasks involving 12 subjects[24] achieved a change of 42.1 meters (SD: 119.0) compared with only a 4.7-meter change following an equal attention upper extremity intervention. The 6MWT is a measure that changes following rehabilitation interventions that target walking.

Interpretability

General Population Values
Gender-specific reference equations are available to determine the percent predicted 6MWT distance for individual healthy adult patients performing the 6MWT for the first time.[34]

Typical Responsiveness Estimates

Individual Patient. Not available

Between Group. Among Individuals with COPD
- Effect size: 0.60[66]
- Minimal clinically importance difference: 54 meters[62]

Among Individuals with Heart Failure
- Effect size: 0.85 (improvement) to 2.13 (deterioration)[37]

Among Individuals with Fibromyalgia
- Reliability change index: 3.48 meters[10]

Comments

Although the purpose of the 6MWT was originally intended to assess exercise tolerance, many clinicians and researchers use it as a measure of functional exercise capacity. Conceptually, functional exercise capacity has been defined as the ability to undertake physically demanding activities of daily living.[35,36]

References

1. Butland RJA, Pang J, Gross ER, Woodcock AA, Geddes DM. Two-, six, and twelve-minute walking tests in respiratory disease. BMJ 1982;284:1607–8.

2. Cooper KH. A means of assessing maximal oxygen intake. Correlation between field and treadmill testing. JAMA 1968; 203:201–4.

3. Solway S, Brooks D, Lacasse Y, Thomas S. A qualitative systematic overview of the measurement properties of functional walk tests used in the cardiorespiratory domain. Chest 2001; 119:256–70.

4. Montgomery PS, Gardner AW. The clinical utility of a six-minute walk test in peripheral arterial occlusive disease patients. J Am Geriatr Soc 1998;46:706–11.

5. Gardner AW, Womack CJ, Sieminski DJ, Montgomery PS, Killewich LA, Fonong T. Relationship between free-living daily physical activity and ambulatory measures in older claudicants. Angiology 1998;49.327–37.

6. McDermott MM, Liu K, Guralnik JM, Martin GJ, Criqui MH, Greenland P. Measurement of walking endurance and walking velocity with questionnaire: validation of the walking impairment questionnaire in men and women with peripheral arterial disease. J Vasc Surg 1998;28:1072–81.

7. Gardner AW, Montgomery PS. Impaired balance and higher prevalence of falls in subjects with intermittent claudication. J Gerontol 2001;56A:M454–8.

8. Mannerkorpi K, Svantesson U, Carlsson J, Ekdahl C. Tests of functional limitations in fibromyalgia syndrome: a reliability study. Arthritis Care Res 1999;12:193–9.

9. Pankoff BA, Overend TJ, Lucy SD, White KP. Reliability of the six-minute walk test in people with fibromyalgia. Arthritis Care Res 2000;13:291–5.

10. Pankoff B, Overend T, Lucy D, White K. Validity and responsiveness of the 6 Minute Walk Test for people with fibromyalgia. J Rheumatol 2000;27:2666–70.

11. King S, Wessel J, Bhambhani Y, Maikala R, Sholter D, Maksymowych. Validity and reliability of the 6 Minute Walk in persons with fibromyalgia. J Rheumatol 1999;26:2233–7.

12. Balfour-Lyn IM, Prasad SA, Laverty A, Whitehead BF, Dinwiddie R. A step in the right direction: assessing exercise tolerance in cystic fibrosis. Pediatr Pulmonol 1998;25:278–84.

13. Gulmans VAM, van Veldhoven NHMJ, de Meer K, Helders PJM. The Six-Minute Walking Test in children with cystic fibrosis: reliability and validity. Pediatr Pulmonol 1996;22:85–9.

14. Vizza CD, Yusen RD, Lynch JP, Fedele F, Patterson A, Trulock EP. Outcome of patients with cystic fibrosis awaiting lung transplantation. Am J Respir Crit Care Med 2000;162:819–25.

15. Stricker H, Domenighetti G, Popov W, Speich R, Nicod L, Aubert JD, et al. Severe pulmonary hypertension: data from the Swiss Registry. Swiss Med Wkly 2001;131:346–50.

16. Miyamoto S, Nagaya N, Satoh T, Kyotani S, Sakamaki F, Fujita M, et al. Clinical correlates and prognostic significance of Six-Minute Walk Test in patients with primary pulmonary hypertension. Am J Respir Crit Care Med 2000;161:487–92.

17. Paciocco G, Martinez FJ, Bossone E, Pielsticker E, Gillespie B, Rubenfire M. Oxygen desaturation on the Six-Minute Walk Test and mortality in untreated primary pulmonary hypertension. Eur Respir J 2001;17:647–52.

18. Fitts SS, Guthrie MR. Six-minute walk by people with chronic renal failure. Am J Phys Rehabil 1995;74:54–8.

19. Boardman DL, Dorey F, Thomas BJ, Lieberman JR. The accuracy of assessing total hip arthroplasty outcomes. J Arthroplasty 2000;15:200–4.

20. Lyles KW, Lammers JE, Shipp KM, Sherman L, Pieper CF, Martinez S, et al. Functional and mobility impairments associated with Paget's disease of bone. J Am Geriatr Soc 1995;43:502–6.

21. Noonan VK, Dean E, Dallimore M. The relationship between self-reports and objective measures of disability in patients with late sequelae of poliomyelitis: a validation study. Arch Phys Med Rehabil 2000;81:1422–7.

22. Visintin M, Barbeau H, Korner-Bitensky N, Mayo NE. A new approach to retrain gait in stroke patients through body weight support and treadmill stimulation. Stroke 1998;29:1122–8.

23. Duncan P, Richards L, Wallace D, Stoker Yates J, Pohl P, Luchies C, et al. A randomized, controlled pilot study of a home-based exercise program for individuals with mild and moderate stroke. Stroke 1998;29:2055–60.

24. Dean CM, Richards CL, Malouin F. Task-related circuit training improves performance of locomotor tasks in chronic stroke: a randomized, controlled pilot trial. Arch Phys Med Rehabil 2000;81:409–17.

25. Schimdt JA, Gruman C, King MB, Wolfson LI. Attrition in an exercise intervention: a comparison of early and late dropouts. J Am Geriatr Soc 2000;48:952–60.

26. King MB, Judge JO, Whipple R, Wolfson L. Reliability and responsiveness of two physical performance measures examined in the context of a functional training intervention. Phys Ther 2000;80:8–16.

27. Lyles KW, Gold DT, Shipp KM, Pieper CF, Martinez S, Mulhausen PL. Association of osteoporotic vertebral compression fractures with impaired functional status. Am J Med 1993;94:595–601.

28. Kadikar A, Maurer J, Kesten S. The Six-Minute Walk Test: a guide to assessment for lung transplantation. J Heart Lung Transplant 1997;16:313–9.

29. Cahalin L, Pappagianopoulos P, Prevost S, Wain J, Ginns L. The relationship of the 6-Min Walk Test to maximal oxygen consumption in transplant candidates with end-stage lung disease. Chest 1995;108:452–9.

30. Janssens JP, Breitenstein E, Rochat T, Fitting JW. Does the 'Oxygen Cost Diagram' reflect changes in six-minute walking distance in follow up studies? Respir Med 1999;93:810–5.

31. Nixon PA, Joswiak ML, Fricker FJ. A six-minute walk test for assessing exercise tolerance in severely ill children. J Pediatr 1996;129:362–6.

32. Troosters T, Gosselink R, Decramer M. Six minute walking distance in healthy elderly subjects. Eur Respir J 1999;14:270–4.

33. Harada ND, Chiu V, Stewart AL. Mobility-related function in older adults: assessment with 6-minute walk test. Arch Phys Med Rehabil 1999;80:837–41.

34. Enright PL, Sherrill DL. Reference equations for the six-minute walk in healthy adults. Am J Respir Crit Care Med 1998; 158:1384–7.

35. Guyatt GH, Thompson PJ, Berman LB, Sullivan MJ, Townsend M, Jones NL, et al. How should we measure function in patients with chronic heart and lung disease? J Chron Dis 1985;38:517–24.

36. **Guyatt GH, Sullivan MJ, Thompson PJ, Fallen EL, Pugsley SO, Taylor DW, et al. The 6-minute walk: a new measure of exercise capacity in patients with chronic heart failure. Can Med Assoc J 1985;132:919–23.**

37. O'Keeffe ST, Lye M, Donnellan C, Carmichael DN. Reproducibility and responsiveness of quality of life assessment and Six Minute Walk Test in elderly heart failure patients. Heart 1998;80:377–82.

38. Roul G, Germain P, Bareiss P. Does the 6-Minute Walk Test predict the prognosis in patients with NYHA class II or III chronic heart failure? Am Heart J 1998;136:449–57.

39. Cahalin LP, Mathier MA, Semigran MJ, Dec GW, DiSalvo TG. The Six-Minute Walk Test predicts peak oxygen uptake and survival in patients with advanced heart failure. Chest 1996;110:325–32.

40. Pinna GD, Opasich C, Mazza A, Tangenti A, Maestri R, Sanarico M. Reproducibility of the Six-Minute Walking Test in chronic heart failure patients. Stat Med 2000;19:3087–94.

41. Zugck C, Kruger C, Durr S, Gerber SH, Haunstetter A, Hornig K, et al. Is the 6-Minute Walk Test a reliable substitute for peak oxygen uptake in patients with dilated cardiomyopathy. Eur Heart J 2000;21:540–9.

42. Opasich C, Pinna GD, Mazza A, Febo O, Riccardi R, Riccardi PG, et al. Six-minute walking performance in patients with moderate-to-severe heart failure. Eur Heart J 2001;22:488–96.

43. Morales FJ, Martinez A, Mendez M, Agarrado A, Ortega F, Fernandez-Guerra J, et al. A shuttle walk test for assessment of functional capacity in chronic heart failure. Am Heart J 1999; 138:291–8.

44. Riley M, McParland J, Stanford CF, Nicholls DP. Oxygen consumption during corridor walk testing in chronic cardiac failure. Eur Heart J 1992;13:789–93.

45. Steele BC, Holt L, Belza B, Ferris S, Lashminaryan S, Bucher DM. Quantitative physical activity in COPD using a triaxial accelometer. Chest 2000;117;1359–67.

46. Langenfeld H, Schneider B, Grimm W, Beer M, Knoche M, Riegger G, et al. The Six Minute Walk—an adequate exercise test for pacemaker patients? Pacing Clin Electrophysiol 1990; 13(12Pt2);1761–5.

47. Guyatt GH, Pugsley SO, Sullivan MJ, Thompson PJ, Berman LB, Jones NL, et al. Effect of encouragement on walking test performance. Thorax 1984;39:818–22.

48. Lipkin DP, Scriven AJ, Crake T, Poole-Wilson PA. Six Minute Walking Test for assessing exercise capacity in chronic heart failure. BMJ 1986;292:653–5.

49. Bernstein ML, Despars JA, Singh NP, Avalos K, Stansbury DW, Light RW, et al. Reanalysis of the 12-minute walk in patients with chronic obstructive pulmonary disease. Chest 1994;105:163–7.

50. Rejeski WJ, Foley KO, Woodard CM, Zaccaro DJ, Berry MJ. Evaluating and understanding performance testing in COPD patients. J Cardiopulm Rehabil 2000;20:79–88.

51. Wijkstra PJ, TenVergert EM, van der Mark TW, Postma DS, Van Altena R, Kraan J, et al. Relation of lung function, maximal inspiratory pressure, dyspnoea and quality of life with exercise capacity in patients with chronic obstructive pulmonary disease. Thorax 1994;49:468–72.

52. Morales FJ, Montemayor T, Martinez A. Shuttle versus Six-Minute Walk Test in the prediction of outcome in chronic heart failure. Int J Cardiol 2000:76:101–5.

53. Rostagno C, Galanti G, Comeglio M, Boddi V, Olivo G, Serneri GGN. Comparison of different methods of functional evaluation in patients with chronic heart failure. Eur J Heart Fail 2000;2:273–80.

54. Faggiano P, D'aloia A, Gualeni A, Lavatelli A, Giordano A. Assessment of oxygen uptake during the 6-Minute Walking Test in patients with heart failure: preliminary experience with a portable device. Am Heart J 1997;134:203–6.

55. Hendrican MC, McKelvie RS, Smith T, McCartney N, Pogue J, Teo KK, et al. Functional capacity in patients with congestive heart failure. J Card Fail 2000;6:214–9.

56. Lucas C, Stevenson LW, Johnson W, Hartley H, Hamilton MA, Walden J, et al. The 6-min walk and peak oxygen consumption in advanced heart failure: aerobic capacity and survival. Am Heart J 1999;138:618–24.

57. Szekely LA, Oelberg DA, Wright C, Johnson DC, Wain J, Trotman-Dickenson B, et al. Preoperative predictors of operative morbidity and mortality in COPD patients undergoing bilateral lung volume reduction surgery. Chest 1997;111:550–8.

58. Haggerty MC, Stockdale-Woodley R, Zu Wallack R. Functional status in pulmonary rehabilitation participants. J Cardiopulm Rehabil 1999;19:35–42.

59. Bowen JB, Votto JJ, Thrall RS, Haggerty MC, Stockdale-Woolley R, Bandyopadhyay T, et al. Functional status and survival following pulmonary rehabilitation. Chest 2000;118:697–703.

60. Belza B, Steele BG, Hunziker J, Lakshminaryan S, Holy L, Buchor DM. Correlates of physical activity in chronic obstructive pulmonary disease. Nurs Res 2001;50:195–202.

61. Bendstrup KE, Jensen JI, Holm S, Bengtsson B. Out-patient rehabilitation improves activities of daily living, quality of life and exercise tolerance in chronic obstructive pulmonary disease. Eur Respir J 1997;10:2801–6.

62. Redelmeier DA, Bayoumi AM, Goldstein RS, Guyatt GH. Interpreting small differences in functional status: the Six Minute Walk Test in chronic lung disease patients. Am J Respir Crit Care Med 1997;155:1278–82.

63. Roomi J, Johnson MM, Waters K, Yohannes A, Helm A, Connolly MJ. Respiratory rehabilitation, exercise capacity and quality of life in chronic airways disease in old age. Age Ageing 1996;25:12–6.

64. Mak VHF, Bugler JR, Roberts CM, Spiro SG. Effect of arterial oxygen saturation on six minute walk distance, perceived effort, and perceived breathlessness in patients with airflow limitation. Thorax 1993;48:33–8.

65. Singh SJ, Morgan MDL, Scott S, Walters D, Hardman AE. Development of a shuttle walking test of disability in patients with chronic airways obstruction. Thorax 1992;47:1019–24.

66. Guyatt GH, King DR, Feenery DH, Stubbing D, Goldstein RS. Generic and specific measurement of health-related quality of life in a clinical trial of respiratory rehabilitation. J Clin Epidemiol 1999;52:187–92.

67. Jones PW, Baveystock CM, Littlejohns P. Relationship between general health measured with sickness impact profile and respiratory symptoms, physiological measures, and mood in patients with chronic airflow limitation. Am Rev Respir Dis 1989;140:1538–43.

68. Knebel AR, Leidy NK, Sherman S. Health related quality of life and disease severity in patients with alpha-1 antitrypsin deficiency. Qual Life Res 1999;8:385–91.

69. Borak J, Chodosowska E, Matuszewski A, Zielinski J. Emotional status does not alter exercise tolerance in patients with chronic obstructive pulmonary disease. Eur Respir J 1998;12:370-3.

70. Paris W, Diercks M, Bright J, Zamora M, Kesten S, Scavuzzo M, et al. Return to work after transplantation. J Heart Lung Transplant 1998;17:430–6.

71. Bittner V, Weiner DH, Yusuf S, Rogers WJ, McIntyre KM, Bangdiwala SI, et al. Prediction of mortality and morbidity with a 6-minute walk test in patients with left ventricular dysfunction. JAMA 1993;270:1702–7.

72. Peeters P, Mets T. The 6-minute walk as an appropriate exercise test in elderly patients with chronic heart failure. J Gerontol 1996;51A:M147–51.

73. Provenier F, Jordaens L. Evaluation of Six Minute Walking Test in patients with single chamber rate responsive pacemakers. Br Heart J 1994;72:192–6.

74. Hazelrigg S, Boley T, Henkle J, Lawyer C, Johnstone D, Naunheim K, et al. Thoracoscopic laser bullectomy: a prospective study with three-month results. J Thorac Cardiovasc Surg 1996;112:319–27.

75. Holden DA, Rice TW, Stelmach K, Meeker DP. Exercise testing, 6-min walk, and stair climb in the evaluation of patients at high risk for pulmonary resection. Chest 1992;102:1774–9.

76. Kessler R, Faller M, Fourgaut G, Mennecier B, Weitzenbaum E. Predictive factors of hospitalization for acute exacerbation in a series of 64 patients with chronic obstructive pulmonary disease. Am J Respir Crit Care Med 1999;159:158–64.

77. Naunheim KS, Hazelrigg SR, Kaiser LR, Keenen RJ, Bavaria JE, Landreneau RJ, et al. Risk analysis for thoracoscopic lung volume reduction: a multi-institutional experience. Eur J Cardiothorac Surg 2000;17:673–9.

This measure can be found in reference 36.

WALK TEST (12-MINUTE) (12MWT)

Developers

C. R. McGavin, S. P. Gupta, and G. J. R. McHardy,[1] Department of Respiratory Diseases, University of Edinburgh, City Hospital, Edinburgh, Scotland (1976)

Purpose

Originally developed to assess exercise tolerance in individuals with chronic bronchitis.[1]

Description

The 12MWT is a performance-based test. Distance walked in 12 minutes is measured and reported in meters or feet. A greater distance indicates a better performance. The 12MWT was derived from Cooper's 12-minute run test for healthy individuals.[2]

Conceptual/Theoretical Basis of Construct Being Measured

None reported.

Groups Tested with This Measure

Individuals with chronic obstructive pulmonary disease (COPD)[1,3–15] and restrictive lung disease,[3] lung resection clients,[16] children with cystic fibrosis,[17] individuals post myocardial infarction,[18] and college students.[19] In addition, the 12MWT has also been used among individuals with pacemakers.[20,21]

Language

English.

Application/Administration

This test is ideally conducted in an enclosed quiet corridor. Patients are instructed to walk from end to end, covering as much ground as possible in 12 minutes. Patients are told that they may rest if they become too short of breath or tired to continue but to resume walking when they are able to do so. At the end of the 12 minutes, patients are told to stop. Distance walked, number of rests, and duration of rest in the 12 minutes are measured. Rating of perceived exertion, dyspnea, oxygen saturation, and heart rate can also be monitored. Encouragement should be standardized with respect to type and timing, and at least two practice walks should be administered before measurements are recorded.[22]

Typical Reliability Estimates

Internal Consistency
Not applicable

Interrater
Not available

Test–Retest
- Significant Increase in distance walked between trials 1 and 2 ($p < 0.001$),[1,3] trials 1 to 3 ($p < 0.05$),[4,11] and trials 1 to 4 ($p < 0.01$)[8] among individuals with respiratory diseases
- ICC: 0.98 for trials 3 and 4 among individuals with COPD[11]
- Coefficient of variation: 4.2% for trial 3 among individuals with COPD,[4] 3.1% with repeated testing on same day and 9.1% biweekly among individuals with COPD,[6] 9.0% for individuals with COPD tested on four occasions at 1-month intervals[15]

Other
Path used for test administration (ie, straight pathway, rectangle pathway, and oval pathway) significantly affects distance walked among healthy college students (ANOVA; $p < 0.05$)[19]

Typical Validity Estimates

Content
No reference to content validity in the literature.

Criterion

Concurrent
- VO_2: $r = 0.49$ to 0.52 among individuals with COPD[1,9]
- VO_2/kg: $r = 0.65$ among individuals with COPD[9]
- VCO_2: $r = 0.38$ among individuals with COPD[9]
- VCO_2/kg: $r = 0.53$ among individuals with COPD[9]
- V_E: $r = 0.53$ among individuals with COPD[1]
- Cycle ergometry performance: $r^2 = 0.51$ among individuals with COPD[8]
- Step ergometry performance: $r^2 = 0.52$ among individuals with COPD[8]
- Workload maximum (W_{max}): $r = 0.68$ among individuals with COPD[5]

Predictive. Not available

Construct—Cross-sectional

Convergent
- Spirometry and pulmonary diffusion capacity: conflicting results ranging from not significant and negligible correlations[1,4,6,8–10] to $r = 0.68$[1,3–6,9,11] in adults with respiratory disease
- 2-minute walk: $r = 0.87$ to 0.94 in adults with respiratory disease[7,9]
- 6-minute walk: $r = 0.96$ to 0.97 in adults with respiratory disease[7,9]
- Subjective ratings of exertion, breathlessness, and oxygen cost: $r = -0.32$ to 0.70 in adults with respiratory disease[1,6,11]
- Functional status questionnaire scores: $r = 0.52$ to 0.70 among individuals with COPD[6,13]
- Health-related quality of life scores: $r = 0.23$ to 0.45 among individuals with COPD[10–12]

Known Groups. Capable of distinguishing between children with cystic fibrosis on an active waiting list for heart-lung transplantation from those either not accepted or on a provisional waiting list ($p < 0.01$)[17]

Discriminant. Refer to conflicting results for convergent construct validity using spirometry.

Construct—Longitudinal/Sensitivity to Change

Convergent
- Change in VO_{2max}: $r = 0.72$ among individuals with COPD[9]
- Change in CO_{2max}: $r = 0.59$ among individuals with COPD[9]
- Change in subjective walking ability: $r = 0.90$ among individuals with COPD[6]
- Change in oxygen cost diagram: $r = 0.64$ among individuals with COPD[6]
- Change in pulmonary diffusion capacity: $r = 0.68$ among individuals with COPD[6]
- Change in depression and anxiety scale scores: $r = -0.51$ to 0.53 among individuals with COPD[14]

Known Groups. Capable of distinguishing change in those who received cardiac rehabilitation from those who received standard hospital care post myocardial infarction ($p < 0.001$)[18]

Discriminant
- Change in spirometry: not significant for individuals with COPD[6,14]
- Change in arterial blood gases: not significant for individuals with COPD[14]

Other Validity Coefficients
- Preoperative 12MWT distance unable to distinguish between patients who had postoperative complications and those without in lung resection patients ($p > 0.05$)[16]
- Post-rehabilitation distance walked < 750 m and > 750 m associated with 68% and 92% 3-year survival rates, respectively, among individuals with COPD[10]

Interpretability

General Population Values (Customary or Normative Values)
Not available. Refer to general population values for the Six-Minute Walk Test.

Typical Responsiveness Estimates

Individual Patient. Not available

Between Group. Not available. Refer to between-group responsiveness estimate for the Six-Minute Walk Test.

Comments

Since this test was developed to assess exercise tolerance, data to support criterion validity were assumed to be other measures of this construct, such as VO_{2max}. However, the data to support criterion validity may be different if the construct being measured is assumed to be something other than exercise tolerance.

References

1. **McGavin CR, Gupta SP, McHardy GJR. Twelve-Minute Walking Test for assessing disability in chronic bronchitis. BMJ 1976;1:822–3.**
2. Cooper KH. A means of assessing maximal oxygen intake: correlation between field and treadmill testing. JAMA 1968; 203:201–4.
3. McGavin R, Artvinli M, Naoe H, McHardy GJR. Dyspnoea, disability, and distance walked: comparison of estimates of exercise performance in respiratory disease. BMJ 1978;2:241–3.
4. Mungall IPF, Hainsworth R. Assessment of respiratory function in patients with chronic obstructive airways disease. Thorax 1979;34:254–8.
5. Alison JA, Anderson SD. Comparison of two methods of assessing physical performance in patients with chronic airway obstruction. Phys Ther 1981;61:1278–80.
6. O'Reilly JF, Shaylor JM, Fromings KM, Harrison BDW. The use of the 12 Minute Walking Test in assessing the effect of oral steroid therapy in patients with chronic airways obstruction. Br J Dis Chest 1982;76:374–82.
7. Butland RJA, Pang J, Gross ER, Woodcock AA, Geddes DM. Two-, six-, and 12-minute walking tests in respiratory disease. BMJ 1982;284:1607–8.

8. Swinburn CR, Wakefield JM, Jones PW. Performance, ventilation, and oxygen consumption in three different types of exercise test in patients with chronic obstructive pulmonary disease. Thorax 1985;40:581–6.

9. Bernstein ML, Despars JA, Singh NP, Avalos K, Stansbury DW, Light RW. Reanalysis of the 12-minute walk in patients with chronic obstructive pulmonary disease. Chest 1994;105:163–7.

10. Gerardi DA, Lovett L, Benoit-Connors ML, Reardon JZ, ZuWallack RL. Variables related to increased mortality following out-patient pulmonary rehabilitation. Eur Respir J 1996;9:431–5.

11. Larson JL, Covey MK, Vitalo CA, Alex CG, Patel M, Kim MJ. Reliability and validity of the 12-minute distance walk in patients with chronic obstructive pulmonary disease. Nurs Res 1996;45:203–10.

12. Ketelaars CAJ, Schlosser MAG, Mostert R, Abu-Saad HH, Halfens RJG, Wouters EFM. Determinants of health-related quality of life in patients with chronic obstructive pulmonary disease. Thorax 1996;51:39–43.

13. Leidy NK, Knebel AR. Clinical validation of the functional performance inventory in patients with chronic obstructive pulmonary disease. Respir Care 1999;44:932–9.

14. Light RW, Merrill EJ, Despars J, Gordon GH, Mutalipassi LR. Doxepin treatment of depressed patients with chronic obstructive pulmonary disease. Arch Intern Med 1986;146:1377–80.

15. Noseda A, Carpiaux J-P, Prigogine T, Schmerber J. Lung function, maximum and submaximum exercise testing in COPD patients: reproducibility over a long interval. Lung 1989;167:247–57.

16. Bagg LR. The 12-min walking distance; its use in the preoperative assessment of patients with bronchial carcinoma before lung resection. Respiration 1984;46:342–5.

17. Whitehead B, Helms P, Goodwin M, Martin I, Lask B, Serrano E, et al. Heart-lung transplantation for cystic fibrosis. 1: Assessment. Arch Dis Child 1991;66:1018–21.

18. Bertie J, King A, Reed N, Marshall AJ, Ricketts C. Benefits and weaknesses of a cardiac rehabilitation programme. J R Coll Physicians Lond 1992;26:147–51.

19. Siler WL, Koch NQ, Frese EM. The path utilized affects the distance walked in the 12 Minute Walk Test. Cardiopulm Phys Ther 1999;10:80–3.

20. Lau C-P, Wong C-K, Leung W-H, Cheng C-H, Lo C-H. A comparative evaluation of a minute ventilation sensing and activity sensing adaptive-rate pacemakers during daily activities. Pace 1989;12:1514–21.

21. Lau C-P, Wong C-K, Tai Y-T, Fong P-C, Li JP-S, Chung FL-W. Ventricular rate-adaptive pacing in the elderly. Eur Heart J 1992;13:908–13.

22. Solway S, Brooks D, Lacasse Y, Thomas S. A qualitative systematic overview of the measurement properties of functional walk tests used in the cardiorespiratory domain. Chest 2001;119:256–70.

This measure can be found in reference 1.

WALK TEST (SELF-PACED) (SPWT)

Developers

E. J. Bassey, P. H. Fentem, I. C. MacDonald, and P. M. Scriven,[1] Department of Physiology and Pharmacology, University Hospital and Medical School, Nottingham, United Kingdom (1976)

Purpose

Although the SPWT was originally developed as an alternative to laboratory methods to evaluate cardiovascular fitness in the elderly, it is also used to evaluate walking efficiency as related to functional performance.

Description

The SPWT is a performance-based test. Various exercise responses can be reported, but primary outcomes include speed of walking and heart rate. Faster walking speeds and lower heart rates indicate better performance.

Conceptual/Theoretical Basis of Construct Being Measured

None reported

Groups Tested with This Measure

Healthy adults,[1-4] elderly individuals,[3,5-7] cardiac clients,[8] and individuals following total knee arthroplasty (TKA).[9]

Language

English

Application/Administration

This test is ideally conducted in an enclosed quiet corridor. The protocol of Bassey et al[1] requires subjects to walk a specified distance (eg, two laps of 128 meters) at three different paces in response to standardized instructions to go "rather slowly," "at a normal pace, neither fast nor slow," and "rather fast, but without overexerting yourself." Time to complete each pace is recorded and used to calculate average speed of walking in meters per second or meters per minute for each pace. In addition, heart rate, rating of perceived exertion, stride/step frequency, and length can also be determined.[1,3,5,10] Oxygen consumption (VO_2) may also be extrapolated using aerobic demand curves, and VO_{2max}

may be estimated using the extrapolated VO_2 and heart rate.[10]

Typical Reliability Estimates

Internal Consistency
Not applicable

Interrater
Not available

Test–Retest
- Variation ±4.7% for normal pace, ±5.2% for fast pace, and +11% for slow pace in older men; no significant difference in younger men[1]
- $r \geq 0.81$ for each pace in men aged 55 to 66; paired t-test indicated no significant difference between tests[4]

Typical Validity Estimates

Content
The developers of the SPWT commented that the SPWT is appropriate as a functional test for an elderly or frail population because in addition to fitness level, walking efficiency also influences performance.[1]

Criterion

Concurrent
- VO_{2max}: $r = 0.25$ to 0.40 in adults at normal and fast paces when other explanatory variables are held constant[4]

Predictive. Not available

Construct—Cross-sectional

Convergent
- Standardized heart rate from bicycle test: $r = 0.79$ with standardized heart rate from SPWT[1]
- Lower Extremity Activity Profile (LEAP) total score: $r = -0.71$ for normal pace and $r = -0.69$ for fast pace in men post TKA; no significant correlation in women ($p > 0.5$) except for difficulty with function subscore: $r = -0.41$ for normal pace[9]
- WOMAC score: $r = -0.55$ for normal speed and $r = -0.54$ for fast speed in men post TKA; no significant correlations in TKA women[9]
- Balance Scale: $r = 0.73$; Functional Assessment Inventory: $r = -0.66$; Falls Efficacy Scale: $r = -0.63$ using modified SPWT in the elderly[6]

- Incapacity Index: $r = -0.56$; knee extensor strength: $r = 0.56$; lower extremity flexibility: $r = 0.42$ to 0.43; outdoor activity: $r = 0.69$ with normal pace in the elderly[5]
- Bruce Protocol Treadmill Time: $r^2 = 0.91$ with self-paced exercise time in patients with heart failure[8]

Known Groups

- Capable of discriminating among persons of different ages ($p < 0.005$)[1,3,4]
- Capable of discriminating elderly individuals with a history of falls from nonfallers ($F_{1,58} = 6.63$, $p = 0.013$)[6] and elderly individuals living independently in the community from those in nursing homes ($p < 0.008$)[5]
- Capable of discriminating individuals of different self-reported activity levels ($p < 0.005$)[2]
- Capable of discriminating cardiac patients with heart failure from those without ($p < 0.001$)[8]

Discriminant. Not available

Construct—Longitudinal/Sensitivity to Change
Not available

Interpretability

General Population Values
(Customary or Normative Values)

- Reference values available for males and females of different age groups (ie, 19 to 39, 40 to 62, and 63+ years) for walking speed, stride length, step frequency, and heart rate[3]
- Reference equations available (based on a non-random sample of healthy subjects aged 20 to 65 years) based on stature, sex, and age[2]

Typical Responsiveness Estimates
Not available

Comments

The results of this measure can be used to determine if a patient is safe for community ambulation. Calculated walking speed at various paces help to decipher if a client is able to walk quickly enough to cross an intersection controlled by traffic lights. Investigations that evaluated or used self-paced walking speed as an outcome were not included in this review; only studies that evaluated or used the SPWT or a specified modified version were included. There are no data to support this measure's ability to detect change in individuals or groups; therefore, it needs to be used as an outcome measure with caution until this measurement property has been tested.

References

1. Bassey EJ, Fentem PH, MacDonald IC, Scriven PM. **Self-paced walking as a method for exercise testing in elderly and young men. Clin Sci Mol Med 1976;51:609–12.**

2. Bassey EJ, MacDonald IA, Patrick JM. Factors affecting the heart rate during self-paced walking. Eur J Appl Physiol 1982;48:105–15.

3. Himann JE, Cunningham DA, Rechnitzer PA, Paterson DH. Age-related changes in speed of walking. Med Sci Sports Exerc 1988;20:161–6.

4. Cunningham DA, Rechnitzer PA, Pearce ME, Donner AP. Determinants of self-paced walking pace across ages 19-66. J Gerontol 1982;37:560–4.

5. Cunningham DA, Paterson DH, Himann JE, Rechnitzer PA. Determinants of independence in the elderly. Can J Appl Physiol 1993;18:243–54.

6. Piotrowski A, Cole J. Clinical measures of balance and functional assessment in elderly persons. Aust J Physiother 1994;40:183–8.

7. Connelly DM, Vandervoort AA. Improvement in knee extensor strength of institutionalized elderly women after exercise with ankle weights. Physiother Can 1995;47:15–23.

8. Ajayi AA, Balogun JA. Symptom-limited, self-paced walking in the assessment of cardiovascular disease in patients with and without heart failure: the predictive value of clinical, anthropometric, echocardiographic and ergonometric parameters. Int J Cardiol 1991;33:233–40.

9. Finch E, Walsh M, Thomas SG, Woodhouse LJ. Functional ability perceived by individuals following total knee arthroplasty compared to age-matched individuals without knee disability. J Orthoped Sports Phys Ther 1998;27:255–63.

10. Noonan V, Dean E. Submaximal exercise testing: clinical application and interpretation. Phys Ther 2000;80:782–807.

This measure can be found in reference 1.

WALK TEST (SHUTTLE) (SWT)

Developers

S. J. Singh, M. D. Morgan, S. Scott, D. Walters, and A. E. Hardman,[1] Department of Respiratory Medicine, Glenfield General Hospital, Leicester, England

Purpose

To assess functional capacity.

Description

The Shuttle Walk Test (SWT) is a 12-level, performance-based, externally paced, progressive intensity field exercise test. The distance walked is reported in meters. A greater distance indicates a better performance. The test was developed from a shuttle running test designed for testing healthy individuals.[2]

Conceptual/Theoretical Basis of Construct Being Measured

None reported.

Groups Tested with This Measure

The SWT has been validated in individuals with chronic airflow obstruction,[3-5] chronic heart failure,[6,7] cardiac disease (myocardial infarction, post coronary artery bypass graft),[8] and rheumatoid arthritis[8] and people awaiting heart transplantation.[9] It has also been used in clients with pacemakers,[10] those undergoing cardiac rehabilitation,[11] and clients with intermittent claudication,[12] advanced cancer,[13] chronic respiratory failure,[14] and fibromyalgia.[15] A modified version (15 levels instead of 12) has been used and validated in adults with cystic fibrosis.[16,17]

Languages

English and Spanish[18]

Application/Administration

Standard instructions for the test are provided on an audiocassette tape. The test requires a quiet corridor or treatment area at least 12 meters in length. Subjects are required to walk to and fro, turning around two cones placed 9 meters apart (shuttle distance = 10 meters), while keeping pace with a prerecorded auditory signal such that they complete a turn as each bleep sounds. Every minute, the audio signal sounds at increasingly shorter intervals. Each shuttle is indicated by a single bleep on the tape, whereas speed increases every minute are indicated with a triple bleep. Walking speed increases from 0.50 m/s at level 1 to 2.37 m/s at level 12. Distance walked is recorded in meters (number of shuttles completed × 10 m/shuttle). No encouragement is provided. The test is terminated when the subject chooses to stop or fails to keep up to the auditory signal after one warning. Attainment of 85% of age-predicted maximal heart rate or oxygen desaturation below a preset limit may also be used as an end point in appropriate subject groups. One practice test is required before a stable estimate is obtained in people with chronic obstructive pulmonary disease (COPD),[1] heart failure,[7] and advanced cancer[13] and those being assessed for heart transplant.[9] No practice test is required in people with pacemakers,[10] chronic respiratory failure owing to thoracic restriction,[14] fibromyalgia,[15] COPD,[18] or cystic fibrosis.[17]

Typical Reliability Estimates

Internal Consistency
Not applicable

Interrater
Not applicable (test is controlled by audiotape)

Test–Retest
- ICC: 0.80[15]
- Bradley et al[17]: SWT 1 (754 m) versus SWT 2 (754 m) (paired t) $p = 0.98$, Pearson's $r = 0.99$, $p < 0.01$)
- Singh et al[1]: SWT 2 (376 m) versus SWT 3 (378 m) (paired t = nonsignificant, $p > 0.05$), Pearson's $r = 0.98$
- Morales et al[7]: SWT 2 (378 m) versus SWT 3 (485 m) (paired t = nonsignificant, $p = 0.33$), Pearson's $r = 0.99$

Typical Validity Estimates

Content
The rationale for this test is that an externally paced, progressive intensity field test eliminates the variable effects of motivation and encouragement seen in self-paced tests and thus more closely approximates the test protocols used in the gold standard laboratory measures of exercise capacity (VO$_{2max}$) than do the standard walk tests.[1,3]

Criterion

Concurrent. VO_{2max}
- $r = 0.70$ to 0.88 in people with COPD[3,4]
- $r = 0.84$ in people with heart failure[6]
- $r = 0.83$ in people with heart failure[7]
- $r = 0.73$ for people being assessed for heart transplant[9]
- $r = 0.95$ for adults with cystic fibrosis (modified shuttle test)[16]

Extrapolated VO_{2max}
- $r = 0.31$ in people with rheumatoid arthritis[8]
- $r = 0.03$ in people after myocardial infarction or coronary bypass graft surgery[8]

Predictive. Not available

Construct—Cross-sectional

Convergent
- 6-Minute Walk Test: $r = 0.68$ in COPD[1]
- Chronic Respiratory Disease Questionnaire (CRQ) (fatigue domain): rho $= 0.68$ in respiratory disability[19]
- CRQ (fatigue domain): $r = 0.23$ in COPD[20]
- LCADL: $r = -0.58$ in severe COPD[21]
- St. George's Respiratory Questionnaire (SGRQ) (activity): rho $= -0.62$ in α_1-antitrypsin deficiency[5]
- SGRQ (activity): $r = -0.35$ in COPD[20]
- 36-Item Short-Form Health Survey (physical functioning): rho $= 0.53$ in COPD[5]
- Treadmill endurance test: $r = 0.73$ in COPD[20]

Known Groups
- Greater distance walked on supplemental oxygen than on room air in COPD ($p < 0.001$)[22]

Discriminant. FEV_1: $r = 0.36$ to 0.65 in people with chronic airflow limitation[3] or with α_1-antitrypsin deficiency[5]

Construct—Longitudinal/Sensitivity to Change

Convergent
- Change in treadmill endurance test: $r = 0.29$ in COPD[20]
- Change in CRQ fatigue domain: $r = 0.23$ in COPD[20]

Known Groups. Not available

Discriminant
- Better correlation with change in treadmill endurance test ($r = 0.29$, $p < 0.01$) than either change in CRQ emotional function ($r = 0.13$, NS), CRQ total ($r = 0.16$, NS), or SGRQ total ($r = -0.07$, NS) in people with COPD[20]

Interpretability

General Population Values (Customary or Normative Values)
Not available

Typical Responsiveness Estimates
Not available

Comments

Although this measure was originally developed to measure exercise tolerance, other constructs were also thought to be reflected (eg, functional capacity or performance, walking ability, lower extremity function). The data to support criterion validity would depend on the construct being measured.

References

1. **Singh SJ, Morgan MDL, Scott S, Walters D, Hardman AE. Development of a shuttle walking test of disability in patients with chronic airways obstruction. Thorax 1992;47:1019–24.**
2. **Leger LA, Lambert J. A maximal multistage 20m shuttle run test to predict VO_{2max}. Eur J Appl Physiol 1982;49:1–12.**
3. Singh SJ, Morgan MDL, Hardman AE, Rowe E, Bardsley PA. Comparison of oxygen uptake during a conventional treadmill test and the Shuttle Walking Test in chronic airflow limitation. Eur Respir J 1994;7:2106–2020.
4. Forte S, Carlone S, Onorati P, DeRocco G, Serra P, Palange P. Shuttle Test vs 6 Minute Walking Test in the evaluation of exercise tolerance in COPD patients. Eur Respir J 1997;10:170S.
5. Dowson LJ, Newall C, Guest PJ, Hill SL, Stockley RA. Exercise capacity predicts health status in α_1-antitrypsin deficiency. Am J Respir Crit Care Med 2001;163:936–41.
6. Keell SD, Chambers JS, Francis DP, Edwards DF, Stables RH. Shuttle walk test to assess chronic heart failure. Lancet 1998; 352:705.
7. Morales FJ, Martinez A, Mendez M, Agarrado A, Ortega F, Fernandez-Guerra J, et al. A shuttle walk test for assessment of functional capacity in chronic heart failure. Am Heart J 1999; 138:291–8.
8. MacSween A, Johnson NJ, Armstrong C, Bonn J. A validation of the 10-meter incremental shuttle walk test as a measure of aerobic power in cardiac and rheumatoid arthritis patients. Arch Phys Med Rehabil 2001;82:807–10.
9. Lewis ME, Newall C, Townend JN, Hill SL, Bonser RS. Incremental shuttle walk test in the assessment of patients for heart transplantation. Heart 2001;86:183–7.
10. Payne GE, Skehan JD. Shuttle walking test: a new approach for evaluating the patient with pacemakers. Heart 1996;75:414–18.
11. Tobin D, Thow MK. The 10m Shuttle Walk Test with Holter Monitoring: an objective outcome measure for cardiac rehabilitation. Coronary Health Care 1999;3:3–17.
12. Walker RD, Nawaz S, Wilkinson CH, Saxton JM, Pockley AG, Wood RF. Influence of upper- and lower-limb exercise training on cardiovascular function and walking distances in patients with intermittent claudication. J Vasc Surg 2000;31:662–9.
13. Booth S, Adams L. The Shuttle Walking Test: a reproducible method for evaluating the impact of shortness of breath on functional capacity in patients with advanced cancer. Thorax 2001; 56:146–50.

14. Schonhofer B, Wallstein S, Wiese C, Kohler D. Noninvasive mechanical ventilation improves endurance performance in patients with chronic respiratory failure due to thoracic restriction. Chest 2001;19:1371–8.

15. Pankoff BA, Hobby KJ, Lucy SD, Overend TJ. Reliability and reproducibility of the Shuttle Walk Test in people with fibromyalgia. Arthritis Rheum 2001;44:S389.

16. Bradley J, Howard J, Wallace E, Elborn S. Validity of a modified shuttle walk test in adult cystic fibrosis. Thorax 2001;54:437–9.

17. Bradley J, Howard J, Wallace E, Elborn S. Reliability, repeatability, and sensitivity of the modified shuttle test in adult cystic fibrosis. Chest 2000;117:1666–71.

18. Elias MT, Fernandez J, Toral J, et al. Reproducibilidad de un test de paseo de carga progressiva (Shuttle Walking Test) en pacientes con enfermedad pulmonary obstructive cronica. Arch Bronconeumol 1997;33:64–8.

19. Singh SJ, Smith DL, Hyland ME, Morgan MDL. A short outpatient pulmonary rehabilitation programme: immediate and longer term effects on exercise performance and quality of life. Respir Med 1998;92:1146–54.

20. Singh SJ, Sodergren SC, Hyland ME, Williams J, Morgan MDL. A comparison of three disease-specific and two generic health-status measures to evaluate the outcome of pulmonary rehabilitation in COPD. Respir Med 2001;95:71–7.

21. Garrod R, Bestall JC, Paul EA, Wedzicha JA, Jones PW. Development and validation of a standardized measure of activity of daily living in patients with severe COPD: the London Chest Activity of Daily Living Scale (LCADL). Respir Med 2000;94: 689–96.

22. Garrod R, Paul EA, Wedzicha JA. Supplemental oxygen during pulmonary rehabilitation in patients with COPD with exercise hypoxaemia. Thorax 2000;55:539–43.

This measure can be found in references 1 and 2. To obtain the audiotape and instructions (cost is CD$80), contact the developers.

WASCANA CLIENT-CENTERED CARE SURVEY-R (WCCS-R)

Developers

Gordon J. G. Asmundson and Sylvia Jones,[1,2] Regina Health District, Regina, Saskatchewan

Purpose

To evaluate the multidimensional concept of client-centered care. The survey can be used to identify areas for quality improvement and can be administered over time to evaluate change within a specific service area.

Description

The WCCS-R is a generic mail-out survey. The original scale was 20 items representing four subscales.[1] This was expanded to 40 items and six subscales (WCCS-II). The scoring of the WCCS-II has been revised again as a result of a factor analysis. The WCCS-R now includes four subscales—client needs and family involvement (7 items), client understanding and participation in care (11 items), physical comfort and emotional support (5 items), and transition/community integration (5 items)—and 12 additional questions, which are examined as individual items only. Items are scored on a 5-point scale with anchors 1 (strongly agree), 3 (hard to decide), and 5 (strongly disagree). Three additional questions allow for qualitative responses about what the service area should "start doing," "stop doing," and "continue to do." Analysis can be done on individual items or subscales. Lower scores reflect a higher rating of client-centered care. It is recommended that a score of greater than 2 be used as an indicator for quality improvement initiatives.

Conceptual/Theoretical Basis of Construct Being Measured

The authors define client-centered care as an approach to care focused on the service providers' incorporation of client-perceived needs, priorities, or expectations into the provision of health care services. The authors state that it is important to examine service delivery from the point of view of those who receive the service and that client-centered care is likely related to but not the same as client satisfaction.[1]

Groups Tested with This Measure

Adult rehabilitation clients with neurologic conditions. With minor changes to the wording, the WCCS-II has been used in a variety of settings and patient populations: medical convalescence, respiratory medicine, renal dialysis, cardiac care, neuroscience, oncology, maternal/newborn, pediatrics, children's rehabilitation, adolescent treatment units, anesthetic care, and community care.[2] The WCCS-II has also been used with clients with rheumatoid arthritis (RA)[3] and lower extremity musculoskeletal conditions who received physiotherapy.[4]

Language

English[2]

Application/Administration

It should be administered by mail 3 to 6 months following the primary period of service delivery. The WCCS-R is a self-report measure; however, family members, friends, or health care providers can also complete it on behalf of the client. Respondents are asked to indicate on the front page how the survey was completed. The item scores are totaled for each subscale and divided by the number of items in the subscale. It requires 10 to 20 minutes to complete. Clients with reading disabilities or poor eyesight may take longer than average. Grade 6 literacy is assumed. No training is needed, but the authors offer an educational session entitled "Understanding and Measuring the Dimensions of Client-Centered Care" to help potential users identify if this survey will meet their needs. A user's manual is available.[2] If a question does not apply, the clients are asked to leave it blank. If clients answer less than 75% of the items, their score is not used in the analysis. When 75% or more of the items are answered, the mean of the item is used to replace the missing value.

Typical Reliability Estimates

Internal Consistency
For the Subscales of the Original WCCS[1]
- Information/understanding: Cronbach's alpha = 0.88

- Community integration: Cronbach's alpha = 0.76
- Respect: Cronbach's alpha = 0.83
- Involvement: Cronbach's alpha = 0.86

For the WCCS-R[2]
- Understanding: Cronbach's alpha = 0.88
- Transition/integration: Cronbach's alpha = 0.85
- Consideration of needs: Cronbach's alpha = 0.92
- Physical/emotional support: Cronbach's alpha = 0.86

Interrater
Not applicable

Test–Retest
Not available

Typical Validity Estimates

Content
Developed through discussions with health care providers and clients with neurologic conditions or injury in an adult rehabilitation setting and further refined to ensure that the measure tapped aspects in the literature that clients reported as important to their care.[1,2]

Criterion
No gold standard available for the construct being measured.

Construct—Cross-sectional

Convergent
- WCCS-II domain score for community integration and years since onset of RA symptoms: $r = 0.48$[3]
- WCCS-II domain score for community involvement and years since onset of RA symptoms: $r = 0.46$[3]
- Domains for community integration, information, and involvement in care and self-efficacy scores: $r = -0.34, -0.42, -0.03$, respectively
- Respect domain and change in health perception: $r = -0.38$
- Community integration domain and change in knowledge: $r = -0.06$

Known Groups. Clients with lower extremity functional conditions who completed their physical therapy (PT) intervention reported significantly higher mean scores for the WCCS-II involvement in care domain than those who did not complete the PT intervention.[4]

Discriminant. In patients with lower extremity musculoskeletal conditions, there were no correlations between WCCS-II domain scores and therapist years of practice or chronicity of disease.[4] Domain scores did not correlate with the intensity of the PT intervention ($r = 0.01$ to 0.18) or with the characteristics of the therapist's practice ($r = 0.01$ to 0.37).[3] In clients with lower extremity musculoskeletal conditions, there was a correlation between the WCCS-II physical domain and improvements in pain scores ($r = 0.13$) and between the information, involvement, respect, and physical domains and improvement in lower extremity function ($r = -0.12$ to -0.16).[4]

Construct—Longitudinal/Sensitivity to Change
Not available

Interpretability

General Population Values (Customary or Normative Values)
Not available

Typical Responsiveness Estimates
Not available

Comment
There are no data to support this measure's ability to detect change in service provision over time; therefore, it needs to be used as an outcome measure with caution until sensitivity to change and responsiveness have been tested.

References

1. Asmundson GJG, Jones S. The Wascana Client-Centered Care Survey: development and psychometric evaluation. Can J Qual Health Care 1996;13:19–21.
2. Asmundson GJG, Jones S. Wascana Client-Centered Care Survey-R: draft user's manual. Regina (SK): Regina Health District; 2001.
3. Asmundson G, Hedley P, Wilkins A, et al. A pilot project to study a new model for physiotherapy practice review, using rheumatoid arthritis as a model. Toronto (ON): College of Physiotherapists of Ontario; 1998.
4. Lineker SC, Wilkins A. Practice review of the physiotherapy management of lower extremity musculoskeletal diseases. Toronto (ON): College of Physiotherapists of Ontario; 2000.

To obtain this measure, contact the developers.

WeeFIM® (Functional Independence Measure for Children)

Developers

Original development team included Carl Granger, Susan Braun, Kim Griswold, Margaret McCabe, Nancy Heyer, Michael Msall, and Byron Hamilton.[1,2] More recent contributions made by Linda Duffy, Kenneth Ottenbacher, Michelle Audet, Roger Fiedler, and Felicia Wilczenski.

Centre for Functional Assessment Research, Uniform Data System for Medical Rehabilitation, 232 Parker Hall, State University of New York South Campus, 3435 Main Street, Buffalo, New York 14214-3007.

Purpose

To measure the severity of disability and changes in functional abilities of children over time and over rehabilitation settings. The developers also state a further purpose: "to weigh the burden of care in terms of physical, technological, and financial resources." The measure was developed for children between the ages of 6 months and 8 years with neurodevelopmental disabilities.

Description

The WeeFIM is an 18-item observational instrument modeled on the adult Functional Independence Measure (FIM). Items sample six domains—self-care, sphincter control, mobility, locomotion, communication, and social cognition—and are organized into two scales: the Motor Scale and the Cognitive Scale. Using a seven-level ordinal scale, individual items are scored based on the amount of assistance required to complete the item tasks. Item scores range from 1 to 7 and total scores from 18 to 126, with highest scores representing the greatest level of functional independence.

Conceptual/Theoretical Basis of Construct Being Measured

Test developers do not specifically define functional independence but specify that the International Classification of Impairment, Disability, and Handicap (ICIDH) and the National Centre for Medical Rehabilitation Research (NCMRR) adaptation of the ICIDH classification system provided the conceptual basis for test development. The WeeFIM is intended to measure function at the level of "disability" in the ICIDH framework and "functional limitations" in the NCMRR framework. "Burden of care" is defined as the type and amount of assistance required by a person to perform daily activities and is thought to be associated with the consumption of social and economic resources.[2,3]

Groups Tested with This Measure

Validated on typically developing children and for children with a range of developmental disabilities.[3,4] In addition, the measure has been used with 5-year-old children with retinopathy of prematurity,[5] children with genetic conditions,[6] and survivors of extremely preterm birth at kindergarten entry.[7]

Language

English

Application/Administration

Administration is by direct observation or by interview of a primary caregiver and is fully described in the WeeFIM guide.[1] The test takes approximately 20 minutes and can be administered by any clinician trained in its use. Missing scores are not allowed. A computer is not required to score the data; however, software is available (WeeFIMware™) to graphically depict the item and domain scores. Training required to use the measure includes review of videotapes, study of the test manual, or attendance at workshops provided by Uniform Data Systems.

Typical Reliability Estimates

Internal Consistency
Cronbach's alpha = 0.90[7]

Interrater
For typically developing children, Pearson's $r = 0.95$ for total WeeFIM scores and a range of 0.74 to 0.96 for domain scores.[8] For children with disabilities, ICC for short delay between tests ranged from 0.82 to 0.94 for items and was 0.97 for total scores.[9] In the long delay condition, ICC for items ranged from 0.73 to 0.90 and was 0.94 for total scores.

Test–Retest

ICC for total scores was 0.98 for children without disabilities and 0.97 for children with disabilities.[9] Item ICCs ranged from 0.90 to 0.99 and subscales from 0.96 to 0.99.

Other

Equivalence reliability of telephone interview administration compared with in-person interview (using the same sample as the test–retest reliability study) was ICC of 0.98 for children without disabilities and 0.97 for children with disabilities.[10] Equivalence reliability of parent interview and direct observation methods of administration (n = 30 children with developmental disabilities) for total WeeFIM scores, ICC = 0.93; for the Cognitive Scale, ICC = 0.75; and for the Motor Scale, ICC = 0.93.[11]

Typical Validity Estimates

Content

A three-phase content validity process is reported.[12] In phase one, four or more experts (of an eight-expert interdisciplinary panel) agreed on placement of items in domains. In the second phase, a content validity index of 0.80 was obtained (CVI calculation reported as method described by Lynn, 1986). In the third phase, none of the subdomains were judged "conceptually adequate" when using the Lynn method of determination. The developers reported that this finding may have been attributable to expert panel members having difficulty with the concept of a minimal data set.

Criterion

No gold standard exists for functional independence in children.

Construct—Cross-sectional

Convergent. Spearman's correlation coefficient between WeeFIM and the Batelle Developmental Screening Test (BDST) total score was 0.92 and between the WeeFIM and the Vineland Adaptive Behavior Scales (VABS) was 0.89. Correlations of WeeFIM total scores with BDST subscales ranged from 0.83 to 0.94 and with the VABS from 0.72 to 0.91.[4] Spearman's correlation coefficient of WeeFIM total score with parents'/teachers' rating on the Amount of Assistance Questionnaire in children with disabilities was 0.91.[13] Time costs of caring for children with severe disabilities correlated ($r = 0.89$) with WeeFIM scores.[14]

Known Groups. WeeFIM distinguished between groups of children with disabilities (n = 30) and children without disabilities (n = 37). Scores of children with moderate to severe impairments fell more than 1 SD below their peers.[8] Rasch analysis also showed scores of children with disability falling below peers without disability and that children with disability were stratified by the severity of motor involvement.[15]

Discriminant. Not available

Construct—Longitudinal/Sensitivity to Change

Not available

Other Validity Coefficients

Correlations of WeeFIM item scores with age in children without disabilities ranged from 0.49 to 0.83.[2]

Sensitivity to change was demonstrated in a 1-year longitudinal study of children with developmental disabilities receiving special services.[16] Four change estimates were reported. The reliability change estimates for the six domains, the two subscales, and the total score were all greater than 2.0 except for the mobility (transfer) domain. The Proportional Change Index for all mean scores was greater than 1.0. The effect size (d index) values ranged from 0.31 to 0.81. P values generated by paired t-tests were all statistically significant at the $p < 0.001$ alpha level.

Interpretability

General Population Values (Customary or Normative Values)

Norms for the WeeFIM are contained in the WeeFIM Guide for children from 6 months to 7 years for each 4-month interval. Norms were calculated using a normative sample (n = 417) of children without developmental delays or in developmental programs.[17]

Typical Responsiveness Estimates

Not available

Comments

An additional recent systematic review of the WeeFIM is available.[18]

References

1. WeeFIM system clinical guide. Buffalo (NY): University at Buffalo; 1993, 1998, 2000.
2. Braun S, Granger, C. A practical approach to assessment in pediatrics. Occup Ther Pract 1991;2:46–51.
3. Msall M, DiGaudio, K, Rogers B, LaForest S, Catanzaro NL, Campbell J, et al. The Functional Independence Measure for Children (WeeFIM): conceptual basis and pilot use in children with developmental disabilities. Clin Pediatr 1994;33:421–30.

4. Ottenbacher K, Msall M, Lyon N, Duffy L, Granger C, Braun S. Measuring developmental and functional status in children with disabilities. Dev Med Child Neurol 1999;41:186–94.

5. Msall M. Severity of neonatal retinopathy of prematurity is predictive of neurodevelopmental functional outcome at age 5.5 years. Pediatrics 2000;106:998–1005.

6. Msall M, Tremont M. Measuring functional status in children with genetic impairments. Am J Med Genet 1999;89:67–74.

7. Msall M, Rogers B, Buck G, Mallen S, Catanzaro N, Duffy L. Functional status of extremely preterm infants at kindergarten entry. Dev Med Child Neurol 1993;35:312–20.

8. Msall M, DiGaudio K, Duffy L. Use of functional assessment in children with developmental disabilities. Phys Med Rehabil Clin North Am 1993;4:517–27.

9. Ottenbacher K, Msall M, Lyon N, Duffy L, Granger C, Braun S. Interrater agreement and stability of the functional independence measure for children (WeeFIM): use in children with developmental disabilities. Arch Phys Med Rehabil 1997;78:1309–15.

10. Ottenbacher K, Taylor ET, Msall M, Braun S, Lane SJ, Granger CV, et al. The stability and equivalence reliability of the Functional Independence Measure for Children (WeeFIM). Dev Med Child Neurol 1996;38:907–16.

11. Sperle P, Ottenbacher K, Braun S, Lane S, Nochajski S. Equivalence reliability of the functional independence measure for children (WeeFIM) administration methods. Am J Occup Ther 1997;51:35–41.

12. McCabe M, Granger C. Content validity of a pediatric functional independence measure. Appl Nurs Res 1990;3:120–2.

13. Ottenbacher K, Msall M, Lyon N, Duffy LC, Ziviani J, Granger CV, et al. Functional assessment and care of children with neurodevelopmental disabilities. Am J Phys Med Rehabil 2000;79:114–23.

14. Curran A, Sharples P, White C, Knapp M. Time costs of caring for children with severe disabilities compared with children without disabilities. Dev Med Child Neurol 2001;43:529–533.

15. McCabe M. Pediatric Functional Independence Measure: clinical trials with disabled and non-disabled children. Appl Nurs Res 1996;9:136–8.

16. Ottenbacher K, Msall M, Lyon N, Duffy LC, Ziviani J, Granger CV, et al. The WeeFIM instrument: its utility in detecting change in children with developmental disabilities. Arch Phys Med Rehabil 2000;81:1317–26.

17. Msall M, DiGaudio K, Duffy L, Laforest S, Braun S, Granger C. WeeFIM: normative sample of an instrument for tracking functional independence in children. Clin Pediatr 1994;33:431–8.

18. Law M, Baum C, Dunn W. Measuring occupational performance: supporting best practice in occupational therapy. Thorofare (NJ): Slack; 2001. p. 138–9.

This measure or ordering information can be found at www.udsmr.org (FIM Website).

WOMAC™ (WESTERN ONTARIO McMASTER OSTEOARTHRITIS INDEX)

Developer

Nicholas Bellamy, Centre of National Research on Disability and Rehabilitation (CONROD), Department of Medicine, C Floor, Clinical Sciences Building, Royal Brisbane Hospital, Herston Road, Brisbane, Queensland 4029, Australia; nbellamy@medicine.uq.edu.au, www.clinimetrics.net.

Purpose

To assess pain, stiffness, and disability in individuals with osteoarthritis (OA) of the hip or knee.[1] The WOMAC™ was initially developed for evaluative research in OA clinical drug trials; it is now used in diverse clinical environments.

Description

The WOMAC is a multidimensional, disease-specific, self-administered health status instrument.[1] Originally, WOMAC items were generated from a structured interview that included both open- and close-ended questions, applied to 100 clients with primary OA of the hip and knee.[2] The WOMAC has three subscales: Pain, Stiffness, and Physical Function. The WOMAC is available in both a 5-point Likert (LK3.1) and 100-mm visual analogue scale format (VAS3.1). The VAS uses terminal descriptors ranging from no difficulty, pain, or stiffness to extreme difficulty, pain, or stiffness. The Likert uses the adjectives none, mild, moderate, severe, and extreme. Summary scores vary according to the version used, with low scores indicating better outcome. In addition, there is also the VA3.0S and LK3.0S, where S represents a signal measurement strategy in which patients identify one item of importance in all three domains. The three items selected then represent the principal focus of subsequent measurement.[3]

Conceptual/Theoretical Basis of Construct Being Measured

None reported.

Groups Tested with This Measure

Hip and knee OA and arthroplasty populations. It has also been used but not validated with clients with fibromyalgia and rheumatoid arthritis.[4]

Languages

Available in 57 languages; however, not all of these have been validated.

Application/Administration

Each questionnaire has an accompanying instruction sheet. Respondents are asked to think about their status over the past 48 hours; however, it can range from 2 to 14 days depending on the need of the study.[5] The time of day that the questionnaire is administered should be kept constant as there is evidence to suggest rhythmic variation in pain on both a daily and a weekly basis.[6] The questionnaire takes 5 to 15 minutes to complete and 5 to 10 minutes to score. Aggregate scores for each dimension are determined by summing the component items for each dimension. Individual subscale scores and a total WOMAC score can be determined by summing each of the dimensions; scores will vary according to the version used.[1] WOMAC scores can be transformed to a 0 to 100 scale to facilitate comparisons with other outcome measures.[5,7]

Typical Reliability Estimates

Internal Consistency

Across various linguistic versions and surgical interventions, the reliability estimates for pain, stiffness, and physical function range from 0.73 to 0.96.[1,8]

Interrater

Not applicable

Test–Retest

Summary values in various studies using OA populations are found in Table 1.[8] Authors acknowledge that scores were somewhat low owing to the varying nature of the disease and time interval between measurements.[1]

TABLE 1

Trial	Global Rating L	Global Rating V	Pain L	Pain V	Stiffness L	Stiffness V	Physical Function L	Physical Function V	Version (L or V) Not Indicated
Drug			0.68	0.64	0.48	0.61	0.68	0.72	
Arthroscopy			0.74		0.58		0.92		✓
German	0.77	0.83	0.79/0.90*		0.43/0.72*		0.93/0.71*		
Swedish			0.88		0.76		0.91		✓
EuroQol			0.65		Not reported		0.80		✓

*Values were cited for clients with hip and knee osteoarthritis.

L = Likert scale; V = visual analogue scale.

Typical Validity Estimates

Content
Items were generated from a structured interview with 100 individuals with primary OA of the hip and knee. The first version of the WOMAC had five subscales: Pain, Stiffness, Physical Function, Social Function, and Emotional Function. Social and Emotional Function were excluded with further testing as they were not as responsive as the Pain, Stiffness, and Physical Function scales.[2,9]

Criterion
No gold standard is available.[1]

Construct—Cross-sectional

Convergent. Construct validity was tested against other indices (Lequesne, Doyle, McMaster Health Index Questionnaire [MHIQ], and the Bradburn Index of Well Being). Index items probing similar constructs in these questionnaires revealed that pain and difficulty often correlated well with one another. Pearson's correlation coefficients for pain, stiffness, and difficulty ranged from 0.20 to 0.62.[1] In a total knee population, Spearman's rank correlation coefficients between the WOMAC's physical functioning dimension and the Health Assessment Questionnaire (HAQ) and the 36-Item Short-Form Health Survey (SF-36) were 0.68 and 0.70, respectively.[10] Other studies evaluating convergent validity with the SF-36 show correlations of 0.75.[11]

Known Groups. WOMAC was able to differentiate between individuals who were satisfied with their TKA compared with those who were not satisfied.[8]

Discriminant. Correlations with unrelated dimensions in the SF-36, Doyle, and MHIQ were found to be low.[1,10]

Construct—Longitudinal/Sensitivity to Change Estimates
Not available

Other Validity Coefficients
Relative efficiency (RE) is a measure of the comparative responsiveness of different measures. When the WOMAC was compared to the Lequesne Knee Index and Doyle Articular Index in the OA population, the RE was similar.[11] Values > 1 indicated that the measure in the numerator was more responsive. When comparing signal measurement of the WOMAC and aggregate scores of the WOMAC, the RE for signal measurement was reported to range from 1.39 to 2.52 for parametric analysis and 1.15 to 1.91 for nonparametric analysis.[3]

Interpretability

General Population Values (Customary or Normative Values)
Not available

Typical Responsiveness Estimates
See Table 2.

Individual Patient. Minimal perceptible clinical improvement was found to be 9.7 mm, 9.3 mm, and 10.0 mm for the Pain, Physical Function, and Stiffness subscales on the WOMAC VA3.1 100-mm normalized VAS.[12]

TABLE 2 Effect Sizes, Standard Response Means, and Mean Change Scores[8]

Intervention or Group	Pain			Stiffness			Physical Function			Global		
	ES	SRM	MCS	ES	SRM	MCS	ES	SRM	MCS	ES	SRM	MCS
THA	1.7–2.6	0.96–1.7	4.4–8.5	1.0–2.2	0.96–1.7	2.4–4.5	1.8–2.9	0.96–1.7	4.8–30.8		2.4	
TKA	0.95–41.0	0.63–1.99	0.8–8.2	0.88–24.0	0.63–1.99	0.7–6.62	1.01–23.9	0.63–1.99	0.8–23.9		2.0	
Drug Intervention*	0.22–0.97	0.08–1.09	0.8–16.49	0.07–.84	0.08–1.09	0.25–8.57	0.17–.82	0.08–1.09	2.96–11.96	0.2–.87		3.3–13.6
Hip/knee patients	0.14–1.5	0.29–1.18	5.3–16.2	0.14–1.5	4.3–21.7	5.3–16.2	0.14–1.5	5.2–13.6	5.3–16.2		5.5–16	
Miscellaneous†	NR		0.14–5.43	0.04–1.3		2.88–3.37	0.0009–1.19		0.01–17.78	0.06–1.2		0.76–20.6

ES = effect size; SRM = standard response mean; MCS = mean change response; NR = not reported.

*Includes both control and treatment groups.

†Miscellaneous includes exercise, manual and physical therapy, acupuncture, and knee braces.

Between Group. Not available

Comments

Using Rasch analysis, recent research identified that it may be possible to reduce the WOMAC, as there appears to be redundancy between the Pain and Function subscales.[13]

References

1. Bellamy N, Buchanan WW, Goldsmith CH, Campbell J, Stitt LW. Validation study of WOMAC: a health status instrument for measuring clinically important patient relevant outcomes to antirheumatic drug therapy in patients with osteoarthritis of the hip or knee. J Rheumatol 1988;15:1833–40.

2. Bellamy N, Buchanan WW. A preliminary evaluation of the dimensionality and clinical importance of pain and disability in osteoarthritis of the hip and knee. Clin Rheumatol 1986;5:231–41.

3. Barr S, Bellamy N, Buchanan WW, Chalmers A, Ford PM, Kean WF, et al. A comparative study of signal versus aggregate methods of outcome measurement based on the WOMAC Osteoarthritis Index. Western Ontario and McMaster Universities Osteoarthritis Index. J Rheumatol 1994;21:2106–12.

4. Wolfe F, Kong SX. Rasch analysis of the Western Ontario MacMaster questionnaire (WOMAC) in 2205 patients with osteoarthritis, rheumatoid arthritis, and fibromyalgia. Ann Rheum Dis 1999;58:563–8.

5. Davies GM, Watson DJ, Bellamy N. Comparison of the responsiveness and relative effect size of the Western Ontario and McMaster Universities Osteoarthritis Index and the short-form Medical Outcomes Study Survey in a randomized, clinical trial of osteoarthritis patients. Arthritis Care Res 1999;12:172–9.

6. Bellamy N, Sothern RB, Campbell J. Rhythmic variations in pain perception in osteoarthritis of the knee. J Rheumatol 1990; 17:364–72.

7. Roos EM, Klassbo M, Lohmander LS. WOMAC osteoarthritis index. Reliability, validity, and responsiveness in patients with arthroscopically assessed osteoarthritis. Scand J Rheumatol 1999;28:210–5.

8. McConnell S, Kolopack P, Davis AM. The Western Ontario and McMaster Universities Osteoarthritis Index (WOMAC): a review of its utility and measurement properties. Arthritis Care Res 2001;45:453–61.

9. Bellamy N, Wells G, Campbell J. Relationship between severity and clinical importance of symptoms in osteoarthritis. Clin Rheumatol 1991;10:138–43.

10. Brazier JE, Harper R, Munro J, Walters SJ, Snaith ML. Generic and condition-specific outcome measures for people with osteoarthritis of the knee. Rheumatology (Oxford) 1999;38:870–7.

11. Bellamy N, Kean WF, Buchanan WW, Gerecz-Simon E, Campbell J. Double blind randomized controlled trial of sodium meclofenamate (Meclomen) and diclofenac sodium (Voltaren): post validation reapplication of the WOMAC Osteoarthritis Index. J Rheumatol 1992;19:153–9.

12. Ehrich EW, Davies GM, Watson DJ, Bolognese JA, Seidenberg BC, Bellamy N. Minimal perceptible clinical improvement with the Western Ontario and McMaster Universities Osteoarthritis Index questionnaire and global assessments in patients with osteoarthritis. J Rheumatol 2000;27:2635–41.

13. Ryser L, Wright BD, Aeschlimann A, Mariacher-Gehler S, Stucki G. A new look at the Western Ontario and McMaster Universities Osteoarthritis Index using Rasch analysis. Arthritis Care Res 1999;12:331–5.

This measure or ordering information can be found at the Website address included in this review.

Glossary

Activity The execution of a task or action by an individual.

Activity limitations Difficulties an individual may have in executing activities.

Bias A systematic difference from the truth.

Body functions The physiologic functions of body systems (including psychological functions).

Body structures Anatomic parts of the body such as organs, limbs, and their components.

Capacity (ICF) An individual's ability to execute a task or an action (i.e. the highest possible level of functioning that a person may reach in a given domain at a given moment).

Ceiling effect The extent to which scores cluster near the more desirable health state extreme on the scale.

Classical test theory The observed score is equal to the true score plus error.

Client The person, group, community, or organization receiving professional services, products, or information.

Coefficient alpha (Cronbach's α) A measure of a test's internal consistency. Conceptually, it represents the average of all split half correlations corrected for test length.

Comparative values The results of an outcome measure administered to a similar client population having low, middle, or high function.

Condition-specific measure Measures composed of items that are most relevant to the condition and of items that are most likely to demonstrate change in the presence of an effective therapeutic intervention.

Conditional standard error of measurement (CSEM) This is an index of the consistency of a measure. The CSEM differs from the SEM in that it acknowledges that error is conditional on the actual score or scores of interest. Like the SEM, it is expressed in the same units as the original measurement.

Construct validity The extent to which a test behaves in accordance with hypotheses concerning how it should behave (eg, on average, patients with low back pain and sciatica should demonstrate greater disability than patients with back pain alone).

Content validity The extent to which a test provides a comprehensive representation of the concept of interest.

Construct The nonobservable attribute, characteristic, or variable of a client or health care system that is hypothesized to be made up of a variety of correlated behaviors and/or be impacted on similarly by other variables or situations.

Cost analysis The appraisal of program costs in relation to program results, using a systematic approach.

Criterion validity The extent to which a test agrees with a gold standard's assessment of the construct of interest.

Cronbach's alpha (coefficient α) A measure of a test's internal consistency. Conceptually, it represents the average of all split half correlations corrected for test length.

Disability (ICF) Any alteration in functioning in terms of performance or capacity—impairments, activity limitations, and participation restrictions.

Disease-specific measure See condition-specific measure.

Effectiveness The extent to which a specific intervention, procedure, regimen, or service, when deployed in the field, does what it is intended to do for a defined population.

Efficacy The extent to which a specific intervention, procedure, regimen, or service produces a beneficial result under ideal conditions.

Evidence-based practice Practice that has a theoretical body of knowledge and uses the best available scientific evidence in clinical decision making and standardized outcome measures to evaluate the service provided.

Face validity The extent to which the test appears to address the construct of interest.

Feasibility analysis Examines the feasibility of the idea for a program.

Floor effect The extent to which scores cluster near the less desirable health state extreme on the scale.

Functioning All body functions, activities, and participation.

Generic measure Those comprehensive measurement tools composed of a number of health-related domains, including social, emotional, role, and physical well-being, that have been developed to measure constructs that are relevant to the general population. Generic measures allow the comparison of health status across a wide variety of conditions and populations.

Goal Attainment Scaling An evaluation method that examines the efficacy of the program in attaining pre-chosen goals.

Handicap (ICIDH) The disadvantage to a given individual, resulting from an impairment or disability, that limits or prevents the fulfillment of a role that is normal for that individual.

Health-related quality of life (HRQL) The value assigned to duration of life as modified by impairments, functional status, perceptions, and opportunities influenced by disease, injury, treatment, and policy.

Health status The level of an individual's physical, mental, affective, and social function; health status is an element of well-being.

International Classification of Functioning, Disability, and Health (ICF) A multipurpose classification of health and health-related states developed by the World Health Organization and designed to provide a unified and standard language and framework. This classification, revised from the original ICIDH, was initially referred to as ICIDH-2. The World Health Assembly adopted ICF as its acronym in May 2001.

Impairments (ICF) Problems in body function or structure such as a significant deviation or loss.

Instrumental activities of daily living Those activities that are required for community living.

Interitem correlation The correlation among items on a test.

Internal consistency One form of reliability the extent to which items on a test are homogeneous. Usually expressed as coefficient alpha or Kuder-Richardson 20 (KR-20).

Interrater reliability The extent to which multiple raters provide consistent rating on a measure.

Intervention Comprises approaches or techniques (rehabilitation strategies) combined together with the aim of normalizing an individual's performance or capacity for activity.

Intraclass correlation coefficient (ICC) as an index of reliability Variance owing to the objects of measurement (usually clients) divided by the total variance.

Item-corrected item total correlation The correlation of an item with the total test score minus the item of interest.

Kappa A chance corrected index of agreement.

Kuder-Richardson 20 (KR-20) A measure of a test's internal consistency. Conceptually, it represents the average of all split half correlations corrected for test length. The Kuder-Richardson formula is appropriate when the items' response options are binary.

Kuder-Richardson 21 (KR-21) This provides a conservative approximation to KR-20. As such, KR-21 will at best be less than or equal to KR-20.

Minimal clinically important difference (MCID) The smallest change that represents an important difference to either the client or the management of the client. It is expressed in the same units as the original measurement.

Minimal detectable change (MDC) This represents an estimate of the smallest change that can be detected for a client, expressed in the same units as the original measurement. Minimal detectable change is based on the standard error of measurement. A confidence level is usually included (eg, 90% CI). In this case, the interpretation is that 90% of stable clients would show a change less than the specified value.

Needs assessment The systematic evaluation of the need for a program, the target audience, and the nature and scope of existing services.

Normative values The results of an outcome measure that has been administered to a healthy population.

Observed score The measured value or score.

Outcome A characteristic or construct that is expected to change as a result of the provision of a strategy, intervention, or program. A successful outcome includes improved or maintained physical function when possible, slows functional decline where the status quo cannot be maintained, and/or is considered meaningful to the client.

Outcome evaluation The systematic evaluation of the impact of a program or intervention to determine whether it meets its objectives.

Outcome measure A measurement tool (instrument, questionnaire, rating form, etc.) used to document change in one or more constructs over time.

Participation (ICF) Involvement in a life situation.

Participation restrictions (ICF) Problems an individual may experience in involvement in life situations.

Patient-specific measure A type of measure composed of items that are most relevant to the individual patient. Because different patients will provide different items, it is generally agreed that patient-specific measures should not be used to make comparisons among patients.

Performance (ICF) What an individual does in his/her current environment (i.e. includes environmental factors).

Performance outcome measures (viewed performance) Measures that test a client's performance of an activity in a specific environment at a particular time.

Process evaluation The systematic evaluation of how a program is operating, focusing on program delivery and usage.

Program Interventions offered to impact globally on an individual's capacity to perform usual activities and participate fully.

Program evaluation The process of systematically gathering, analyzing, and reporting data about a program and using that information to guide decision making.

Program logic model The use of a flowchart, table, or map to present the main components of a program, such as the objectives, underlying assumptions, and short-term and long-term outcomes.

Psychometric (measurement) properties The reliability and validity, including responsiveness and sensitivity to change, of a measurement tool.

Quality of life A personal assessment of the good or satisfactory characteristics of life.

Regression toward the mean On average, repeated measurements on persons who demonstrate extreme scores will yield subsequent values closer to the group mean.

Rehabilitation A goal-oriented and time-limited process aimed at enabling an impaired person to reach an optimum mental, physical, and/or social function level, thus providing the person with the tools to change his/her own life. It can involve interventions intended to compensate for a loss of function or a functional limitation.

Reintegration The reorganization of physical, psychological, and social characteristics so that an individual can resume well-adjusted living after an incapacitating illness or trauma.

Reliability The consistency of a measure. Classical test theory defines reliability as the variance among sub-

jects (usually clients in the clinical setting) divided by the total variance.

Responsiveness The ability of a measure to assess clinically important change over time. This term is often used interchangeably with sensitivity to change.

Scaling A set of procedures used to assign numeric weights to items in a measure to reflect the severity of disability implied.

Self-report outcome measures Questionnaires or interviews completed by the client or someone acting on behalf of the client (caregiver).

Sensitivity to change The capacity of a measure to assess change over time. This term is often used interchangeably with responsiveness.

Specific outcome measures Measures designed for a specific client population (related to disease, condition, region, or patient) that can be used only to compare clients within that particular group.

Standard error of measurement (SEM) An index of the consistency of a measure. It is expressed in the same units as the original measurement.

Standardized measure A published measurement tool, designed for a specified purpose in a given population, with detailed instructions provided on administration and scoring and the results of reliability and validity testing published in peer-reviewed journals.

Strategy A rehabilitation modality, approach, or technique that seeks to normalize body structure or function.

Test–retest reliability The extent to which multiple applications of a test provide consistent results.

True score (sometimes referred to as consensus score) A conceptual score that would be obtained by averaging an infinite number of repeated measures on a patient.

Utility The value, between 0 and 1, representing the strength of preference an individual has for a given multidimensional health state.

Validity The extent to which a measure assesses what it is intended to measure.

Weighted kappa A chance corrected agreement that provides partial credit for minor disagreements. When the quadratic weighting method is used (ie, the weights are based on the square of the discrepancy between categories), the point estimate provided by weighted kappa is equal to the point estimate determined by the intraclass correlation coefficient.

APPENDIX

Information Extraction Form for Measurement Studies

This form was developed to assist persons in their search for scientific information about the measurement properties of instruments. This form is to be used only the first couple of times an individual critiques a measurement study. Such studies are sometimes complicated, with several components. For novice reviewers, it is easiest to read in sections and extract information in a brief narrative form. The reviewer can, if necessary, consult reference sources related to the development and testing of measures and then judge the quality of the section recorded. This form is to be used in conjunction with the *Critical Appraisal Form for Measurement Studies* (page 273). Both forms are designed for critiquing published articles that report the conceptualization, development, and psychometric testing of a new measure. Both forms assume that the reader has prior knowledge about the development of measures and about clinical research.

The form was developed as a tool for a graduate-level course, Measurement in Rehabilitation, taught at McGill University by Sharon Wood-Dauphinee. Dr. Wood-Dauphinee has been gracious enough to share this with us and permit it to be included in this book. It is included with the view that, when readers wish to review articles on measurement properties of measures, they will have a guide that they can use to judge the scientific value of the material presented.

Although there are many critical appraisal forms, there is not one for appraising the measurement literature. As such, this is Dr. Wood-Dauphinee's adaptation of common principles of appraisal to the situation of measurement studies. Content was drawn from many sources. In particular, the forms used by the Quebec Task Forces on Spinal Disorders and Whiplash-Associated Disorders provided the format and general ideas for the appraisal form.

The extraction form provides a list of data elements that the critical reader of measurement research should extract from an article on the measurement properties of an instrument. Once the relevant information has been extracted, the reviewer would then judge the scientific value of the information using the *Critical Appraisal* form.

This form is only for extracting information about the quality of the measurement development and is not for use when judging the overall quality of the article, which would include areas such as style or clarity of results.

INFORMATION EXTRACTION FORM FOR MEASUREMENT STUDIES

I. **Reference of Article**

Author(s), Title, Journal, Volume, Pages, and Year of Publication

II. **Descriptive Information for Introductory Section**

1. What was covered in the literature review?
2. What was the rationale for developing the measure?
3. What were the objectives of the study?
4. For whom is this measure intended?

III. **Descriptive Information for General Methodologic Issues**

1. Which important terms (constructs) were defined? (*eg, function, independence, quality of life, disability, and so on*)

2. What type of measure was being developed? (*eg, evaluative, discriminative, predictive*)
3. How is the measure or test administered? (*eg, viewed performance, self-administered, proxy administered, interview administered*)
4. How is the measure scored? (*eg, categorical score, single cumulative score, subscale scores, weighted score, algorithmic score*)
5. In which languages was the measure developed or translated? (*The issue of cultural adaptation and validation of measures to other languages is an extensive methodologic undertaking on its own and will not be covered here.*)

IV. Descriptive Information for Content Development

1. What construct was being measured?
2. What was the conceptual framework for the measure?
3. What sources of information were used to develop the content of the measure? (*eg, patients, family members, friends, professionals, literature*)
4. What processes were used to develop the items comprising the content? (eg, *literature review, interviews, focus groups, mail questionnaires*)
5. What information was provided about item performance? (ie, *prevalence of responses, means, frequencies, correlations, kappas, missing data*)
6. On whom were these data collected?
7. What was the data collection process?
8. By which criteria were items reduced? (*eg, proportion of data missing, item reliability value, magnitude of interitem correlations*)
9. Which statistical analyses were performed to assess the criteria?

V. Descriptive Information for Reliability Section

1. Which types of reliability were being assessed? (*eg, test–retest, interrater, intrarater, internal consistency*)
2. What were the sources of patient subjects? (eg, *inpatients from different rehabilitation services, people with stroke on a stroke unit, community sample*)
3. What were the inclusion and exclusion criteria?
4. How many patients were included?
5. What was the distribution of severity across patients?
6. Who were the raters/interviewers? (*eg, therapists, nurses, lay individuals*)
7. How were they trained?
8. How many raters were there?
9. How many subjects were assigned to each rater?
10. How were the subjects assigned to raters? (*eg, randomly assigned, by convenience*)
11. What designs were used to obtain the rater reliability information? (*eg, how many ratings, time between ratings*)
12. Which ratings were compared? (*eg, all possible pairs, convenient pairs*)
13. Which statistical tests were used? (*eg, Pearson's r, intraclass correlation coefficient [ICC], kappa, Kendal's tau, coefficient alpha, etc*)
14. What were the results of these statistical tests?

VI. Descriptive Information for Validity Section

1. What types of validity were being assessed? (*eg, content, criterion, construct*)
2. What were the sources of patients? (*eg, inpatients from different rehabilitation services, people with stroke on a stroke unit, community sample*)

3. What were the inclusion and exclusion criteria?
4. How many patients were included?
5. Who were the evaluators/interviewers? (eg, therapists, nurses, lay individuals)
6. What other measures were selected for validation purposes?
7. Were these comparative measures described in terms of their psychometric properties?
8. Were the data collected cross-sectionally, longitudinally, or both?
9. Were the hypotheses being tested stated in terms of a priori magnitudes and directions?
10. Which statistical tests were used? (eg, correlations, t-tests, analysis of variance, regression, factor analysis)
11. What were the results?

VII. Descriptive Information for Sensitivity to Change/Responsiveness Section

1. What was the source of subjects? (eg, inpatients from different rehabilitation services, people with stroke on a stroke unit, community sample)

2. What were the inclusion and exclusion criteria?
3. How many subjects were included?
4. Who were the evaluators? (eg, therapists, nurses, lay individuals)
5. How were they trained?
6. What was the study design? (eg, within a clinical trial, prospective cohort)
7. Was the minimal important difference discussed in relation to the measure?
8. Which statistical tests were used? (eg, effect sizes, paired t-test, receiver operating characteristic curve, correlation of change scores, regression)
9. What were the results?

VIII. Descriptive Information for Discussion and Conclusion

1. Did the authors relate the results to the hypotheses?
2. Did they relate findings to previous studies?
3. What were the suggestions for further studies related to the development of the measure?
4. What directions were given about the immediate use of the measure?
5. What were the conclusions of the authors?

Critical Appraisal Form for Measurement Studies

This form is to be used in conjunction with the *Information Extraction Form for Measurement Studies* (page 277). Both forms are designed for critiquing published articles that report the conceptualization, development, and psychometric testing of a new measure.

I. **Reference of Article**: Author(s), Title, Journal, Volume, Pages, and Year of Publication

II. **Methodologic Issues for Introductory Section**

Criteria	Y	S	N	NC	NR	NA	Comments
Adequate literate review							
Reasonable study rationale							
Objectives clearly stated							
Target population discernible							

Y = yes; S = somewhat; N = no; NC = not clear; NR = not reported; NA = not applicable.

III. **General Methodologic Issues**

Criteria	Y	S	N	NC	NR	NA	Comments
Terms clearly defined							
Type of measure declared							
Ethical issues addressed							
Methods of test administration reported							
Tactics for scoring reported							

Y = yes; S = somewhat; N = no; NC = not clear; NR = not reported; NA = not applicable.

IV. **Methodologic Issues Related to Content**

Criteria	Y	S	N	NC	NR	NA	Comments
Concepts clearly defined							
Conceptual framework provided							
Adequate sources of information for content development							
Process of item generation acceptable							

IV. *Continued*

Criteria	Y	S	N	NC	NR	NA	Comments
Process for data collection satisfactory							
Adequate data collection							
Stated criteria for item reduction							
Process for item reduction acceptable							
Appropriate statistical tests							
Content reaffirmed							

Y = yes; S = somewhat; N = no; NC = not clear; NR = not reported; NA = not applicable.

V. Methodologic Issues for Reliability Sections

Reliability being assessed: test–retest ___, interrater___, intrarater ___, internal consistency ___.

Criteria	Y	S	N	NC	NR	NA	Comments
Study setting(s) described and adequate							
Sources of patients described and adequate							
Appropriate spectrum of subjects in terms of severity							
Sample size preplanned to provide sufficient power							
Sources of raters/ interviewers described							
Subjects randomly assigned to raters if all subjects not tested by all raters							
Same information about subjects provided to each rater							
Ratings are independent							
Time between ratings appropriate							
Calibration of instruments described							
Statistical analyses appropriate							

Y = yes; S = somewhat; N = no; NC = not clear; NR = not reported; NA = not applicable.

VI. Methodologic Issues for Validity Sections

Validity being assessed: concurrent criterion validity _____, predictive criterion validity_____, construct validity_____.

Criteria	Y	S	N	NC	NR	NA	Comments
Study setting(s) described and adequate							
Source(s) of patients described and adequate							
Patient sample size(s) preplanned to provide sufficient power							
Sources of raters/interviewers described							
Training of raters/interviewers adequate							
Data collection procedures explained and adequate							
Validation measures rationalized and described adequately							
Specific hypotheses proposed							
Statistical analyses appropriate							

Y = yes; S = somewhat; N = no; NC = not clear; NR = not reported; NA = not applicable.

VII. Methodologic Issues for Sensitivity to Change/Responsiveness Section

Criteria	Y	S	N	NC	NR	NA	Comments
Setting of study described and adequate							
Source of patients described and adequate							
Patient sample size preplanned to provide sufficient power							
Source of raters/interviewers described							
Training of raters described							
Data collection procedures explained and adequate							
Statistical analyses appropriate							

Y = yes; S = somewhat; N = no; NC = not clear; NR = not reported; NA = not applicable.

VIII. Presentation Issues for Results Section

Criteria	Y	S	N	NC	NR	NA	Comments
Patient groups described adequately							
All patients accounted for							
Raters/interviewers described adequately							
Clear and detailed presentation of findings							
Missing data taken into account							
Withdrawals reported, explained, and reasonable							
Conclusions supported by results							

Y = yes; S = somewhat; N = no; NC = not clear; NR = not reported; NA = not applicable.

IX. Reviewer's Conclusions and Assessment of the Article

1. Strengths of the paper

2. Weaknesses of the paper

3. Scientific merit (place X between appropriate brackets)

   Very good   (   )

   Good   (   )

   Scientifically acceptable   (   )

   Scientifically unacceptable   (   )

Index

WHO, 4, 7
ICIDH
  WHO, 7, 76
Idiopathic pulmonary fibrosis
  HRQL, 224
Impact evaluation
  definition of, 53t
Impairments
  definition of, 271
  ICF description of, 8t
  measures for, 67
Infants
  cocaine-exposed
    motor scale, 78
  delayed motor development, 78
  gross motor performance, 159
  motor performance, 237
  motor scale, 78
Information extraction
  measurement studies, 274–276
Instrumental activities of daily living
  definition of, 271
Interitem correlation
  definition of, 271
Intermittent claudication
  exercise test, 261
  quality of life, 125
Internal consistency, 29
  definition of, 271
International Classification of Functioning,
    Disability and Health (ICF)
  definition of, 271
  terminology of, 8t
  WHO, 4, 7
International Classification of the Consequences
    of Disease, Impairment, Disability and
    Handicap (ICIDH)
  WHO, 7, 76
Interpretability, 22, 36–40
Interrater reliability, 29–30
  definition of, 271
Interstitial fibrosis
  dyspnea, 121
Interstitial lung disease
  dyspnea, 123
Interval scales, 26
Interventions, 10
  definition of, 271
Intraclass correlation coefficient (ICC), 70
  as an index of reliability
    definition of, 271
Item-corrected item total correlation
  definition of, 271

J
Journal articles
  reference for, 274
Juvenile arthritis
  health status, 81

K
Kappa
  definition of, 271
Key words, 20
Knee replacement, 114
  balance, 71
Known group validity, 31
(KR-20) Kuder-Richardson 20
  definition of, 271
(KR-21) Kuder-Richardson 21
  definition of, 271
Kuder-Richardson 20 (KR-20)
  definition of, 271
Kuder-Richardson 21 (KR-21)
  definition of, 271

L
Language, 5
LEAP (Lower Extremity Activity Profile), 164–166
LEFS (Lower Extremity Functional Scale), 46,
    167–168
Libraries, 20–21
Literature review
  coverage of, 274
Literature searches, 19–21
Longitudinal validity, 31, 32–36
Longitudinal validity coefficients, 33, 34
Long-term care
  upper extremity, 110
Low back pain, 85, 180, 186
  daily activities, 221
  functional disability, 198
  functional status, 206
  quality of life, 125, 175
Lower extremity, 140, 264
  amputations
    balance, 242
    health status, 81
    normal living, 201
  functional reach, 150
  functional status, 190
  measures for, 69
  pain, 180
  sarcomas
    reintegration to normal living, 201
  traumatic injuries, 165
Lower Extremity Activity Profile (LEAP), 164–166